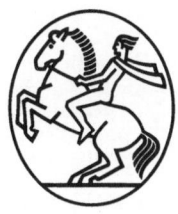

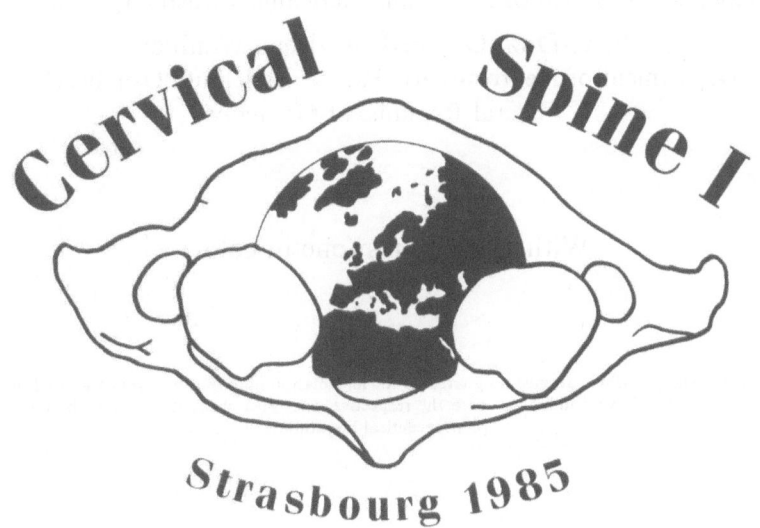

Cervical Spine I

Strasbourg 1985

Edited by P. Kehr and A. Weidner

Springer-Verlag Wien GmbH

Professor Pierre Kehr, M.D.
Hôpital chirurgical orthopédique Stéphanie, Strasbourg, France
Priv.-Doz. Dr. med. Andreas Weidner
Department of Neurosurgery, Paracelsus-Klinik, Osnabrück,
Federal Republic of Germany

With 178 Figures (one in color)

Library of Congress Cataloging-in-Publication Data. Cervical spine I. 1. Vertebrae, Cervical—Wounds and injuries—Congresses. 2. Vertebrae, Cervical—Diseases—Congresses. 3. Vertebrae, Cervical—Surgery—Congresses. I. Kehr, Pierre. II. Weidner, Andreas, 1943– . III. Title: Cervical spine 1. [DNLM: 1. Cervical Vertebrae—congresses. WE 725 C4195 1985]. RD531.C48. 1987. 617'.375. 86-29759.

ISSN 0930-8725
ISBN 978-3-7091-8884-2   ISBN 978-3-7091-8882-8 (eBook)
DOI 10.1007/978-3-7091-8882-8

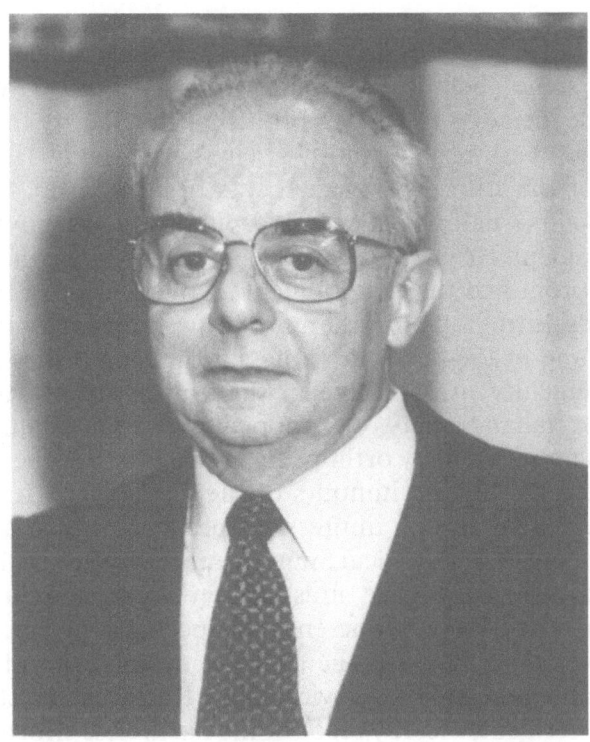

MarioBoni

Preface

Cervical Spine Research Society
European Branch

"The Cervical Spine Research Society is an organization of individuals interested in clinical and research problems of the cervical spine. Its purpose is for the exchange and development of ideas and philosophy regarding the diagnosis and treatment of cervical spine injury and disease. The composition of the membership should reflect the varying specialities and disciplines dealing with the cervical spine; biochemical, engineering, neurology, neurosurgery, radiology, orthopedic surgery and others", wrote J. William Fielding, New York City, one of the Society's founding members.

In 1984 the membership list contained 118 names. The overwhelming majority of members came from the United States, four from Canada and 9 Europeans, amongst them Mario Boni. He was the organizer, in conjunction with the members of the Cervical Spine Research Society, of a splendid "International Meeting for the updating on pathology and surgery of the cervical spine" held in Pavia (Italy) in May 1982. It was from this meeting that the idea of a European branch of the Society first originated, with the purpose of establishing multi-disciplinary meetings in Europe. The first meeting of the European branch was organized by A. Weidner in September 1984 in Osnabrück (Federal Republic of Germany). Mario Boni was elected president. He was not only the initiator but also the driving force who tirelessly promoted the development of the European branch.

Mario Boni's death in 1986 at the age of 64 was a great loss to us. He was born in Rome and in 1964 became Professor of Orthopedics and Traumatology in the Faculty of Medicine in the University of Pavia. He was President of the Italian Society of Orthopedics and Traumatology and was an honorary member of many orthopedic societies in Europe and America. He was awarded the highest honours of the Republic of Italy. He was a highly intelligent man and an impressive speaker. His last address at the Strasbourg meeting of the Cervical Spine Research Society in 1985 included the statement: "All knowledge must follow from a multi-disciplinary analysis of the various topics inherent in a specific problem. One is not a *cervical surgeon* simply because one operates on the cervical spine."

The European branch of the Cervical Spine Research Society elected him as its Honory President, thereby recognizing his tireless efforts on behalf of the Society.

According to the constitution a joint meeting of the Cervical Spine Research Society and the European branch takes place every three years. The first combined meeting was organized by Pierre Kehr in Strasbourg (France) in June 1985. More than 130 specialists in Orthopedics, Neurosurgery, Traumatology, Neurology, Anatomy, Rheumatology, Radiology and others from every part of Europe, America and Japan participated. This was convincing proof of the great interest which exists in Europe in research into injuries and diseases of the cervical spine. The main topic was the lower cervical spine, although some of the papers also dealt the upper cervical spine, with the result that altogether a good overview was provided of our present state of knowledge of diseases of the cervical spine.

Important as the spoken word and personal contact are, they suffer from the disadvantage that only a few can participate. This book contains virtually all the papers which were read and makes them accessible to all those interested in the cervical spine. We are grateful to the authors for their efforts.

We Europeans use a variety of languages to express ourselves. English is the native language of only a minority. Translation obscures individual modes of expression but we have tried to retain these as much as is possible, for which we ask your indulgence. We are indebted to Mrs. Danielle Gantz (Strasbourg) and Mrs. Alison Trainer (Glasgow) for their assistance with the preparation of the English text.

The publication of this book would not have been possible without the help of our secretaries to whom we express our thanks.

Our publisher Springer-Verlag (Wien—New York) has been most mindful of our wishes, generous with advice and lavish in the production of this volume. In Dr. Sepp Weingärtner of Springer-Verlag we have had a most competent collaborator and we are grateful for his willingness also to publish the next combined meetings. The next meeting will be organized by R. Louis in Marseille (France) in 1987. We hope that this will be a further step along the road to a strong European branch of the Cervical Spine Research Society.

Strasbourg and Osnabrück, December 1986

Pierre Kehr, Andreas Weidner

Membership List

ARGENSON, CLAUDE, M.D., Professor, Orthopedics, founding member, Nice, France.

BRAAKMAN, R., M.D., Professor, Neurosurgery, founding member, Rotterdam, The Netherlands.

CANADELL, JOSÉ, M.D., Professor, Orthopedics, founding member, Pamplona, Spain.

CAPESIUS, PIERRE, M.D., Radiology, Luxembourg, Luxembourg.

CHERUBINO, PAOLO, M.D., Professor, Orthopedics, secretary, Pavia, Italy.

DALLE ORE, G., M.D., Professor, Neurosurgery, founding member, Verona, Italy.

DENARO, VICENZO, M.D., Professor, Orthopedics, Pavia, Italy.

DIRHEIMER, YVES, M.D., Rheumatology, Strasbourg, France.

EVANS, D. K., M.D., Professor, Orthopedics, founding member, Ranmoor Sheffield, England.

FINESCHI, GIANAFRANCO, M.D., Professor, Orthopedics, founding member, Roma, Italy.

FUENTES, JEAN-MARC, M.D., Neurosurgery, Murviel les Montpellier, France.

GUTMANN, GOTTFRIED, M.D., Non-surgical therapy, Bad Sassendorf, Federal Republic of Germany.

HOHMANN, DIETRICH, M.D., Professor, Orthopedics, founding member, Membership Committee, Erlangen, Federal Republic of Germany.

JUNG, ADOLPHE, M.D., Professor, Orthopedics, honorary member, Strasbourg, France.

KEHR, PIERRE, M.D., Professor, Orthopedics, founding member, President 1985/86, Strasbourg, France.

KORRES, DEMETRE S., M.D., Professor, Orthopedics, Athens, Greece.

LOGROSCINO, CARLO, M.D., Professor, Orthopedics, founding member, Membership Committee, Roma, Italy.

LOUIS, RENÉ, M.D., Professor, Orthopedics, founding member, Membership Committee, Marseille, France.

MAGERL, FRIEDRICH, M.D., Orthopedics, St. Gallen, Switzerland.

MARTI, RENÉ, M.D., Professor, Orthopedics, Amsterdam, The Netherlands.

O'BRIEN, JOHN, M.D., Professor, Orthopedics, founding member, London, England.

RODEGERDTS, UDO, M.D., Professor, Orthopedics, founding member, Treasurer, Bremerhaven, Federal Republic of Germany.

ROY-CAMILLE, RAYMOND, M.D., Professor, Orthopedics, Paris, France.

VIEIRA, JOSÉ-MARIA, M.D., Professor, Orthopedics, founding member, President 1986/87, Lisboa, Portugal.

WACKENHEIM, AUGUST, M.D., Professor, Radiology, Research Committee, Strasbourg, France.

WEATHERLEY, CHRIS, M.D., Professor, Orthopedics, Oswestry, England.

WEIDNER, ANDREAS, M.D., Priv.-Doz., Neurosurgery, founding member, Editor, Osnabrück, Federal Republic of Germany.

Contents

1. Biodynamics of the Cervical Spine

2. Diagnostic Evaluation

3. Traumatic Instability and Management

4. Degenerative Lesions and Management

List of Contributors

BANCALE, R., M.D., Università di Bari, Istituto di Clinica Ortopedica, I-70124 Bari, Italy.

BAUER, RUDOLF, M.D., Professor, Direktor der Orthopädischen Universitätsklinik, Anichstraße 35, A-6020 Innsbruck, Austria.

BENOIST, M., M.D., Hôpital Beaujon, 100 boulevard du Général Leclerc, F-92110 Clichy, France.

BONI†, M., M.D., Professor, Honorary President, CSRS—European Branch, Clinica Ortopedica dell'Università di Pavia, Viale Taramelli, 3, I-27100 Pavia, Italy.

BOYER, P., M.D., Service de Neurochirurgie, Hôpital de Hautepierre, Centre Hospitalier Universitaire, F-67098 Strasbourg, France.

BUCHHEIT, F., M.D., Professor, Service de Neurochirurgie, Hôpital de Hautepierre, Centre Hospitalier Universitaire, F-67098 Strasbourg, France.

BURKE, STEPHAN W., M.D., Professor, Hospital for Special Surgery, 535 East 70th Street, New York, NY 10021, U.S.A.

CAPESIUS, PIERRE, M.D., 2, rue de Strasbourg, L-1025 Luxembourg, Grand Duché du Luxembourg.

CARRET, J. P., M.D., Centre Hospitalier Lyon-Sud, Jules-Courmont—Sainte-Eugénie, Clinique chirurgicale orthopédique et traumatologique, F-69310 Pierre-Bénite, France.

CASPAR, WOLFHARD, M.D., Neurochirurgische Universitätsklinik, D-6650 Homburg (Saar), Federal Republic of Germany.

CLARK, CHARLES R., M.D., Professor, University of Iowa, Department of Orthopaedic Surgery, Iowa City, IA 52242, U.S.A.

COOK, STEPHEN D., Ph.D., Director—Biomaterials Laboratory, Department of Orthopaedic Surgery, Tulane University Medical School, New Orleans, LA 70112, U.S.A.

CORREIA MARTINS, M. A., M.D., Rua Camilo 62, P-4490 Povoa de Varzim, Portugal.

CUSICK, J. F., M.D., Professor, Medical College of Wisconsin, Department of Neurosurgery, 8700 West Wisconsin Avenue, Milwaukee, WI 53226, U.S.A.

DEBURGE, A., M.D., Professor, Hôpital Beaujon, 100 boulevard du Général Leclerc, F-92110 Clichy, France.

DENARO, VINCENZO, M.D., Professor, Istituto di Clinica Ortopedica e Traumatologica, Università di Pavia, Viale Taramelli, 3, I-27100 Pavia, Italy.

DESCHAMPS, G., M.D., Université Claude Bernard, Laboratoire d'Anatomie, 8, avenue Rockefeller, F-69373 Lyon Cedex 08, France.

DI GUGLIELMO, L., M.D., Professor, Institute of Radiology, University of Pavia, Viale Taramelli, 3, I-27100 Pavia, Italy.

DIMNET, J., M.D., École Centrale de Lyon, 36, avenue Guy de Collongue, F-69130 Ecully, France.

DIRHEIMER, YVES, M.D., Cabinet de Rhumatologie, 40, rue du Tivoli, F-67000 Strasbourg, France.

EDMUNDS, J. OLLIE, JR., M.D., Professor, Orthopaedic Surgery, Tulane University School of Medicine, New Orleans, LA 70112, U.S.A.

EPSTEIN, JOSEPH A., M.D., 410 Lake Ville Road No. 100, New Hyde Park, NY 11042, U.S.A.

EPSTEIN, NANCY E., M.D., 410 Lake Ville Road No. 100, New Hyde Park, NY 11042, U.S.A.

FIELDING, J.-W., M.D., Professor, St. Luke's/Roosevelt, Amsterdam Avenue at 114th Street, New York, NY 10025, U.S.A.

FINESCHI, G., M.D., Professor, Direttore Istituto di Clinica Ortopedica, Università Cattolica, Largo A. Gemelli, 8, I-00168 Roma, Italy.

FISCHER, L. P., M.D., Professor, Clinique de Chirurgie Orthopédique, Hôpital Edouard Herriot, place d'Arsonval, F-69374 Lyon Cedex 08, France.

FRANCIS, WILLIAM R., M.D., 1709 Dryden, Suite 920, Houston, TX 77030, U.S.A.

FRENCH, H. GRAEME, M.D., Orthopaedic Surgery, Tulane University School of Medicine, New Orleans, LA 70112, U.S.A.

FUENTES, JEAN-MARC, M.D., Centre de Neurochirurgie, Clinique Rech, avenue Charles Flahault, F-34100 Montpellier, France.

GONON, G. P., M.D., Université Claude Bernard, Laboratoire d'Anatomie-Faculté de Médecine, Grange-Blanche, 8, avenue Rockefeller, F-69373 Lyon Cedex 08, France.

GROB, D., M.D., Klinik für Orthopädische Chirurgie, Kantonsspital, CH-9007 St. Gallen, Switzerland.

HAWKINS, RICHARD, M.D., 50 Central Avenue, Suite 107, London, Ontario N6B 2E8, Canada.

HENSINGER, ROBERT, M.D., Section of Orthopaedic Surgery, Box 54, University Hospital, Ann Arbor, MI 48109, U.S.A.

HIRABAYASHI, KIYOSHI, M.D., Professor, Department of Orthopaedic Surgery, School of Medicine, Keio University, 35 Shinanomachi, Shinjuku, Tokyo 160, Japan.

HUSAG, L., M.D., Leitender Arzt, Kantonsspital Aarau, Neurochirurgische Klinik, CH-5001 Aarau, Switzerland.

HYMAN, ROGER A., M.D., Professor, Chief, Division of Neuroradiology, North Shore University Hospital, Cornell University Medical College, 300 Community Drive, Manhasset, NY 11030, U.S.A.

ITOH, TATSUO, M.D., Department of Orthopaedic Surgery, Toyama Medical and Pharmaceutical University, 2630 Sugitani, Toyama 930-01, Japan.

JEANNERET, BERNARD, M.D. (Klinik und Poliklinik für Orthopädische Chirurgie, Inselspital, CH-3010 Bern). Present address: Klinik für Orthopädische Chirurgie, Kantonsspital, CH-9007 St. Gallen, Switzerland.

JESEL, M., M.D., Professor, Service d'Électromyographie, Clinique Neurologique, C.H.U. Strasbourg, 1, place de l'Hôpital, F-67091 Strasbourg Cedex, France.

KAISER, MARC C., M.D., Academisch Ziekenhuis Vrije Universiteit, Neuroradiologie, de Boelelaan 1117, P.O. Box 7057, NL-1007MB Amsterdam, The Netherlands.

KEHR, PIERRE, M.D., Professeur à la Faculté de Médecine de Strasbourg, Hôpital chirurgical orthopédique Stéphanie, F-67026 Strasbourg Cedex, France.

KIWERSKI, JERZY, M.D., Professor, Head of Rehabilitation Clinic, Warsaw Medical Academy, Wierzejewskiego 12, PL-05-510 Konstancin, Poland.

KORRES, D. ST., M.D., Professor, 10, rue Heyden, GR-10434 Athens, Greece.

KRAUSE, D., M.D., Service de Radiologie, Hôpital de Hautepierre, Centre Hospitalier Universitaire, F-67098 Strasbourg, France.

LANG, G., M.D., Professor, Hôpital de Hautepierre, Centre Hospitalier Universitaire, F-67089 Strasbourg, France.

LEMAIRE, J. P., M.D., Department of Orthopaedic Surgery, Section of Spine Surgery, Hôpital du Bocage, boulevard de Lattre de Tassigny, F-21000 Dijon, France.

LIND, BENGT, M.D., Department of Orthopaedic Surgery I, Sahlgren Hospital, S-41345 Göteborg, Sweden.

LOGROSCINO, C., M.D., Professor, Clinica Ortopedica, Università Cattolica, Largo A. Gemelli, 8, I-00168 Roma, Italy.

LOUIS, RENE, M.D., Professor, Service de chirurgie vertebrale, Hôtel-Dieu, 6, place Daviel, F-13002 Marseille, France.

MAGERL, F., M.D., Klinik für Orthopädische Chirurgie, Kantonsspital, CH-9007 St. Gallen, Switzerland.

MAITROT, D., M.D., Professor, Service de Neurochirurgie, Hôpital de Hautepierre, Centre Hospitalier Universitaire, F-67098 Strasbourg, France.

MAZEL, CH., M.D., Hôpital de la Pitié, 83, boulevard de l'Hôpital, F-75634 Paris Cedex 13, France.

MESTDAGH, HENRI, M.D., Professor, Centre Hospitalier et Universitaire de Lille, Service de Traumatologie et Orthopédie D, Hôpital B, F-59037 Lille Cedex, France.

MISASI, M., M.D., Professor, Direttore Clinica Ortopedica, Università degli Studi di Napoli, Via S. Pansini, 5, I-80131 Napoli, Italy.

MYKLEBUST, JOEL B., Ph.D., Medicine College of Wisconsin, Department of Neurosurgery, 8700 West Wisconsin Avenue, Milwaukee, WI 53226, U.S.A.

NAKANO, NOBORU, M.D., Nakano Orthopaedic Hospital, West 15, South 7, Chuoku, Sapporo 064, Japan.

NAKANO, TOHRU, M.D., Nakano Orthopaedic Hospital, West 15, South 7, Chuoku, Sapporo 064, Japan.

NORDWALL, ANDERS, M.D., Professor, Göteborgs Universitet, Department of Orthopaedic Surgery I, Sahlgren Hospital, S-41345 Göteborg, Sweden.

NORTHRUP, BRUCE, M.D., Thomas Jefferson University, Department of Neurosurgery, 1025 Walnut Street, Philadelphia, PA 19107, U.S.A.

ORSINI, G., M.D., Ospedale "San Giovanni Battista", Divisione di Ortopedia e Traumatologia, I-Torino, Italy.

OSTERHOLM, J. L., M.D., Thomas Jefferson University, Department of Neurosurgery, 1025 Walnut Street, Philadelphia, PA 19107, U.S.A.

O'BRIEN, J. P., M.D., Professor, 149, Harley Street, London WIN 2DE, England.

PIERCE, DONALD S., M.D., Massachusetts General Hospital, Harvard Medical School, Boston, MA 02114, U.S.A.

PIPINO, F., M.D., Professor, Direttore Istituto di Clinica Ortopedica, Università di Bari, I-70124 Bari, Italy.

PROBST, CH., M.D., Professor, Kantonsspital Aarau, Neurochirurgische Klinik, CH-5001 Aarau, Switzerland.

RAYNOR, R. B., M.D., Department of Neurosurgery, St. Vincent's Hospital, New York University Medical School, 112 East 74th Street, New York, NY 10021, U.S.A.

REYNOLDS, MARY C., M.D., Department of Orthopaedic Surgery, Tulane University School of Medicine, 1430 Tulane Avenue, New Orleans, LA 70112, U.S.A.

ROY-CAMILLE, R., M.D., Professor, Hôpital de la Pitié, 83, boulevard de l'Hôpital, F-75634 Paris Cedex 13, France.

SAILLANT, G., M.D., Professor, Hôpital de la Pitié, 83, boulevard de l'Hôpital, F-75634 Paris Cedex 13, France.

SEEMANN, P.-S., M.D., Klinik für Orthopädische Chirurgie, Kantonsspital, CH-9007 St. Gallen, Switzerland.

SHERK, HENRY H., M.D., Division of Orthopaedics, Medical College of Pennsylvania, 3300 Henry Avenue, Philadelphia, PA 19129, U.S.A.

SICK, H., M.D., Professor, Institut d'Anatomie, Faculté de Médecine, Université Louis Pasteur, F-67000 Strasbourg, France.

SILBOHM, HANS, M.D., Department of Orthopaedic Surgery I, Sahlgren Hospital, S-41345 Göteborg, Sweden.

SOLINI, A., M.D., Professor, Ospedale "San Giovanni Battista", Divisione di Ortopedia e Traumatologia, I-Torino, Italy.

STAUFFER, E. SH., M.D., Professor, Southern Illinois University, School of Medicine, P.O. Box 3926, Springfield, IL 62708, U.S.A.

STEIB, J. P., M.D., Hôpital chirurgical orthopédique Stéphanie, F-67026 Strasbourg, France.

STRELI, RUDOLF, M.D., Ärztlicher Leiter des AUKH, Blumauerplatz 1, A-4020 Linz, Austria.

TONGIO, J., M.D., Professor, Service de Radiologie, Hôpital de Hautepierre, Centre Hospitalier Universitaire, F-67096 Strasbourg, France.

TRANQUILLI LEALI, P., M.D., Clinica Ortopedica, Università Cattolica, Largo A. Gemelli, 8, I-00168 Roma, Italy.

TRENSZ, T., M.D., Hôpital chirurgical orthopédique Stéphanie, F-67026 Strasbourg, France.

ULRICH, CHRISTOPHER G., M.D., The Charlotte Radiological Group, P.A., Wendover Building, Suite 102, 3535 Randolph Road, Charlotte, NC 28211-1089, U.S.A.

ULRICH, CHR., M.D., Klinikum für Unfallchirurgie, Hand-, Plastische und Wiederherstellungschirurgie der Universität Ulm, Steinhövelstrasse 9, D-7900 Ulm, Federal Republic of Germany.

VAUTRAVERS, PH., M.D., Service d'Électromyographie, Clinique Neurologique, C.H.U. Strasbourg, 1, place de l'Hôpital, F-67091 Strasbourg Cedex, France.

VICHARD, PH., M.D., Professor, Centre Hospitalier et Universitaire de Besançon, Service d'Orthopédie—Traumatologie, Hôpital Jean Minjoz, boulevard Fleming, F-25030 Besançon Cedex, France.

WACKENHEIM, A., M.D., Professeur à la Faculté de Médecine de Strasbourg, 4, rue Dotzinger, F-67000 Strasbourg, France.

WEATHERLEY, C. R., M.D., Orthopaedic Hospital, Oswestry, Shropshire, England.

WHITE, III, AUGUSTUS A., M.D., Department of Orthopaedic Surgery, Beth Israel Hospital, Boston, MA 02115, U.S.A.

WHITECLOUD, III, TH. S., M.D., Department of Orthopaedic Surgery, Tulane University School of Medicine, 1430 Tulane Avenue, New Orleans, LA 70112, U.S.A.

WÖRSDÖRFER, O., M.D., Priv.-Doz., Klinik für Unfallchirurgie, Hand-, Plastische und Wiederherstellungschirurgie der Universität Ulm, Steinhoevelstrasse 9, D-7900 Ulm, Federal Republic of Germany.

1. Biodynamics of the Cervical Spine

1.1. Anatomo-Clinical Correlations in Cervical Spondylosis

M. Boni and V. Denaro, Pavia, Italy

Before addressing the clinical manifestations and therapy of cervical arthrosis it is first necessary to:

1. define arthrosis;

2. study the alterations of the spinal column, particularly of the cervical region, provoked by arthrosis;

3. correlate the various clinical syndromes to the pathological situations from which they are derived;

4. furnish coherent therapeutic indications for the different clinical syndromes.

Arthrosis can be defined as the constellation of alterations provoked by relative functional overload, acting mainly on cartilage but also on other articular structures. Relative functional overload may be the result of an ultrafunctional load placed on normal cartilage or a normal load placed on previously altered cartilage.

The final result is a series of lesions which create a vicious circle involving the metaplasm (collagen and proteoglycans). While cellular changes cause modifications in the synthesis and degradation of collagen or proteoglycans, alterations in the pericellular environment diminish mechanical protection and increase cellular exposure to the effects of mechanical action (even in situations of normal functional load). In response to this degenerative process, chondrocytes and other cells of the surrounding tissues tend to proliferate in an attempt at repair (Fig. 1).

The full expression of arthrosis is seen in an anarchic, irregular biochemical, morphological and ultrastructural mixture of these elements. Analogous changes occur in the vertebrae; especially in the interhypophyseal articulations, intervertebral discs and uncovertebral articulations.

Within the vertebral column—especially in the cervical spine—it is important to distinguish between lesions due to ageing and those secondary to arthrosis. The cervical region is the most mobile portion of the spinal column, and consequently it is here that the earliest disc degenerations are encountered. By the fourth decade of life horizontal or radial fissures begin to develop in the intersomatic disc and the nucleus polposus becomes

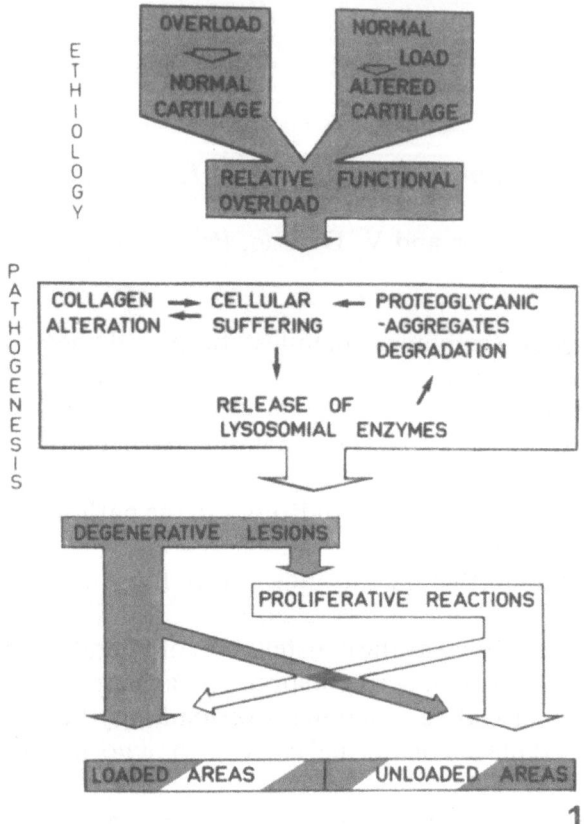

Fig. 1. Effect of relative functional overload

unrecognizable (Figs. 2 a, b). With age these fissures grow and the disc becomes thinner (Figs. 3 a, b). Even in subjects over 80 years of age these alterations in disc morphology (although severe) are not correlated with the lesions encountered in arthrosis (Figs. 4 a, b).

At this point a question arises. What is the pathogenesis of cervical arthrosis and how does it present itself clinically?

Cervical arthrosis can involve the intersomatic disc (discoarthrosis) the unco-vertebral articulation (uncoarthrosis), or the interhypophyseal articulation (hypophyseal arthrosis).

Discoarthrosis is most common and is often associated with uncoarthrosis. Hypophyseal arthrosis may develop independently leading to cases of severe hypophyseal arthrosis in association with normal or near normal disc structure. This fact is of importance to the discussion of the pathogenesis and therapy of cervico-brachialgic syndromes.

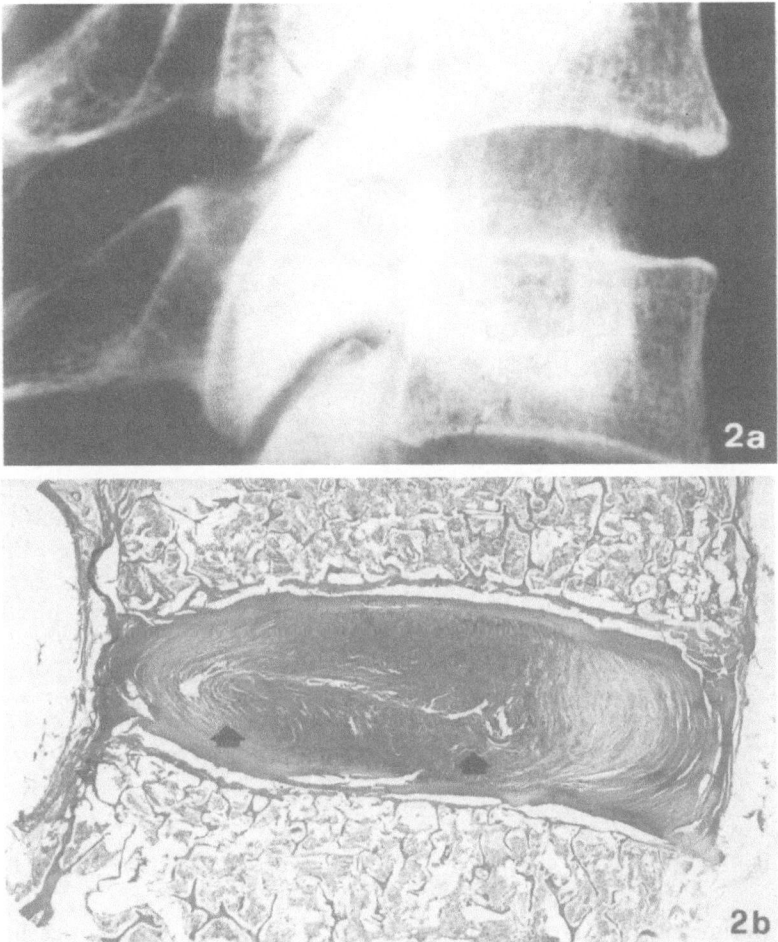

Fig. 2. Specimen from 53-year-old man at the level of C5–C6. Note initial degeneration of the disc (horizontal and radial fissures). The nucleus polposus is not recognizable

As stated above, cervical arthrosis occurs most frequently at the intervertebral disc (Fig. 5), where it principally causes the thinning of the disc and the formation of osteophytes in addition to altering the first order framework of the vertebral bodies.

The anatomopathologic changes of the central portion of the disc, the annulus fibrosus, and the cortical margins are well known. We will concentrate briefly on osteophyte formation. Osteophytes have different characteristics according to their location at the anterior or posterior margins of the vertebral body.

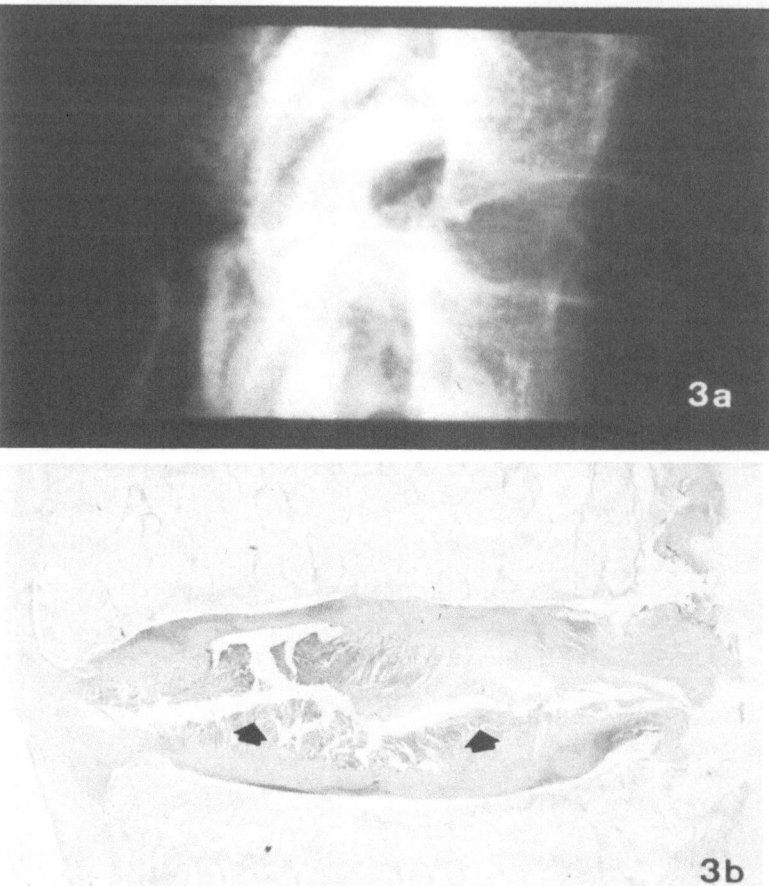

Fig. 3. Specimen from 61-year-old man at the level of C 5–C 6. Notice how the number of fissures increases progressively with age, with a concomitant decrease in the thickness of the disc

As a consequence of relative functional overload, discoarthrosis is frequently seen in the cervical spine secondary to the habitual reduction of cervical lordosis (increasingly a result of desk work, driving, reading and watching television). In these situation the head must be held in anterior inclination. To keep the head in equilibrium its weight is countered by a contraction of the cervico-nuchal extensor musculature. With increased anterior inclination and decreased cervical lordosis there is an increase in anterior leverage and a concomitant increase in the tone and work of the extensor muscles. The result is an overloading of the occipito-atlantal articulation and the entire cervical spine. Furthermore in arthrosis the cervical musculature may be already abnormally contracted, thereby

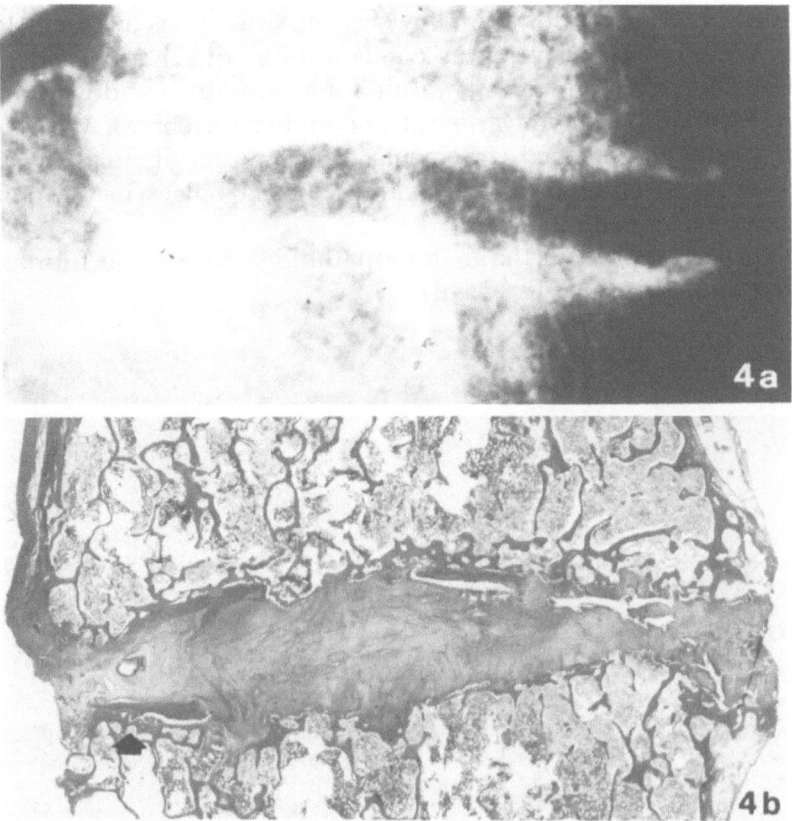

Fig. 4. Specimen from 83-year-old man at the level of C6–C7. Note that with increasing age the disc becomes even thinner and degenerated, but no posterior protrusions or osteophytes are normally observed

further increasing the load placed on the rigid, flexed spine. One may thus deduce, that functional overload can cause disc degeneration and osteophyte formation at any level.

From this theoretical reconstruction we can conclude that there exists a direct force acting on the disc in the cranio-caudal and postero-anterior directions. This force can be considered as the resultant of two vectors, one antero-posterior and the other cranio-caudal.

We can theorize that anterior osteophytes should form on the anterior vertebral border under the anterior longitudinal ligament, and are largely in the forward direction. Posterior osteophytes should be directed in a vertical direction parallel to the posterior aspect of the vertebral bodies.

This hypothesis is clinically fully confirmed. Anterior osteophytes of superior vertebrae are directed anterior-inferiorly, while those of inferior vertebrae are directed anterior-superiorly (Figs. 6 a–f).

At the posterior vertebral rim however the situation is different (Fig. 7). Posterior osteophytes develop as condensations of sclerotic bone at the posterior edge of the intervertebral disc and are directed downwards (in overlying vertebrae) or upwards (in underlying vertebrae). With growth they cause to be detached (fragments of the posterior annulus) and to become trapped and shifted backwards causing bulges in the posterior longitudinal ligament.

This process represents the anatomopathologic basis of the formation of so-called hard hernias (Figs. 7 a–d).

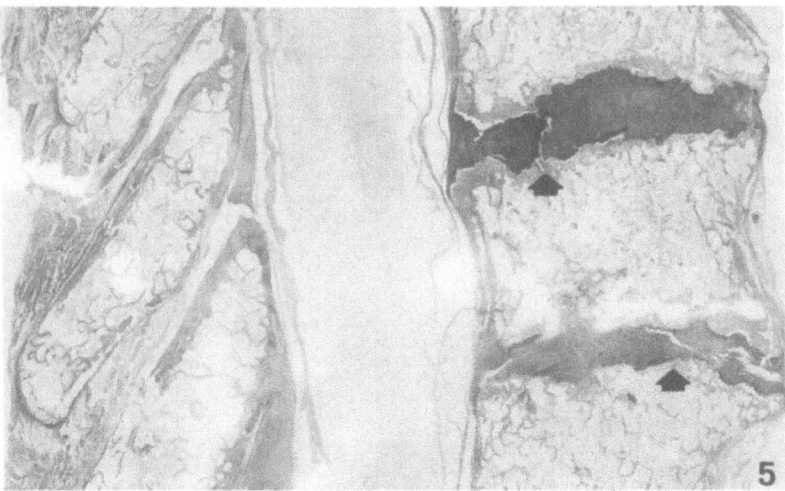

Fig. 5. Specimen from subject with initial arthrosis showing how during the pathogenetic evolution of cervical spondylosis the intersomatic disc is very frequently the first structure to undergo pathologic changes

Hard hernias are statistically more frequent than soft hernias. The latter consist of trapped disc fragments which protrude under the longitudinal ligament, or more frequently are expelled into the vertebral canal. In our observation of 137 cases of various ages, this situation was never encountered.

Unco-vertebral degeneration usually parallels disco-arthrosic degeneration. Thinning of the disc causes the corresponding surfaces of contiguous vertebrae to draw nearer. Initial osseous sclerosis is followed by the deformation of the uncus which then curves laterally to finally form the osteophytes characteristic of uncoarthrosis (Figs. 8 a–d). It has been said that uncoarthrosis sometimes results in compression of the vertebral artery with consequent functional disturbances, organic lesions or irritation of the perivascular sympathetic plexus (Figs. 8 e, f).

It must be remembered that the anatomical changes seen in advanced age, such as cervical spine shortening and disc thinning, do not coincide with shortening of the vertebral artery. On the contrary, certain adaptations, such as bone reabsorption, take place and permit the continued normal functioning of the vertebral artery.

These examples may be extreme but we are all familiar with the bends that occur in the 2nd portion of the vertebral artery which have no pathologic significance.

At times compression of the vertebral artery does occur with resulting deformation of its lumen. In this case the pathology has an organic basis readily confirmed by current diagnostic tests.

Arthrosis of the interhypophyseal articulations (Figs. 9 a, b) is similar to that seen in other diartric joints, with cartilaginous degeneration, formation of large osteophytes and deformation of the articular facets. The facets may then protrude forward restricting the canal and causing alterations of the joint capsule, the synovium (with local or referred pain) and extrinsic nerve root compression (causing' cervico-brachialgia and peripheral radicular signs).

In the intervertebral articulation we must also consider the yellow ligaments which form an elastic syndesmosis. Although they do not degenerate in arthrosis, they can hypertrophy and therefore contribute to posterior stenosis of the canal (Fig. 10).

It is also worth noting that ossification of the anterior longitudinal ligament, and more rarely but much more seriously, of the posterior longitudinal ligament (OPLL according to Japanese authors) may occur.

Considering the alterations encountered in vertebral arthrosis, we can now outline the correlated clinical syndromes (Fig. 11).

Discoarthrosis may result in:

1. anterior osteophytosis (almost always asymptomatic);

2. disc degeneration with algogenic nociceptive reactions (the posterior longitudinal ligament is rich in afferent nerve fibers whose stimulation results in cervicoalgia with characteristic pain radiation);

3. formation of posterolateral protrusions (hard or soft hernias) which cause cervico-brachialgia with peripheral signs that follow nerve root distribution;

4. formation of medial (more common) or posterior protrusions which cause medullar symptoms (spondylotic myelopathy);

5. associated syndromes such as radiculo-myelopathy.

Unco-vertebral arthrosis can provoke more or less complex syndromes such as headache, radiculopathy, Neri-Barré-Lieou types syndromes, syndromes of the superior quarter of the trunk, etc.

Hypophyseal arthrosis may cause cervicoalgia, cervico-nuchalgia and cervico-brachialgic syndromes.

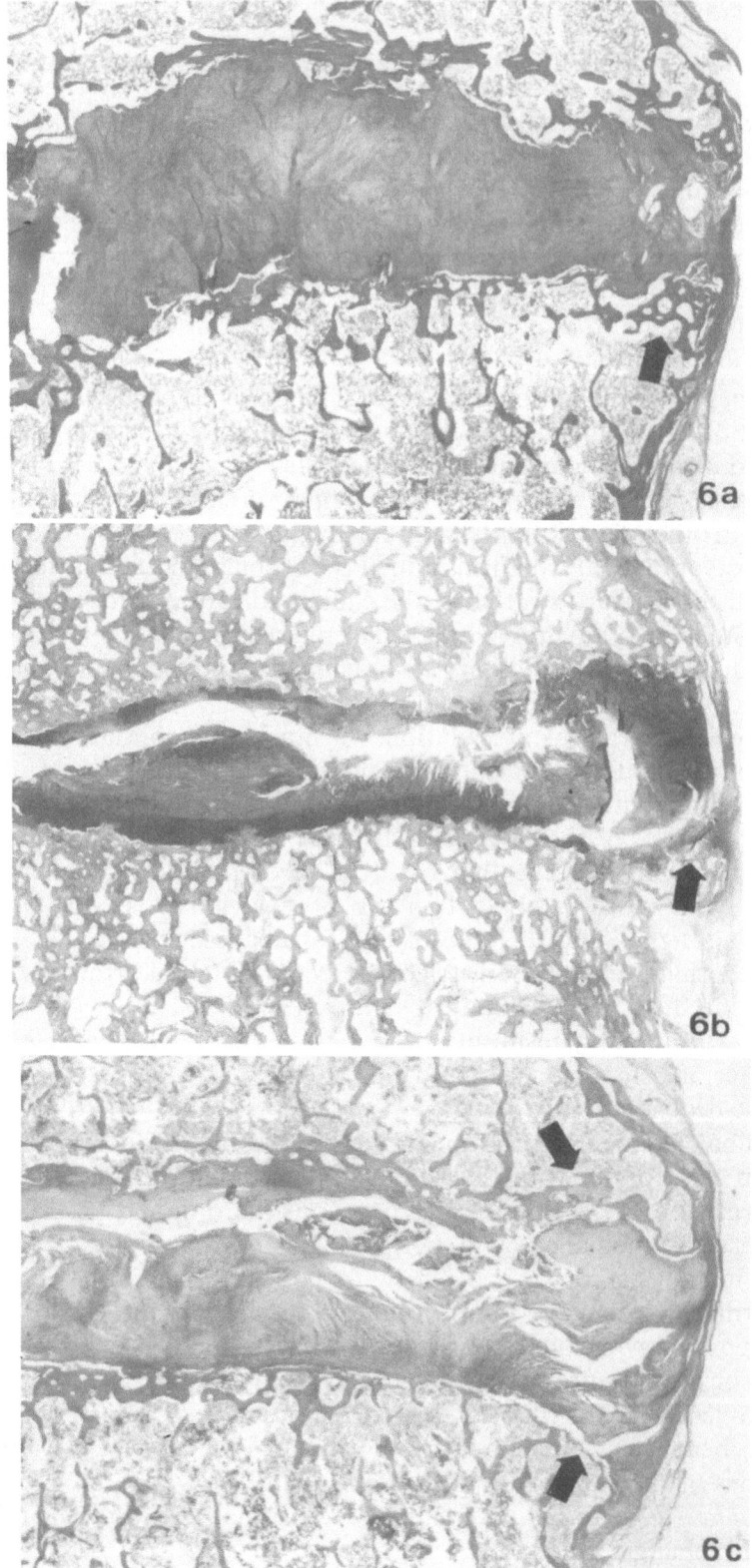

Fig. 6. Series of specimens of discoarthrosis in progressive stages of increasing arthrosis and formation of anterior osteophytes. a), b) At the anterior angles of the vertebral bodies, the bone becomes sclerotic just beneath the anterior longitudinal

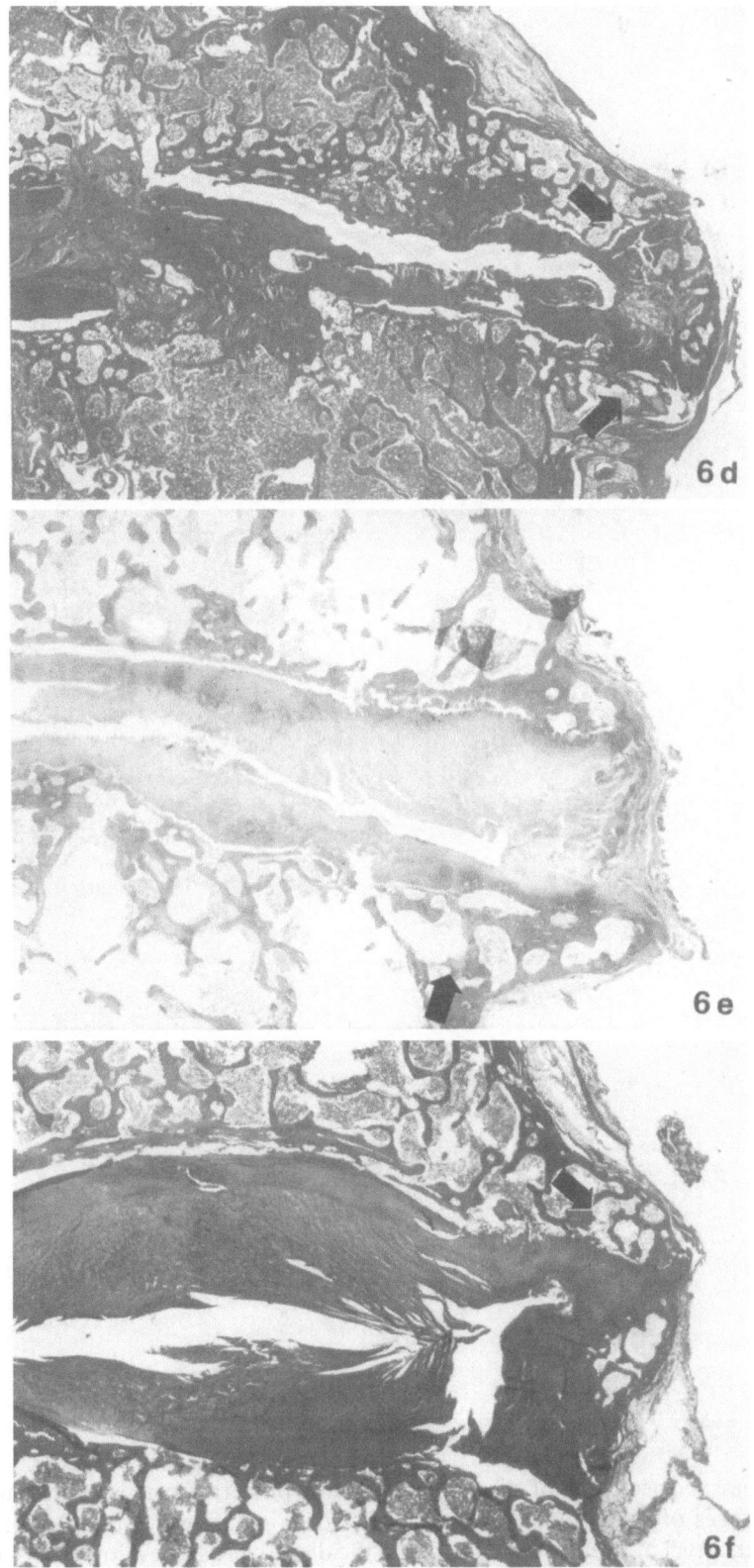

ligament. c), d) Sclerosis becomes more intense, and sclerotic bone accumulates with the formation of the osteophytic spurs, which direct forward. e), f) Finally, they converge, pushing the anterior longitudinal ligament

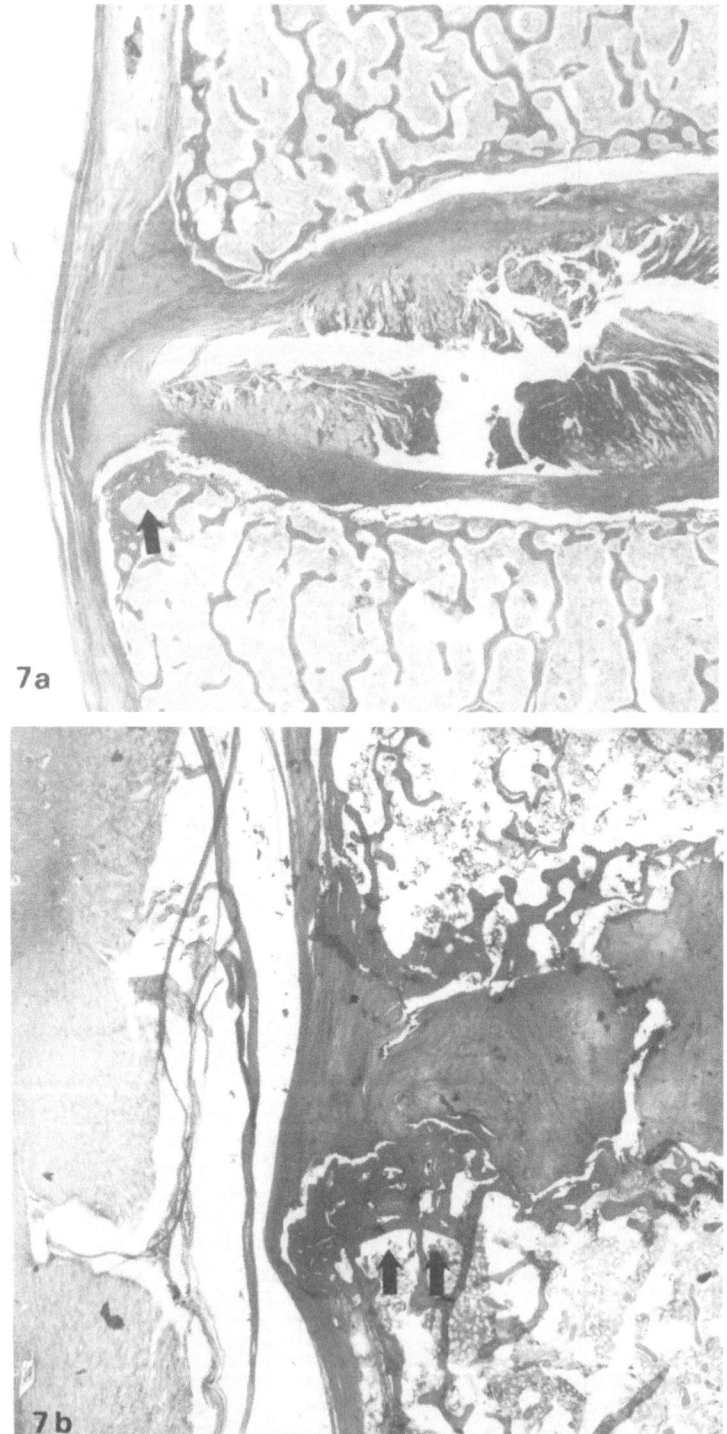

Fig. 7. Series of specimens of discoarthrosis with posterior osteophytic spurs in different stages of development. At the posterior edge of two adjacent vertebral bodies, at the level of the posterior border of the disc, sclerosis develops. With time, it becomes more intense, and sclerotic bone accumulates (a, b), with the formation of spurs. The protruding fragments of the disc remain isolated and are pushed

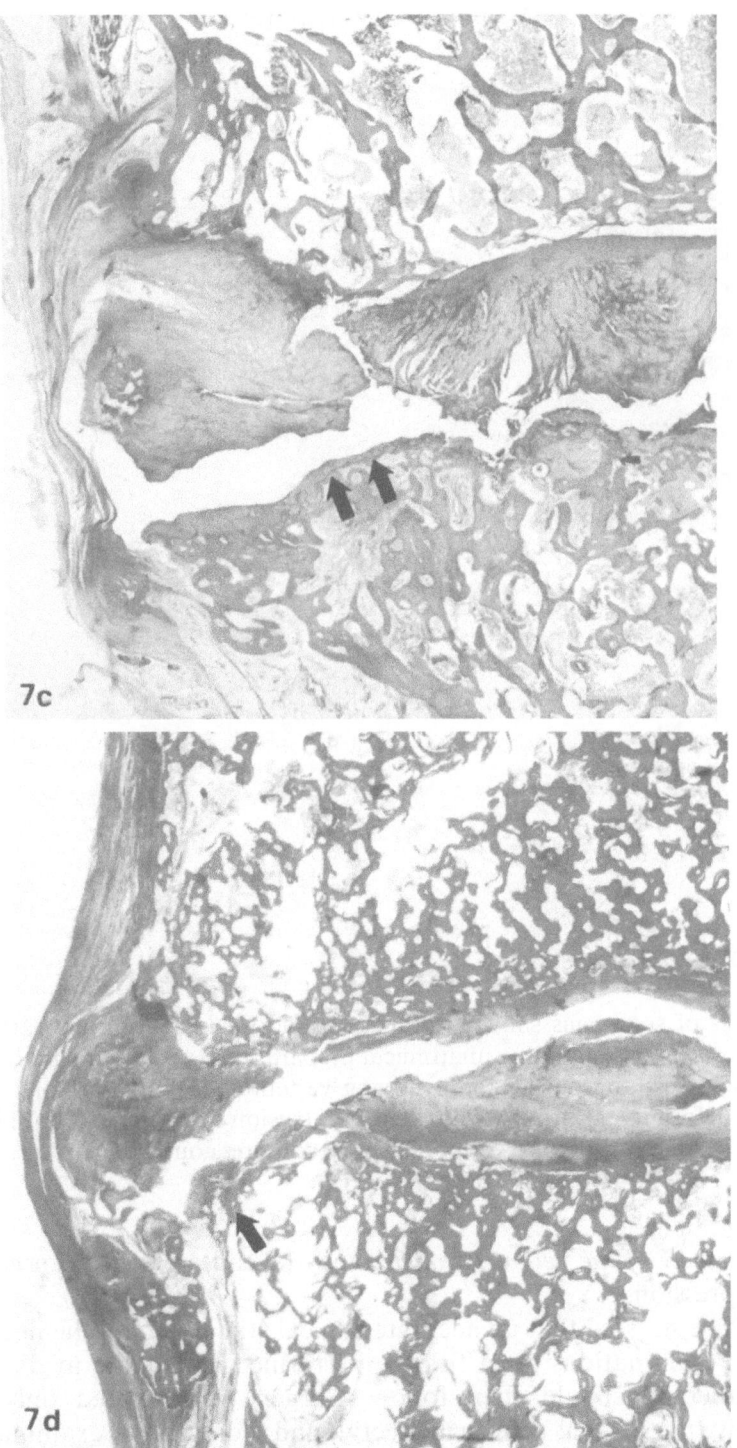

7c

7d

backwards by the compressive action of the disc (due to its increased thickness), together with the posterior osteophytic spurs (c). The posterior spurs are partly composed of osteophytes and partly of sequestered fragments of the posterior portion of the annulus (d)

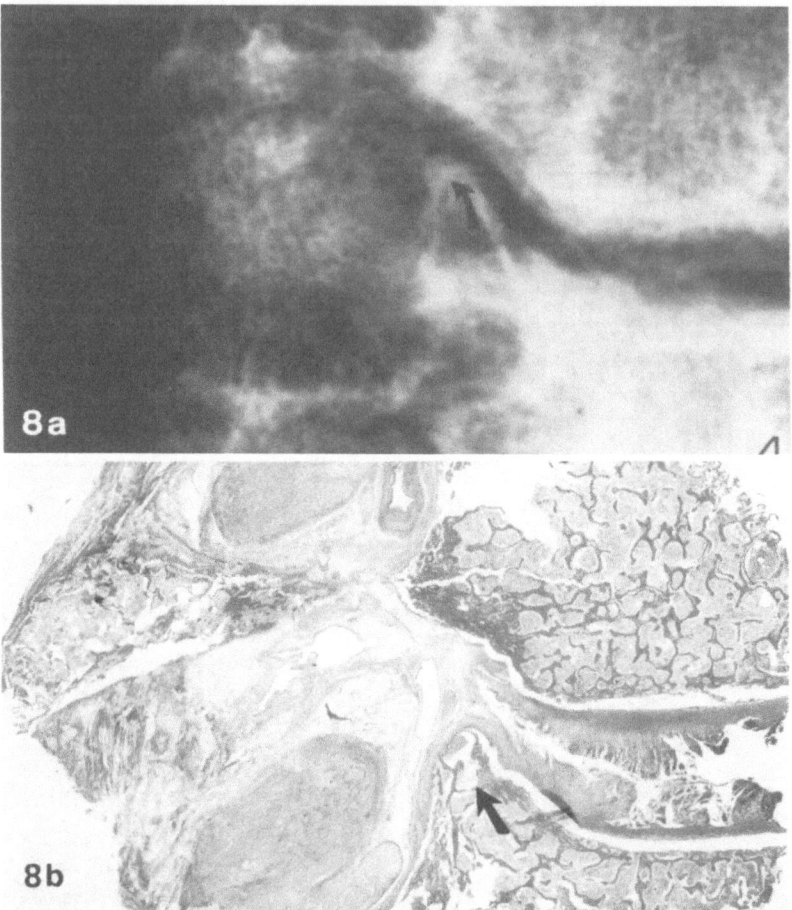

Fig. 8. Series of specimens showing different stages of increasing uncoarthrosis:
radiographs and corresponding anatomical preparations. a), b) The disc becomes
thinner, the uncus approaches the overlying vertebral body. c), d) Later on, an
increase of deformity takes place with lateral protrusion of the uncus. e), f) This can
provoke vertebral artery compression

Hypertrophy of the yellow ligaments may be cause of posterior cervical
cord compression.

It must be stressed that an accurate clinical study with all the necessary
diagnostic examinations must first be performed. Adequate medical and
physical therapy should then follow. Surgery is indicated only after
conservative therapy has proven ineffective and radiographic examinations,
myelography, CT, electromyography and scintigraphy have indicated
extrinsic compression.

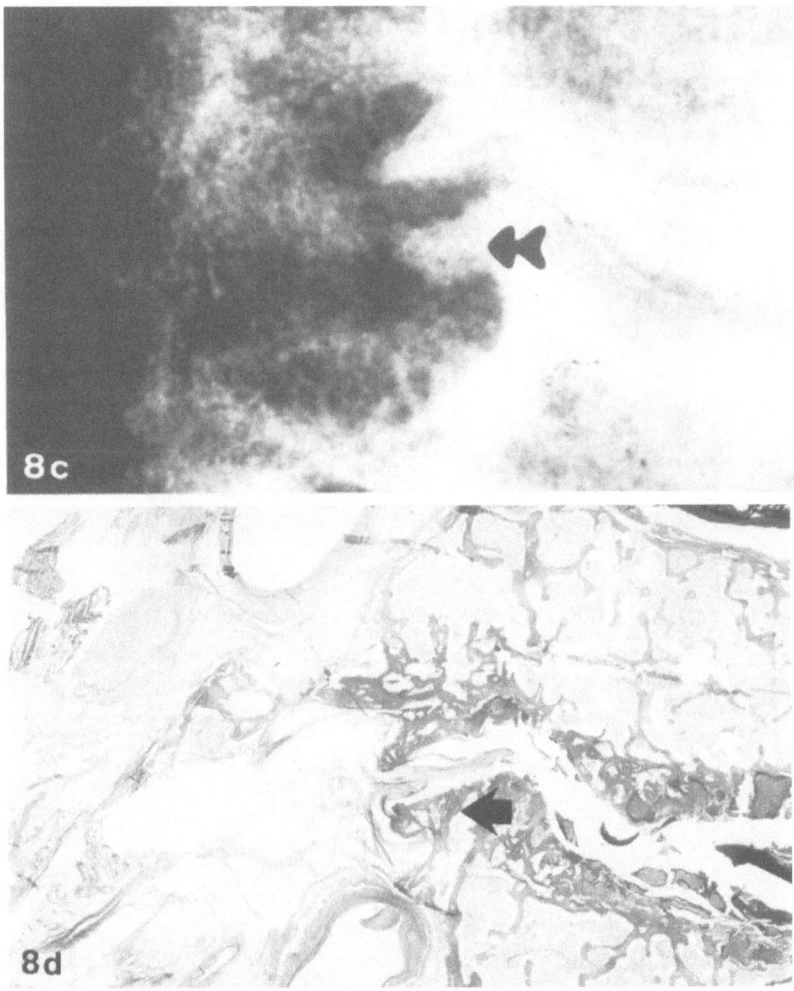

The surgical approach to the cervical spine may be posterior, anterior or lateral. As a general rule the anterior approach is used in the case of anterior lesions, and likewise, the posterior approach is employed for posterior lesions.

The posterior surgical procedures for enlargement of the vertebral canal or removal of lateral disc protrusions are exceptions to this rule.

Many different surgical techniques [2, 3, 4] have been proposed.
The anterior approach may be used for:
discectomy without arthrodesis
    with or without removal of osteophytes
    microdiscectomy
    decompression with curette according to Louis

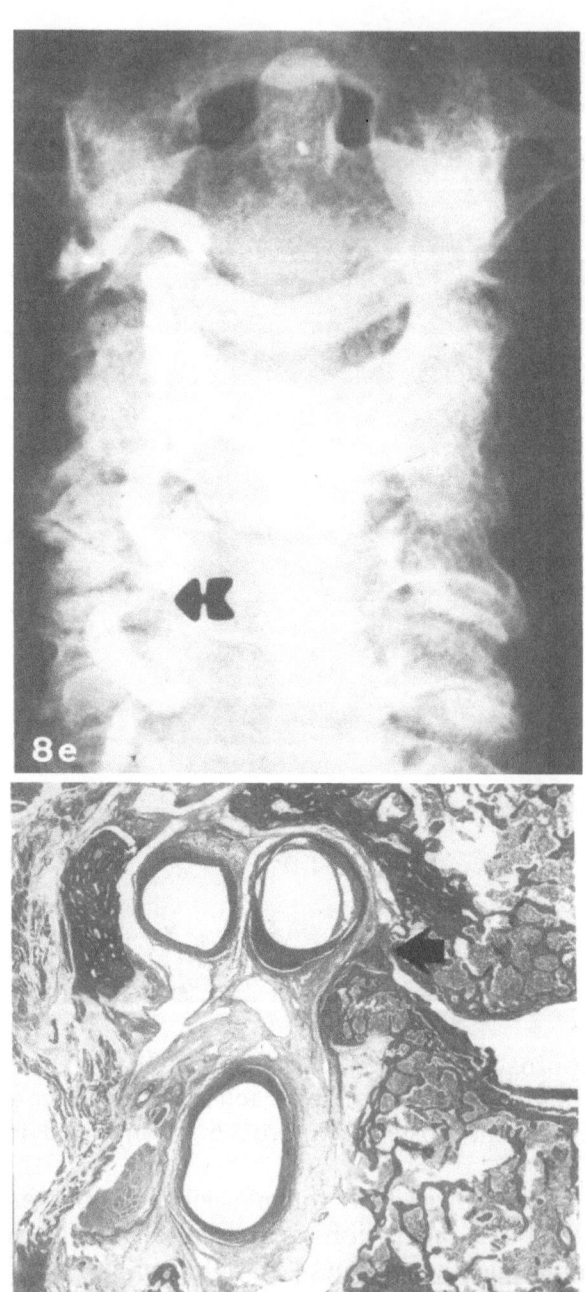

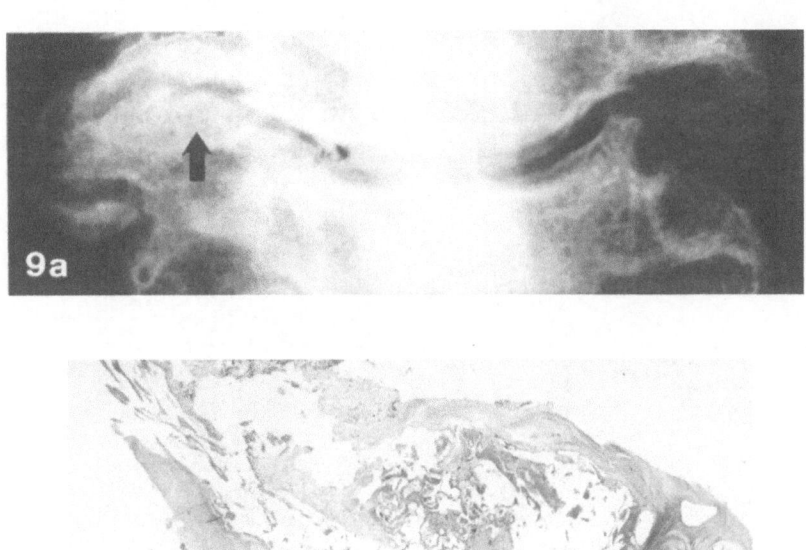

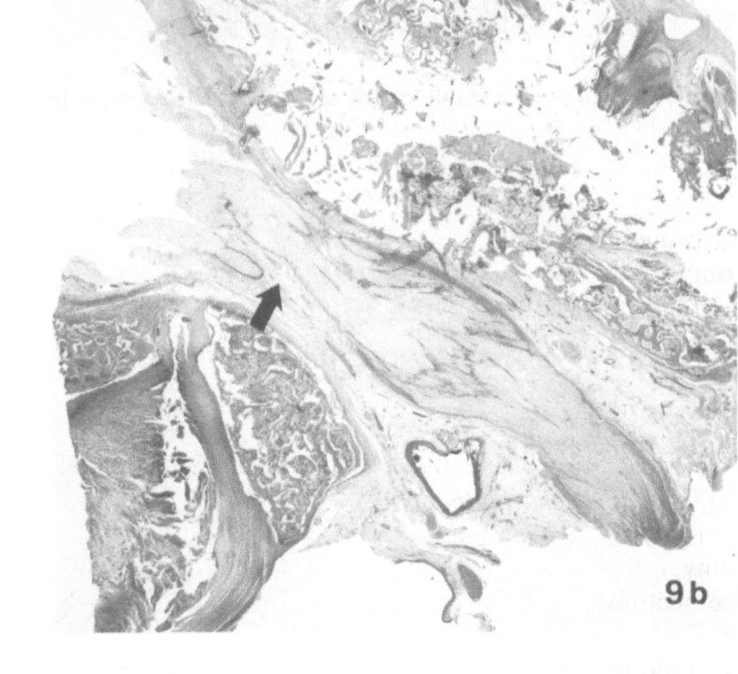

Fig. 9. Specimen showing interhypophyseal arthrosis which has developed independently of discoarthrosis; a) X-ray, b) anatomical preparation from the same patient. Note the well conserved disc and marked degeneration of the articular facets

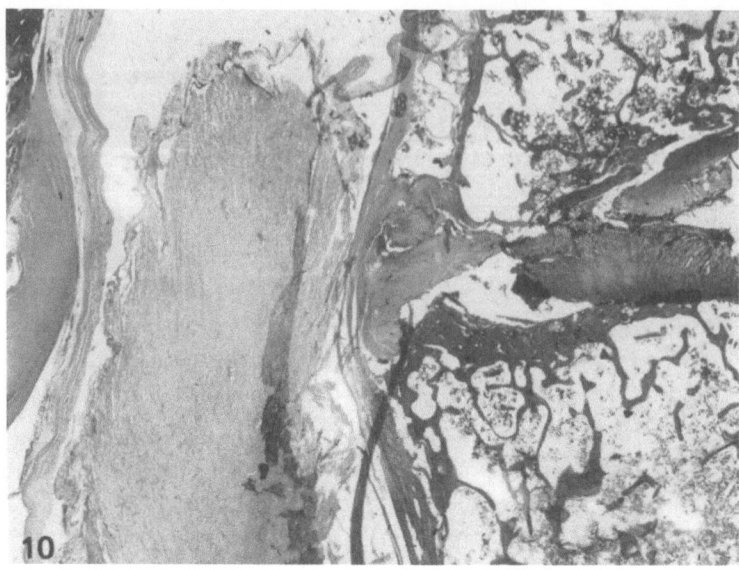

Fig. 10. Specimen showing an example of hypertrophy of the yellow ligaments

discectomy with arthrodesis
    Smith-Robinson
    modified Magerl procedure
    Bailey-Badgley
    Cloward
    modified Cloward
multiple subtotal somatectomy

The antero-lateral approach may be used for:
    transversectomy;
    uncusectomy;
    uncuforaminectomy;
    Kehr technique;
    Verbiest technique.

The posterior approach can be used to perform:
    decompressive laminectomy;
    hemilaminectomy;
    facetectomy;
    enlargement of the vertebral canal with various techniques
    (Hirabayashi).
    We prefer the anterior approach for treatment of the following

INTERAPOPHYSEAL JOINT DEGENERATION

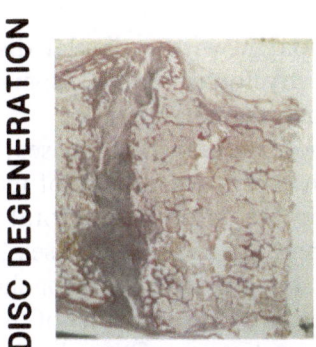

Radiculopathy causing cervicobrachialgia
Cervicoalgia

DISC DEGENERATION

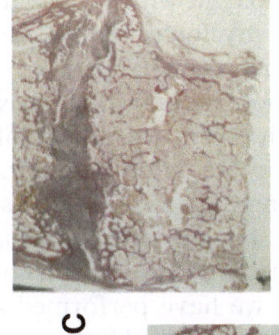

Cervicoalgia
Cervicodorsalgia

LATERAL OSTEOPHYTOSIC PROTRUSION

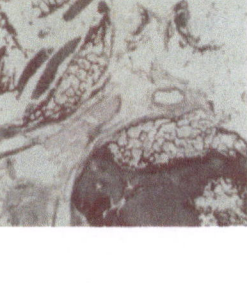

Radiculopathy and radiculomyelopathy

CENTRAL OSTEOPHYTOSIC PROTRUSION

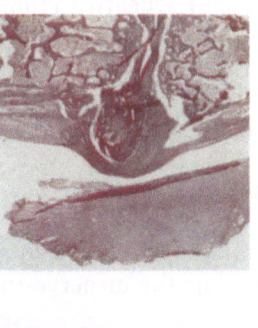

Spondylotic myelopathy

YELLOW LIGAMENT HYPERTROPHY

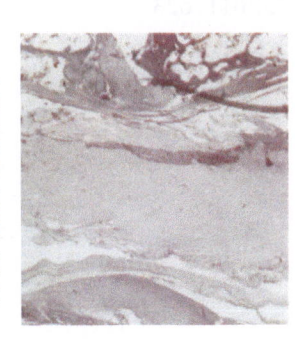

Posterior stenosis

UNCO-VERTEBRAL DEGENERATION

Radiculopathy
Neri - Barré - Lieou and correlated syndromes
IVB

Fig. 11. Clinical syndromes

syndromes:

cervicobrachialgia with radicular distribution;

spondylotic myelopathy and associated syndromes;

certain cervico-cephalalgia,

and we use in the large majority of cases [1] the Cloward procedure, at one or two levels (with several variations of technique). However, since 1969, we have been using the multiple subtotal somatectomy, for more extensive lesions involving 3 or more levels (see 2.10, page 124).

Concerning the posterior approaches (in cases of posterior stenosis, laminar-hypertrophy, hypertrophy of the yellow ligaments, dismorphism of the peduncles) we have performed a laminectomy and more recently we have used the method of Hirabayashi [2].

In conclusion, each author must have an eclectic knowledge of many techniques to be able to evaluate their limits and to be able to adapt them to each specific pathology or clinical case.

It is important to underline that recognition of the anatomopathologic background of each case is one of the surest elements for guidance in the proper choice of surgical procedure.

References

1. Boni M, Denaro V (1982) Traitement chirurgical des cervicarthroses. Révision à distance (2–13 ans) des 100 premiers cas opérés par voie antérieure. Rev Chir Orthop 68: 269–280
2. Hirabayashi K *et al* (1980) Operative treatment for cervical spinal disc lesions. Eighth Annual Meeting Cervical Spine Research Soc. Palm Beach, December 10–13, 1980
3. Jung A *et al* (1975) Névralgies cervico-brachiales. Rev Chir Orthop 61 [Suppl] 2: 7–26
4. Verbiest H *et al* (1966) Anterolateral surgery for cervical spondylosis in cases of myelopathy or nerve-root compression. J Neurosurg 25: 611–623

1.2. Stability and Instability of the Cervical Spine

R. Louis, Marseille, France

Most theories about instability are based on anatomo-pathologic data such as:

— The posterior vertebral body wall theory (Decoulx and Rieunau 1958 [1]).

— The posterior ligamentous complex theory (Holdsworth 1963 [3]).

— The middle segment theory (Roy-Camille 1979 [9]).

— The three-column spine concept (Denis 1983 [2]).

None of these theories can explain the mechanism of normal stability. We started our studies with investigations on fresh and normal cadaveric spines before analyzing clinical cases. Consequently, in 1975, I described a three-column spine concept, different from that of Denis [5].

Firstly it is necessary to define stability and instability. Stability of the spine is the means by which the vertebral structures maintain their cohesion in all physiological positions. Instability or loss of stability is a pathological process which can lead to displacement of vertebrae beyond their normal physiological limits.

It is necessary to consider spinal stability in both the vertical axis and the horizontal plane.

Vertical Axis Stability (Fig. 1)

In order to study this, one must consider the morphology of the individual vertebrae and the structure of the spine as a single unit.

Vertebral morphology. From the atlas to the sacrum it is possible to identify those structures in the complex morphology of the vertebrae that resist the forces of gravity.

Overall architecture of the spine. The juxtaposition of the various vertebral structures makes it possible to follow the lines of load-bearing forces from the cranium to the pelvis. The cranium transfers its weight to the spine through the two pillars of the atlas lying in the same coronal plane. The two pillars become three columns in the body of the axis, which is a crossroads for the transmission of the forces. These are then transmitted down the three columns, which are arranged in a triangle with an anterior apex. The larger anterior column takes on the aspect of a quadrangular pyramid formed by the alternating vertebral bodies and intervertebral discs down to the sacral base. The two posterior columns lying in a coronal plane are formed by the successive articular processes. This three-column structure of the spine, like a three-legged stool, provides the simplest and most efficient system of stability.

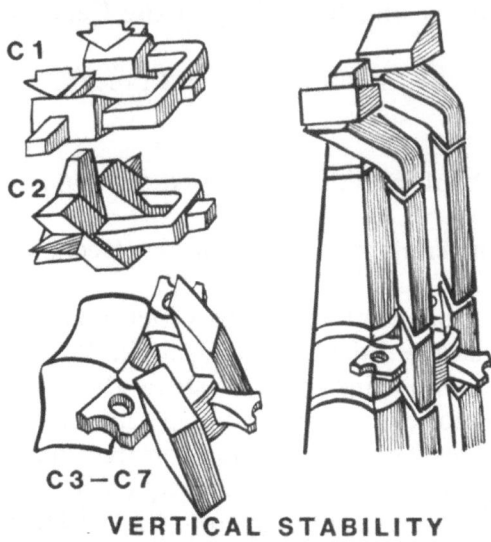

Fig. 1. Illustrations of the morphology of vertebrae and overall architecture of the spine showing the vertical columns which are two at the C 1–C 2 level and three from C 2 to the sacrum

Transverse Stability (Fig. 2)

When the spine is subjected to forces perpendicular to its axis, the points of weakness are located in the intervertebral motion segments. At all spinal levels the same mechanism stabilizes the spine: the coupling of bony stops and ligamentous brakes.

The Coupling of Bony Stops and Ligamentous Brakes

Any extreme vertebral motion is blocked by the coupling action of bony stops and ligamentous brakes. During flexion: the bony stops or buttresses are either in the C 1–C 2 motion unit—the dens against the anterior arch or between C 2–C 3 and L 5–S 1 motion units—the articular processes and the anterior edge of end-plates against each other similarly. The ligamentous brakes are in the C 1–C 2 motion unit—the transverse ligament, the posterior atlantoaxial membrane and the articular capsules of the lateral atlantoaxial joints or between C 2–C 3 and L 5–S 1 motion segments, the ligamentous brakes are all the ligaments located posterior to the annulus fibrosus, the posterior longitudinal ligament, the articular capsules, the ligamenta flava, and the inter- and supra-spinous ligaments.

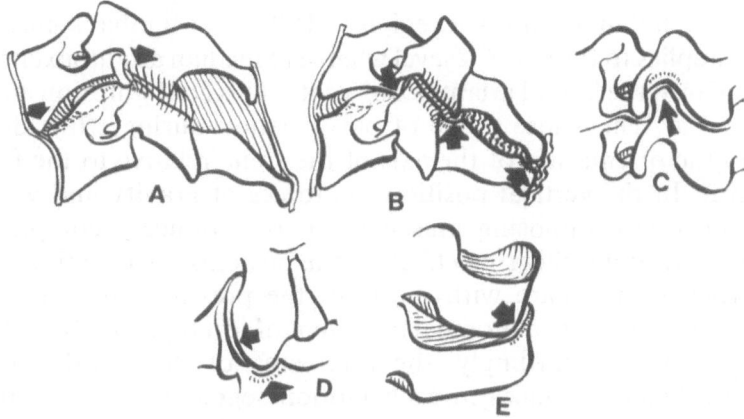

HORIZONTAL STABILITY

Fig. 2. Illustrations of the transverse instability of the spine during flexion-extension at the lower cervical region and during inclination-rotation. Dark arrows show the bony buttresses combined with ligamentous brakes for stabilizing vertebrae during excessive motion

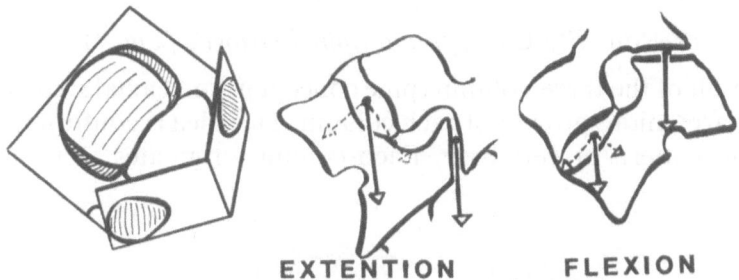

EXTENTION   FLEXION

Fig. 3. Illustration of the articular orthogonal triangulation concept. On the left, upper view of the three joints of a cervical motion segment. At each level the posterior articulations lie in a plane which opposes that of the intervertebral disc: this is approximately 45° in the cervical area. On the right: the cervical motion segments are shown during extension and flexion of the spine. Arrows indicate the direction of weight-bearing forces acting upon the disc and the posterior joints. When the disc resists compression forces the posterior facets resist shearing forces and vice-versa

The Articular Orthogonal Triangulation Theory (Fig. 3)

Each mobile spinal segment is formed by a set of three joints located at each angle of a triangle and lying in nearly perpendicular planes. These three joints are the intervertebral disc and the two zygapophyseal joints. With the exception of the bi-articular atlanto-occipital segment, all the mobile spinal segments are tri-articular. At each level the posterior articulations lie in a opposite plane to that of the intervertebral disc: this is approximately 45° in the cervical area, 60° in the thoracic region and 90° in the lumbar spine. This concept also applies to the C 1–C 2 level where the median atlantoaxial joint is perpendicular to the lateral atlantoaxial joints. This configuration creates an orthogonal system whose mode of participation during effort differs according to the orientation of the axis of the spine relative to the forces acting upon it. In the vertical position the forces of gravity and weight-bearing coupled with opposing muscular forces produce a compressive effect on the discs and a shearing effect on the posterior articulations. The posterior articulations share with the discs the pressure applied to the vertebrae, there thus exists a modulated system of leverage involving these different structures. Accordingly, the total area of the discal and zygapophyseal articular surfaces in each motion segment increases in the cranio-caudal direction to meet the increasing physical constraints.

Discussion and Clinical Relevance

The clinical relevance will be considered in relation to the development of the spine, adaptation to wear and spinal instability.

The Stability Concept and Spinal Growth (Fig. 4)

As a result of the three-column spine concept normal axial spine growth needs an harmonious growth of each column. This idea is confirmed by the ossification pattern of vertebrae. Each column originates from a single

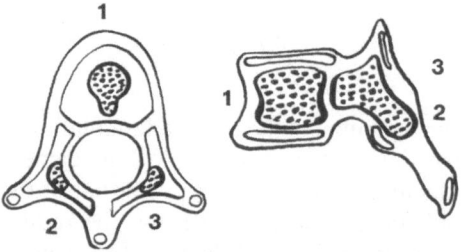

Fig. 4. Ossification pattern of vertebra. There are three single primary ossification centers: one for each vertical column (1, 2, 3)

primary ossification center: the centrum for the anterior column and the two vertebral arch centers for the two posterior columns. As a consequence of this and to avoid deformity it is important when operating on the (growing) spine of a child to perform a symmetrical fusion of all three columns for any limited disease requiring stabilization.

Adaptation of the Spine to Wear (Fig. 5)

My stability concept permits an understanding of constraints to which the spine is submitted: axial pressure along the three columns, pressure on the bony buttresses, the shearing effects on the ligamentous and discal brakes. When a joint acts in extreme positions, signs of early wear are usually noted. Subsequently, vertebral hyperflexion or hyperkyphosis increase the load on the anterior part of the intervertebral discs, the end-plates of the vertebral bodies and the superior part of the articular facets where osteophytes will be located. Hyperextension or hyperlordosis transfer forces towards the posterior arch and to the posterior part of the intervertebral disc. Lateral flexion with rotation increases the load on the part of the discs (uncarthrosis) and the homolateral posterior articulation with neocontact between the cervical transverse processes and the tips of the superior articular facets (Fig. 5).

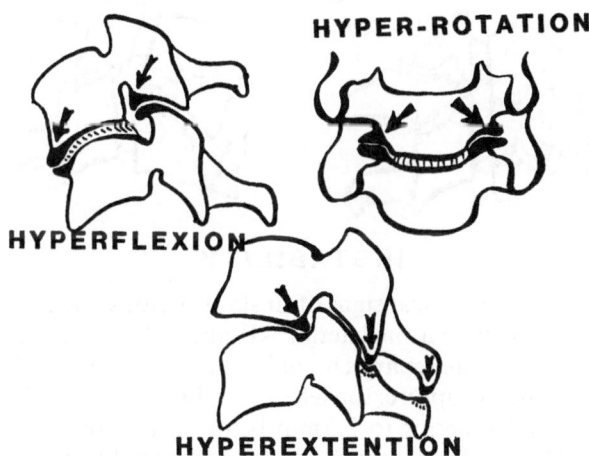

Fig. 5. Drawings showing how the spine adapts to wear in different conditions: hyperflexion or kyphosis, hyperextension or hyperlordosis and inclination-rotation such as scoliosis or uncarthrosis. Osteophytes and bony condensation appear where constraints are excessive at bony stop zones. In addition, stretched ligamentous brakes result in firstly spinal sprain, secondly spondylotic instability

Spinal Instability (Fig. 6)

As a result of these biomechanical data and of anatomo-pathological observations I proposed in 1975 [5] an instability theory with classification of lesions in order to determine therapeutic indications. Each vertical column ruptured is given a score of + 1, so the Chance fracture (slice fracture of the three columns in their bony structures) and the bilateral dislocation (horizontal shear through a motion segment) would score + 3.

The score for an incomplete lesion of the vertebral body and the fracture of pedicles or laminae are scored + 0.5. The fracture of transverse or spinous processes is scored + 0.25. The lack of substance in a vertical column is assessed as + 2. This is the case with severe compression fractures that have been reduced by a conservative method; so the vertebral body substance

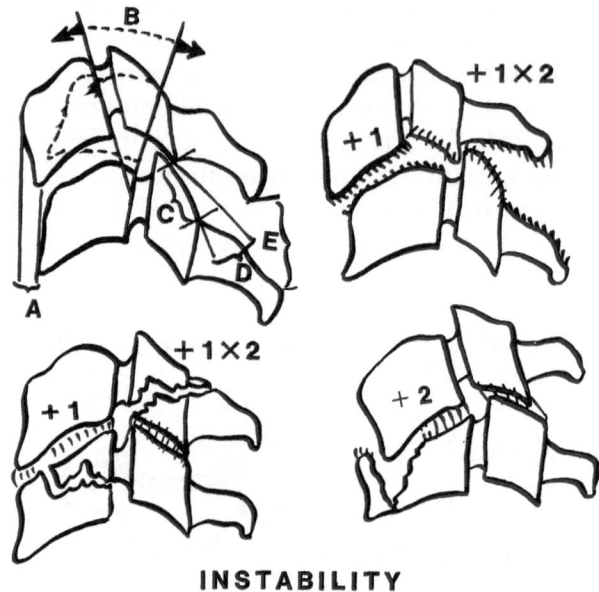

INSTABILITY

Fig. 6. Illustration of radiological signs of unstable lesions due to severe sprains or spondylosis. These are shown on lateral, AP and CT-scan dynamic roentgeno-grams. These severe signs are separately sufficient to confirm instability due to disc and ligament loosening or rupture: top left *A* vertebral body translation superior to 3.5 mm above C 4 and superior to 2.5 mm below C 4, *B* flexion-extension range superior to 11°, *C* loss of facet contact superior or equal to 50%, *D* loss of facet parallelism, *E* interspinous widening. In addition, classification and scoring of severe traumatic lesions of the spine. Each vertical column is given a score of + 1. The lack of substance of a vertical column is assessed as + 2: coronal fracture of the vertebral body with tilt of the subadjacent vertebra. A lesion is unstable when the final score is superior or equal to + 2

contains several gaps which yield a recurrence of the kyphotic deformity despite prolonged immobilization. Otherwise, a coronal fracture of the vertebral body sometimes produces a loss of substance under the antero-inferior edge of the vertebra above, automatically inducing a further kyphotic focus. Consequently, an unstable lesion corresponds to a score equal or superior to + 2. Unstable lesions might be separated in two groups. Firstly a "temporary bony instability" such as Chance fracture for instance with bony lesions being likely to heal after reduction and immobilization without surgery. Secondly, a "permanent ligamentous instability" such as a bilateral dislocation involving ligament and disc lesions which are likely to yield weak scar so that surgical stabilization and fusion are advocated. Permanent ligamentous instability due to lesions of the stabilizing factors (bony stops and ligamentous brakes) corresponds to a motion spinal segment working loose either from injury or spondylosis.

Diagnosis of ligamentous instability, when not obvious, necessitates dynamic roentgenograms displaying one or several of the following signs: vertebral body translation superior to 3.5 mm above C4 and to 2.5 mm below C4 (Fig. 6 top left, A), flexion-extension range superior to 11° (Fig. 6 top left, B), loss of facet contact superior or equal to 50% (Fig. 6 C), loss of facet parallelism (Fig. 6 top left, D), and interspinous widening (Fig. 6 top left, E).

The history of patients suffering from spinal pain demonstrates that pain is preceeded by "spinal sprains" due to excessive or violent movements of some motion segments which can later lead to degenerative changes with fibrous and articular damage.

References

1. Decoulx P, Rieunau G (1958–1959) Rapport à la 23° Réunion Annuelle de la Société Nationale Française de chirurgie Traumatologique. Rev Chir Orthop 44: 244, 45: 237
2. Denis F (1983) The three-column spine and its significance in the classification of acute thoracolumbar spine injuries. Spine 8: 817
3. Holdsworth FW (1963) Fractures, dislocations and fracture-dislocations of the spine. J Bone Joint Surg 45 B: 6
4. Kirkaldy-Willis WH, Farfan HF (1982) Instability of the lumbar spine. Clin Orthop 165: 110
5. Louis R, Bonsignour JP, Ouiminga R (1975) Réduction orthopédique contrôlée des fractures du rachis. Rev Chir Orthop 61: 323
6. Louis R, Goutallier D (1977) Fractures instables du rachis. Rev Chir Orthop 63: 5–415
7. Louis R (1982) Chirurgie du rachis. Springer, Berlin Heidelberg New York Tokyo
8. Nicoll EA (1949) Fractures of the dorso-lumbar spine. J Bone Joint Surg 31 B: 376
9. Roy-Camille R (1979) Rachis cervical traumatique non neurologique. Masson, Paris
10. White A, Panjabi M (1978) Clinical biomechanics of the spine. JB Lippincott Company, Philadelphia, USA

1.3. Biodynamics of the Lower Cervical Spine

F. Pipino and R. Bancale, Bari, Italy

This is a study of the biodynamics of the lower cervical spine in relation to the global function of the spine. The lower cervical spine has therefore been investigated with reference to both the maintenance of the neutral posture, and to its responses to various functional stresses.

I. The theory of opposed pyramids and the dynamic modalities of the lower cervical spine. In a schematic representation of the spinal column as a whole, the spine could be thought of as a structure made of two truncated pyramids with opposite vertices and an intersposed fulcrum (discs L 3–L 4–L 5). The upper pyramid—to which the head and the upper limbs both converge—represents predominantly the dynamic part of the system, since it is controlled mostly by muscles. The lower pyramid—stiffer—prevalently controlled by ligaments, is instead intended to distribute loads to the lower limbs. Obviously the theory of opposed pyramids is just a graphic representation of the work of the spinal column as a whole. It is not intended to overcome the idea of *motor segment* which, in a metameric vision of the spine, fully preserves its validity. From a strictly anatomical-functional point of view, we regard as valid the distinction, on a longitudinal plane, between *fore* vertebral section (discs, vertebral bodies, fore and hinder longitudinal ligaments) and *hinder* vertebral section (facet joints, vertebral arches and hinder ligaments). The two sections regulate the vertebral work in a different way through their fundamental anatomical-functional structures. The nucleus polposus—understood as a precompressed hydraulic chamber—is at the same time the bearing system of the axial loads, and the fulcrum of the intervertebral movement.

The posterior joints are the sliding track of the movement. The neuromuscular control system is the real starter of the movement and controls its initation; the propioceptives nervous impulses, in fact, condition the changes in muscular work during the various kinematic moments. The brakes are bony structures, capsules and ligaments, which control the movement. The *lower* cervical spine is therefore one of the anatomo-functional areas of the upper pyramid. In relation to the *quality* of the movement it may be thought of as a polyarticular functional unit. In fact from the anatomical point of view we notice the following characteristics: the vertebral bodies have the same morphology; spatial arrangement and the shape of the facet joints is almost the same; the intervertebral discs are nearly the same size and ligaments and muscles are in common. That entails, from a biodynamic point of view, that the kinetic modalities of the sector are the same for all motor segments and, above all, that the work produced is homogeneous and interchangeable. Concerning the *quantity* of work made by each motor segment in the pyramid, there are specific differences. In fact in relation to the flexion-extension movement, the sector C 4–C 6 is certainly the structure that, seen in the dynamic modulus of the upper pyramid, plays a primary role in securing the sagittal movement. The upper cervical spine and the thoracic spine take also part in such a movement but with smaller potentiality. On the other hand, the above mentioned C 4–C 6 sector plays a less important role in rotation movements. In that such dynamism is the apanage of the upper cervical spine and of the thoracic spine, whereas it gradually diminishes in the lower cervical spine. Nevertheless it has to be taken into account that the movement of any single motor segment is always the result of one main movement in connection to other matched movements.

In conclusion, as far as *sagittal* movements are concerned, the dynamic behaviour of the lower cervical spine may be compared to that of a fulcrum in a flexible system with stiffer ends in relation to the central part which is very mobile. On the contrary, *rotation* movements may be schematically visualized as a spiral with wide coils at the top of the figure in order to represent the high rotatory potentiality of the upper cervical spine, and smaller ones from C 3 to C 7 which become wider again toward the thoracic spine.

II. The functional interdependence between lower and upper cervical spine. In a dynamic analysis of the lower cervical spine the posture of the upper cervical spine is not to be neglected; during the movement in fact, the posture of the upper cervical spine conditions the dynamic possibilities of the lower cervical spine. Such functional interdependence has been summarized in four points: 1) the ventral flexion is much bigger if the upper cervical spine first and then the lower cervical spine bend successively; 2) the rotatory movement of the lower cervical spine takes place only after that C 1 has rotated round C 2; 3) when the head is turned or bended, the flexion of the cervical spine is smaller; 4) in cases of flexion-extension movements without any involvement by the upper cervical spine—*i.e.* without bending or stretching the head—it happens that: while *flexing*, the lower cervical spine bends and the upper cervical spine stretches; while *stretching* the neck, the lower cervical spine stretches and the upper cervical spine bends.

Such reciprocal biodynamic interferences demonstrate what the opposed pyramids theory schematically represents: the cervical spine finds its working scheme in itself as a whole, whereas having located in the cervical spine particular functional areas signifies the acknowledgement of the existence of specific kinetic modalities.

III. The functional interference between lower cervical spine and biological status. In the lower cervical spine the possibility and the range of motion depend on the biological status of the capsules, discs, and ligaments. The indirect evidence of such functional interdependence has been given by the entity and location of arthrosic degenerations in the fore and hinder vertebral sections. After a X-ray screening performed on individuals older than 50 years, we could verify that [where according to the X-ray views (standard and dynamic) it could be diagnosed either "normal disc" or "laxity" with initial appearance of hypermovement also in absence of clear instability] serious arthrosic degenerations occur at the expenses of the hinder section. On the contrary in degenerative discopathies with fore fixity, in the hinder section arthrosic degenerations were always of minor importance. This phenomenon may be interpreted according to the pyramids theory. The lower cervical spine is to be considered as a part of the kinematic pyramid, which presents between the fore and hinder section an exchange of kinetic work usually defined as movement. On the contrary in the lower—static—pyramid there is an exchange of work mostly understood as load support between the two vertebral sectors.

IV. The question of cervical lordosis. Biodynamically thinking, is cervical lordosis a real entity? Cervical lordosis, lumbar lordosis, and to a lesser degree thoracic kyphosis, exist in normal individuals in the sense that they take place at rest and in standing postures when observed horizontally. We know that such sinuous shape of the cervical spine on the sagittal plane is biomechanically useful because it increases the endurance of the structure. However, such curves are liable to continuous changes both in their dimensions and in their conformation in connection to the functional requirements and space changes, which the spine undergoes during working and social life. We have studied such dynamics adjustment of the spine on individuals varying in age from 20 to 50 years, who have undergone a series of tests. As an essential qualification, none of them had any pathology of the cervical spine or any other complaint which could have altered the results of the tests. The tests consisted in recreating in a laboratory setting some of the most common working and social situations, and by taking swift and matched X-rays of the cervical spine and photograms of the subject. Keeping the "anatomic posture" as a reference point we were able to notice that in the global dynamics of the cervical spine, the lower cervical spine is the vertebral section which most modifies its disposition. Such changes have very rarely produced an increase of the lordosis; in almost all subjects under examination we found a steady tendency towards a decrease in the height of lordosis with values under 11.8 mm, a fugure which notoriously indicates the standard value of such height.

We can therefore conclude that the lower cervical spine has to be seen—from a biodynamical point of view—as a polyarticular functional unit expressing its kinetic potentiality chiefly in the ventral flexion.

1.4. Kinematic Study of the Inferior Cervical Spine in Sagittal Plane

J. P. Gonon, Lyon, G. Deschamps, Lyon, J. Dimnet, Ecully,
and L. P. Fischer, Lyon, France

Using a refined kinematic method, it is possible to precisely determine the rotation centers of the cervical vertebra when they are moving on a sagittal plane. These measures are directly applicable to kinesiology and to pathology.

1. Material and Method

The study material uses a series of 5 to 7 dynamic X-ray carried out from the maximum extension to the maximum flexion of the head.

According to the principals of the articular kinematic [1, 2] the study technique uses an automatic acquisition of the coordinates of the anterior and posterior angles of the cervical vertebral bodies. Each cervical vertebra is represented by a rectangle delimited by:

— a straight line, joining the anterior and posterior angles of the inferior vertebral margin,

— a straight line, tangent to the superior vertebral margin,

— two straight lines perpendicular to the former and tangent to the anterior and posterior edges of the vertebral body (Fig. 1).

Defined this way, the center of the rectangle is the intersection of the diagonals. On a straight line passing through this center and parallel to the tangents on the superior and inferior margins of the vertebral body, two points are chosen equidistant on both sides from this center. Thus a direction is appointed to the moving vertebra.

The fixed mark for the calculation of the instant centers of rotation is the seventh cervical vertebra, dependant of the verticality and horizontality marks provided by the edges of the radiographic film.

The calculator program stores the coordinates of each cervical vertebra for each position of movement, checks the evenness of movement and supplies the geometrical (global and segmentary amplitudes) and kinematic results.

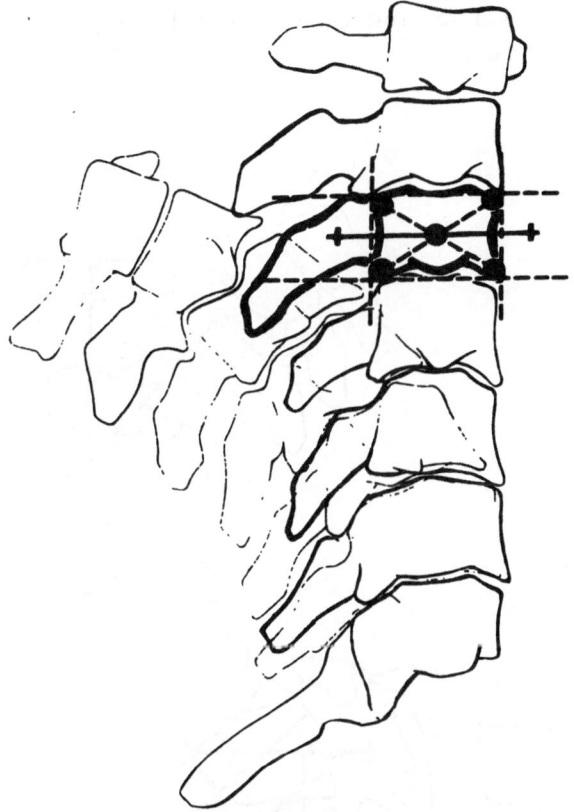

Fig. 1. Shot of the coordinates: tangent on the superior vertebral margin, tangent on the inferior vertebral margin and rights perpendicular to the previous lines

Absolute Instant Centers of Rotation (Fig. 2)

The absolute instant centers of rotation are the centers of rotation of each cervical vertebra in relation to the seventh cervical vertebral considered as fixed during the movement of flexion—extension. They are represented by a mark with a rectangle of doubt explaining the error on this mark. The absolute instant centers of rotation can be regrouped in a circle of whose center and radius are known.

Relative Instant Centers of Rotation (Fig. 2)

The relative instant centers of rotation represent the rotation centers of each cervical vertebral in relation to the subjacent vertebra between two successive positions of the movement of flexion—extension. The trajectory of the relative instant centers of rotation is contained in a rectangle the size of which is known.

This study was carried out on 10 normal living subjects and on 10 pathological subjects.

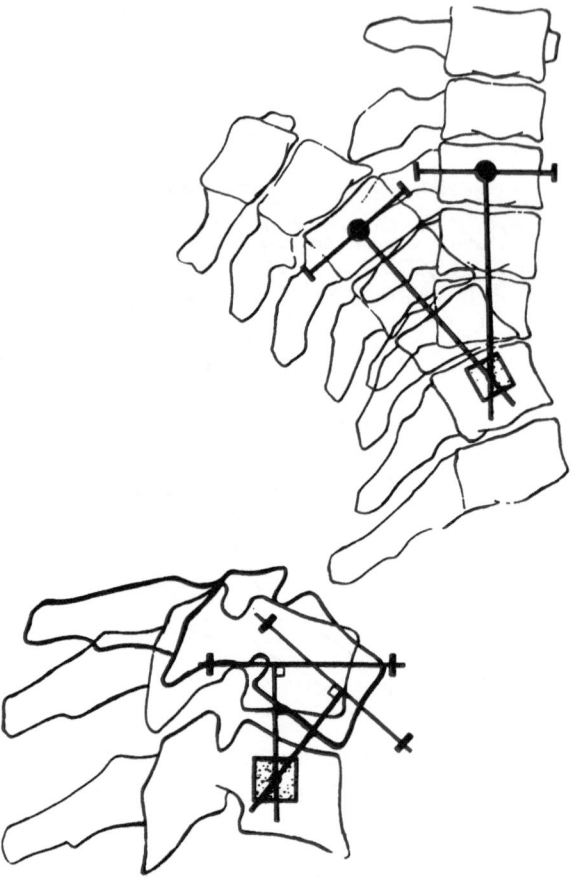

Fig. 2. Above: localization of the absolute instant center of rotation with its error rectangle. Below: localization of the relative instant center to a couple of vertebra, with its error rectangle

II. Results

A. Normal Subjects

The geometrical results show that the maximum mobility zone on the sagittal plane is situated between the fourth and sixth cervical vertebra.
Kinematic results (Figs. 3 and 4).

In each case, the absolute instant centers of rotation of each vertebra in relation to the seventh cervical vertebra stand out in a circle centered on the sixth cervical vertebra in the intermediary position.

In the normal subject, the instant centers of rotation of each cervical vertebra in relation to the subjacent (relative instant centers of rotation) are grouped in a rectangle standing out in the middle part of the discal zone and over and under the vertebral bodies.

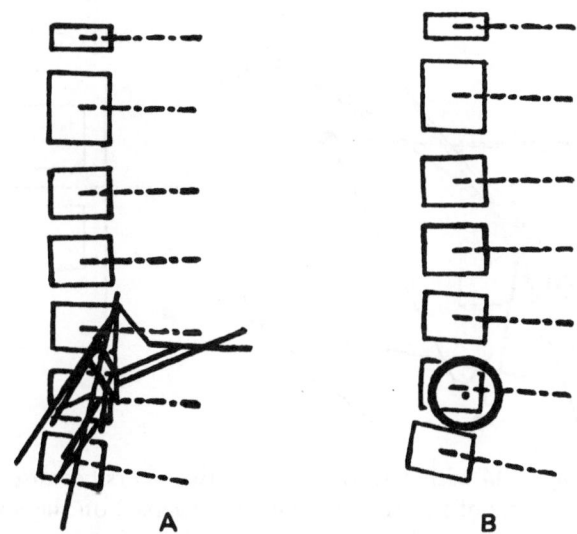

Fig. 3. Normal subject: absolute instant centers of rotation. A) Trajectory of the absolute instant centers of rotation. B) Regrouping circle of the absolute instant centers of rotation standing out on the sixth cervical vertebra in the intermediary position

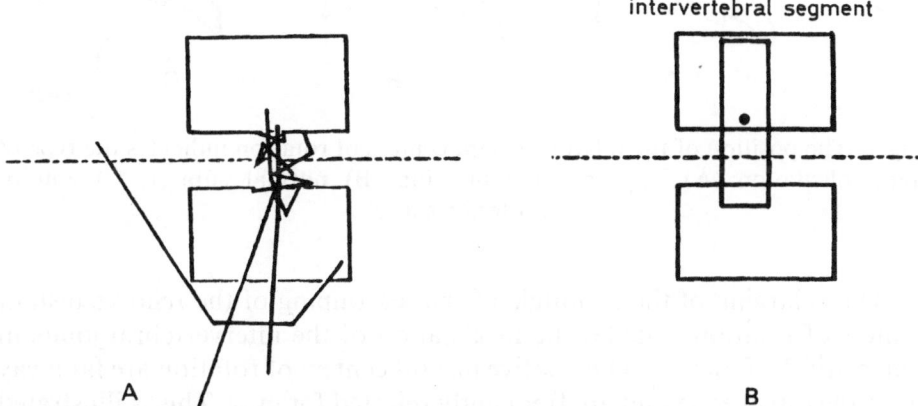

Fig. 4. Normal subject: relative instant centers of rotation. A) Trajectory of the relative instant centers of rotation. B) Regrouping rectangle of the relative instant centers of rotation standing out on the middle part of the intervertebral disc and the over and subjacent vertebral bodies

B. Pathological Subjects

The kinematic study of dynamic X-rays in flexion—extension is useful for the diagnosis of pathological cases (cervical sprain sequels) and the estimation of functional consequences of cervical arthrodesis.

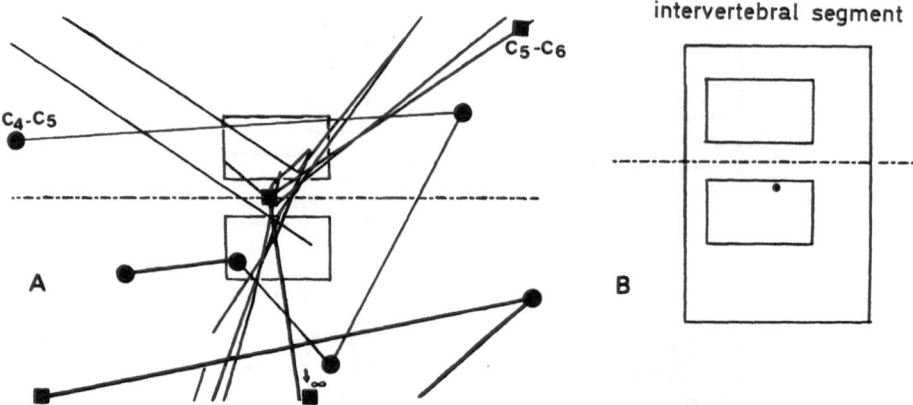

Fig. 5. Male subject aged 44 with arthrodesis since two years because of luxation. The relative instant centers of rotation are widely dispersed on the levels C 5–C 6 and C 4–C 5 with an enlargement of the regrouping rectangle

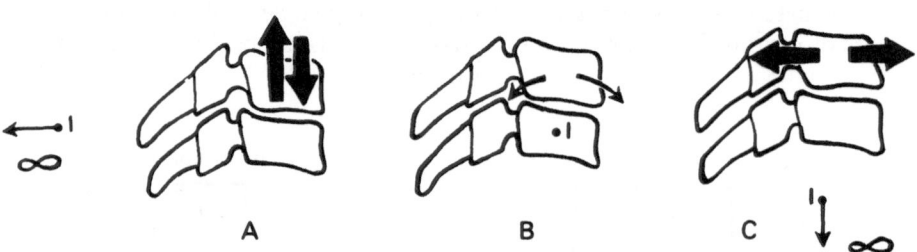

Fig. 6. The position of the relative instant centers of rotation indicates the type of hypersolicitation: A) Traction—compression, B) normal subject, C) antero-posterior shear

The enlarging of the rectangle of the regrouping of the relative instant centers of rotation, enables the localization of the intervertebral joints in kinematic dysfunction. The relative instant centers of rotation are far away from the discal zone and are frequently rejected for ever. This is illustrated by Fig. 5 showing the dispersion of the relative instant centers of rotation to the two years and carried out on a 44-year-old man for C 6–C 7 dislocation.

The position of the relative instant centers of rotation enables us to know the type of hypersolicitation: traction—compression or shear (Fig. 6).

III. Discussion

This method can be carried out on the living subject, simple and repetitive. It is precise in the error margin carried out on the reading of points and within the limits of a perfect evenness of movement. In reality this error margin is weak if the program doesn't take into account the "no-plane" X-rays, and if the measures are repeated several times for each vertebra and then averaged.

The study of relative instant centers of rotation state the results given by Lysell [3] and Penning [4]. They seem very interesting for determining the localization and type of functional abnormality when standard X-rays are not very explicit.

References

1. Dimnet J, Fischer LP, Gonon GP, Carret JP (1976) A technique for joint center analysis using a stored program calculator. J Biomech 9: 771–778
2. Fischer LP, Gonon GP, Dimnet J, Carret JP (1978) Radiographic studies of lateral flexion in the lumbar spine. J Biomech 11: 143–150
3. Lysell E (1969) Notion in the cervical spine—an experimental study on autopsy specimens. Acta Orthop Scand [Suppl] 123
4. Penning L (1978) Normal movements of the cervical spine. AJR 130–137

1.5. Instability in Cervical Arthrosis

A. Deburge and M. Benoist, Clichy, France

Instability is not a main feature of cervical arthrosis. Anterior and posterior osteophytes, and disc narrowing usually cause a marked stiffness of this vertebral segment. In a review on cervical instability, Bailey [1] reports no less than nine causes of instability but does not mention arthrosis.

On the other hand, instability in the lumbar spine is considered as a significant factor in the pathophysiology of arthrosis. A degenerative spondylolisthesis is often observed at the L 4–L 5 level, the wearing of the articular facets, which is maximum at this level, is the main cause of slipping. However, this slipping is rarely severe, and, if the patient is not operated on, does not increase significantly in time [4].

Nevertheless instability is sometimes seen in cervical osteoarthritis but little emphasis has been put on this possibility. Ehni [3], one of the few authors to have mentioned it, notes that the slipping is rare at the cervical spine in osteoarthritis, and usually takes place at C 5–C 6 or C 6–C 7 level. This is not in agreement with our findings. In our experience, instability in cervical arthrosis differs from that seen at lumbar spine level.

In our 7 cases, only one was comparable to the lumbar degenerative spondylolisthesis: the slipping was at C 7–T 1; at this level both the posterior and anterior arthrosis were marked. In all the other cases, the slipping was located at C 3–C 4 or C 4–C 5. In each case, there was no disc narrowing at the level of the slipping but the interapophyseal arthrosis was severe. Conversely, the intersomatic arthrosis was severe at the level below the slipping. In two cases there was slipping both at C 3–C 4 and C 4–C 5 (Table 1). All the slippings were reducible in hyperextension.

Table 1. *Level of Slipping in Seven Cases.* (Slipping in C 3–C 4 and C 4–C 5 in two cases.)

C 3–C 4	3
C 4–C 5	5
C 5–C 6	—
C 6–C 7	—
C 7–D 1	1

Instability in cervical arthrosis raises two questions: Is instability responsible for the symptoms and what is the pathophysiology?

The *symptoms* were varied in our cases:

In the four cases severe neck pain was the only symptom; cervico-brachialgia with motor deficit of the shoulder muscles was observed in one case; in the remaining two cases there were signs of cord compression. Slipping is only one of the possible causes of compression and pain, and it is difficult to affirm the relationship between the slipping and symptoms, particularly when there was only neck pain present.

In one case however, reported earlier [2], instability seemed to be the direct cause of symptoms. The patient, a 65-year-old woman, had been complaining for six months of severe neck pain before signs of cord compression appeared with flexion of the neck. The standard X-rays showed a marked anterior arthrosis below C 5, and a marked posterior arthrosis above this level. With neck flexion, there was a very important marked anterior displacement of C 4, which was completely reduced in extension. The symptoms disappeared after stabilization by anterior fusion.

In other cases, the responsibility of the instability was doubtful. However, when a myelopathy develops in a narrow cervical canal with osteoarthritis changes, slipping is probably an additional factor of compression.

The *pathophysiology* of cervical osteoarthritic spondylolisthesis is not clear [4]. We express the hypothesis that the slipping occurring in the upper vertebrae of the lower cervical spine (C 3 to C 5) is caused by the absence of intersomatic arthrosis facing a severe posterior arthrosis. Therefore, as the lower cervical vertebrae are stiffened by anterior arthrosis, the stress is displaced onto the upper vertebrae and the slipping occurs.

However, this hypothesis is not fully satisfying. Cervical arthrosis is usually predominant at the two or three lower levels; in spite of that, instability rarely occurs above. Besides, the long term follow-up of anterior cervical fusions shows that in spite of a completely rigid lower cervical segment, there is no slipping at the levels above.

One must realize that stiffness of the lower cervical vertebrae is not sufficient to create instability at the levels above, and that an additional factor is necessary, which may be a *preexisting* cervical hyperlordosis.

References

1. Bailey RW (1978) Instability of the cervical spine. Instructional course lectures. A.A.O.S. Vol XXVII. Mosby, St. Louis, pp 159–172
2. Deburge A (1984) Instabilité du rachis cervical par arthrose. Une forme particulière de spondylolisthésis dégeneratif. Rev Chir Orthop 70: 387–399

3. Ehni G (1984) Cervical arthrosis. Year Book Medical Publishers, pp 58–59
4. Fitzgerald JAW, Newman PH (1976) Degenerative spondylolisthesis. J Bone Joint Surg 58-B: 184–192
5. Kirkaldy Willis WH, Farfan HF (1982) Instability of the lumbar spine. Clin Orthop 165: 110–123

1.6. Lower Cervical Spine:
Biomechanical and Clinical Combined Approach

G. F. Fineschi, C. A. Logroscino, and P. Tranquilli Leali, Roma, Italy

Introduction

The increasing rate of road accidents and the introduction of new surgical procedures have given support to the present trends in the field of cervical spine surgery.

Analyzing the lesion produced by a car accident it is evident that the head and the trunk easily achieve a different speed, due to a difference in inertial mass. An impact vector will therefore be generated on the lower cervical spine, which is the transition point between a mobile segment (cervical) and a rigid one (thoracic).

Furthermore the surgeon should select the best treatment taking into consideration the different approaches (anterior, posterior and combined) and the different instrumentations (rods, plates, etc) according to the indications particular to each patient.

The multiplicity of the indications meets with a lack of knowledge about spine mechanics and spine-instrumentation interactions.

For these reasons a computer assisted procedure was developed in our department with the aim of increasing the information retrieval tools for the surgeon regarding the geometry and space behaviour of the patient spine.

Materials and Methods

A Digital PDP 11/23 computer with graphic facilities and a digitizer HP 9874 A were used to develop a procedure [4] structured in the following headings:

Acquisition. Marker points (no. 13) which are able to describe the morphology of the vertebra are input by means of the digitizer from standard A.P. and Lat. X-ray films. For testing the system a calibration frame (Fig. 1) was realized and an anatomical specimen was used to simulate different spatial configurations of the cervical spine.

Geometric Compute and Display. The cartesian coordinates are scaled and the main geometric parameters (Cobb angles, proximal and distal end

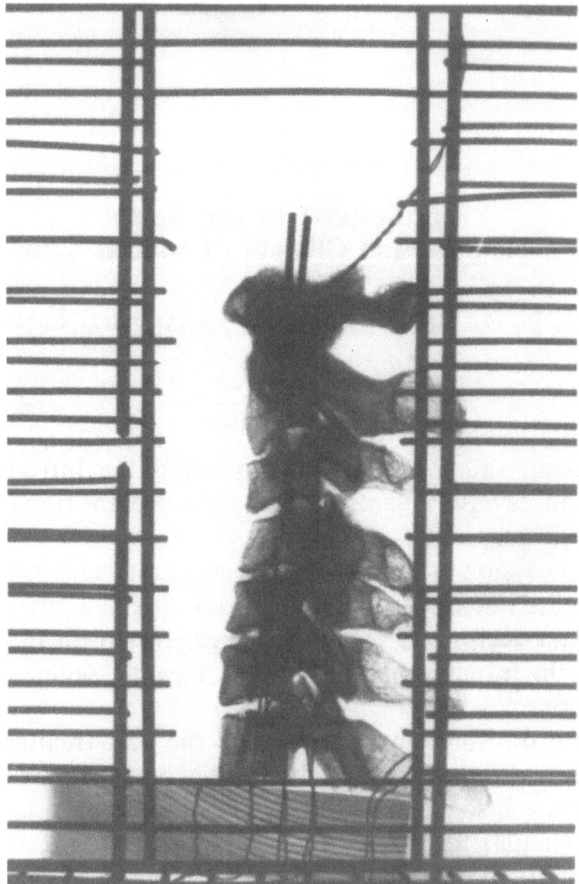

Fig. 1. Calibration frame and the spine model

vertebrae, rotations, tilts, asymmetries of the disc and of the body) are computed and stored while the A.P. and Lateral views are displayed online. Then the top-view of the centers of the vertebrae is also displayed.

Three-dimensional modelling. A theoretical model of the vertebra is scaled and orientated and a three-dimensional model of the vertebral column is generated.

This model can be interactively observed from every point of view the operator requires.

Stress analysis. The three-dimensional model can be also analyzed using a finite elements program. Consequently it is possible to have some piece of information—at least qualitative—about loads, forces and moments acting on every spine model.

The procedure was applied on experimental models simulating a normal, a kyphotic, a lordotic and a dislocated (C 5–C 6) cervical spine.

Results

In Fig. 2 is reported the graphic display of a quite normal (*N*) configuration of the cervical spine together with the centers profiles. The computer output of the lateral views relative to the pathological conditions studied is shown in Fig. 3. These configurations are: dislocation C 5–C 6 (*D*); lordosis (*L*); kyphosis (*K*).

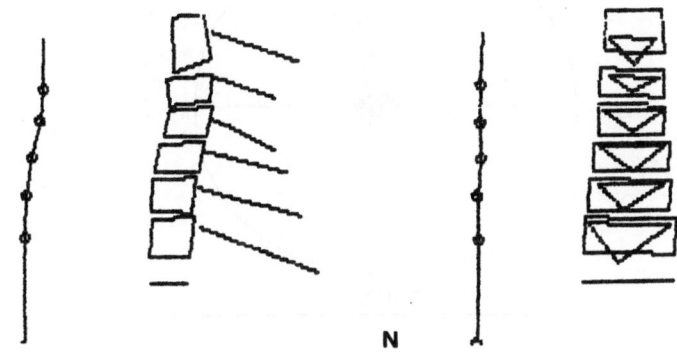

Fig. 2. Data acquired from the X-ray films can be displayed on a graphic printer. A line connecting the centers of the vertebrae is also printed out

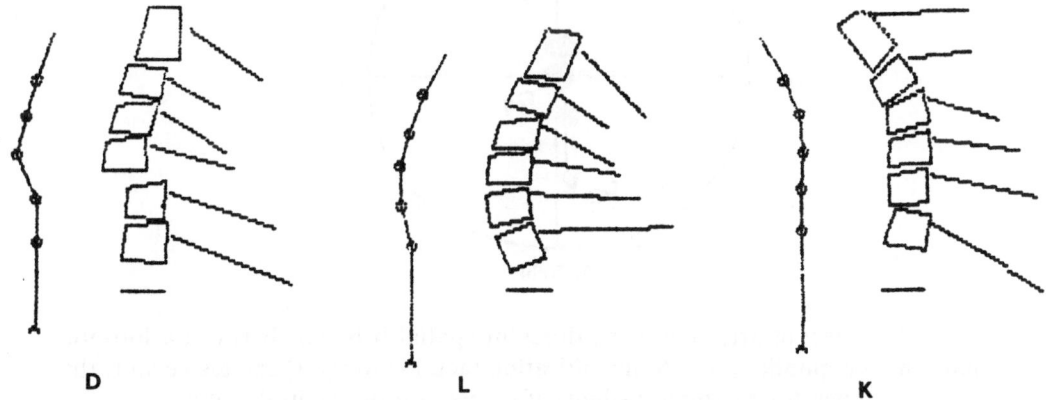

Fig. 3. Lateral views under three different conditions: a dislocation C 5–C 6 (left); a lordotic spine (center); a kyphotic spine (right)

By comparison between the top view of a lordotic and a kyphotic spine (Fig. 4) a clearly different spatial behavior is shown and further information about the related mechanical equilibrium are obtained. In Fig. 5 is reported the 3-D model of the dislocated spine from two different viewpoints.

A finite element elaboration can be applied to this type of model. Being this model significantly exemplified, only the beams connecting the vertebrae and simulating the disc were considered for the discussion. In fact the observation of forces and moments on the anterior and posterior (left

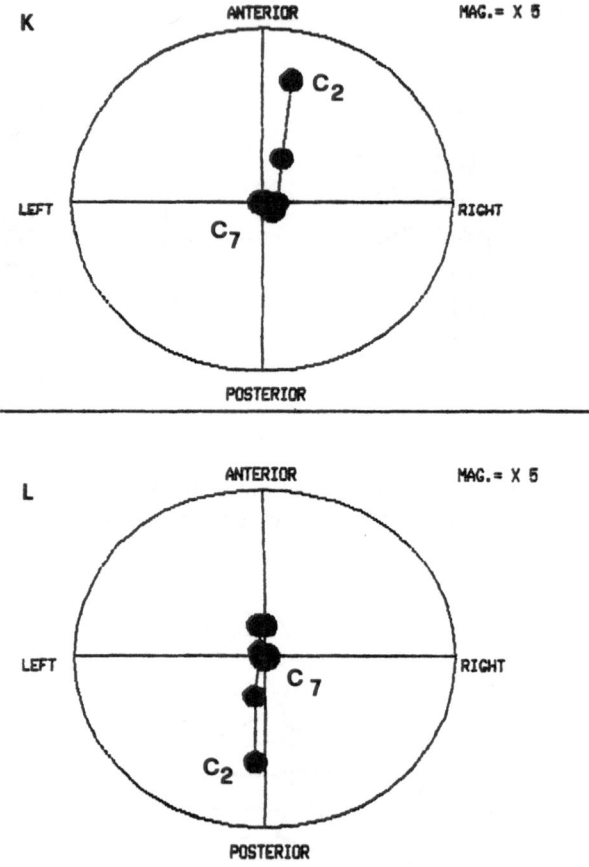

Fig. 4. Top view clearly shows the different spatial behavior between a lordotic spine and a kyphotic spine. A magnification factor (top right) can also enable the operator to amplify slight differences on the sagittal plane

and right) beams give some interesting informations, *e.g.* in Fig. 6 is reported the distribution of the A.P. shearing force Y. It is evident that in the kyphotic spine an increase of positive shearing stress on the anterior components is present, while in the lordotic spine and opposite loading can be seen.

Considering that the experimental values are plotted sequentially (C 7, C 6, C 5, C 4, C 3, C 2) it is also shown that Y shearing components are higher on the top of the kyphotic spine (C 3) and on the bottom of the lordotic one (C 6).

If we analyze better the moments on each disc beam (ant. left, post. left, post. right, ant. right) looking at the force applied at each extremity (up = C.S.; down = C.I.) of the disc beams, it is observed that when C.I. and C.S. are equal or slightly different there is no applied moment on the beam. The comparative analysis of the different spatial conditions (Figs. 7 a–d) give an idea of moments on disc model and therefore of the quality and of the direction of the applied stresses.

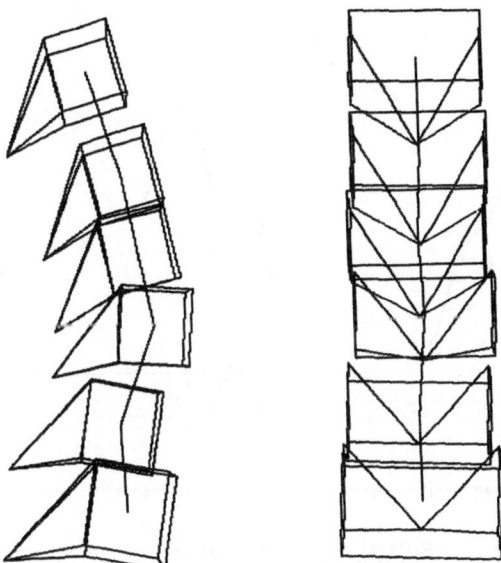

Fig. 5. The three-dimensional model of the dislocated spine is shown from the lateral and frontal viewpoint. The operator can interactively change the view point to better read the spatial behavior of the spine; of a great help is the use of the color screen monitor

In Fig. 8 is reported the behavior of shearing force Y by using the well-known theory of the three functional columns. It is also shown that the force distribution can change according to the different configuration of the spine.

Discussion

The two first headings of the procedure (acquisition, geometric compute and display) represent powerful tools for the surgeon. In fact by these means it is possible to rapidly screen the geometrical parameters of the spine, saving time and reducing the imprecision of subjective evaluation.

Furthermore the related data base is worthwhile for monitoring the patients and for further statistical evaluation of the clinical series [2, 3].

The 3-D and stress analysis headings are in fact instructional tools because the static analysis is carried out on a theoretical vertebra without taking into account many components as muscles, ligaments, posterior joints, etc.

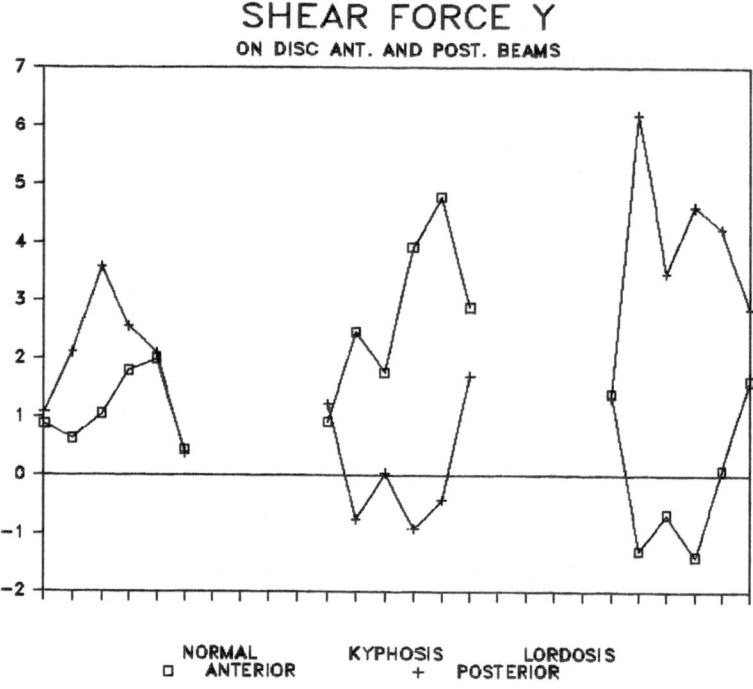

Fig. 6. Shear force Y (anterior-posterior): a positive increase in anterior loadings in kyphosis and an opposite condition in lordosis are shown

In any case the qualitative information gives a description of the level, the direction and versus of the applied stresses. The comparative evaluation of the different conditions (lordosis, kyphosis, etc) gives a good idea of the related biomechanical patterns. These patterns are clearly different and give a very good description of a 3-D phenomenon as for instance the lordosis. Furthermore they can give more precise informations than standard X-rays films about the consequences of loadings about each configuration on each single patient.

The study of applied moments on disc beams (Fig. 7) is a tentative approach to understand which are the risk areas in degenerative osteoarthritis and to find a correlation between spatial configuration and disc changes.

All these considerations could be also useful in planning the approach and instrumentation, but for this further step we need to develop a more precise procedure especially the acquisition phase. In fact the standard X-rays films do not give enough accuracy and repeatibility. The use of the calibration frame can reduce the errors but it is not always applicable in clinical cases. For these reasons we are also working on CAT scan and magnetic resonance to increase the number and the quality of the morphological information.

The standard X-ray films are at present unable to face all the needs of the spine surgeon and less visual (subjective) techniques are developing [1]. Obviously there are many problems to be solved, anyway the diagnostic tools are turning out from "imagery" to "data".

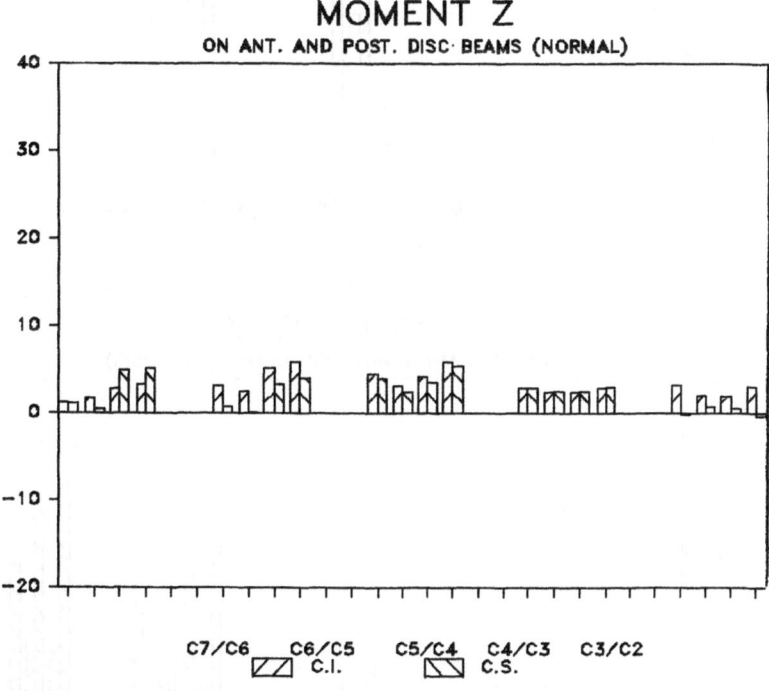

Fig. 7. a) Z Moment on the normal model: the quite equal range of the inferior and superior force components, their same direction (sign) and the overall low level of values (if compared with the subsequent situation) show the absence of applied moments on the beams. b) Z Moment on a lordotic spine: appearance of significant moments on the anterior beams (first two couple of stacked bars of each group of the four couples used to describe the beams simulating the intervertebral discs. c) Z Model on the kyphotic spine: appearance of significant moments on the posterior beams, particularly at the C 4–C 5 intervertebral disc. d) Z moment on a dislocated spine: relevant moments on the anterior beams of the C 6–C 5 disc; smaller moments propagate on higher levels

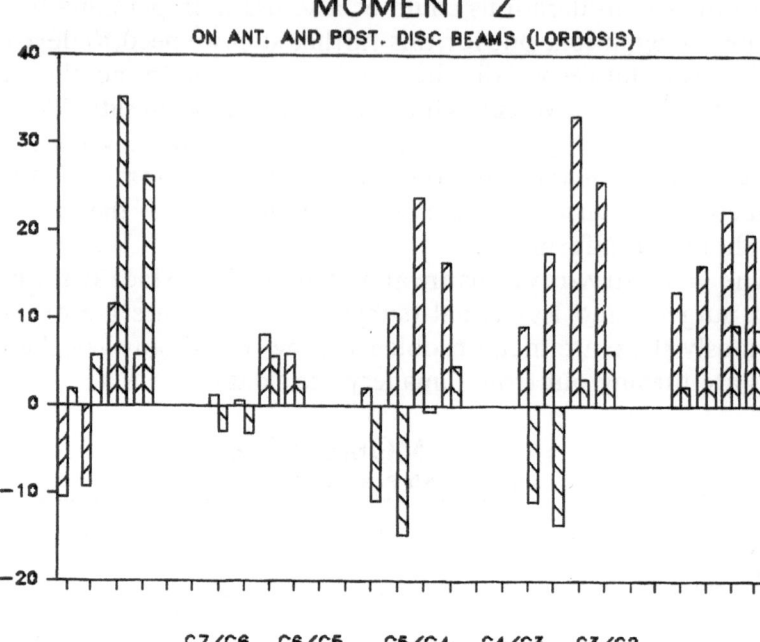

Fig. 7b

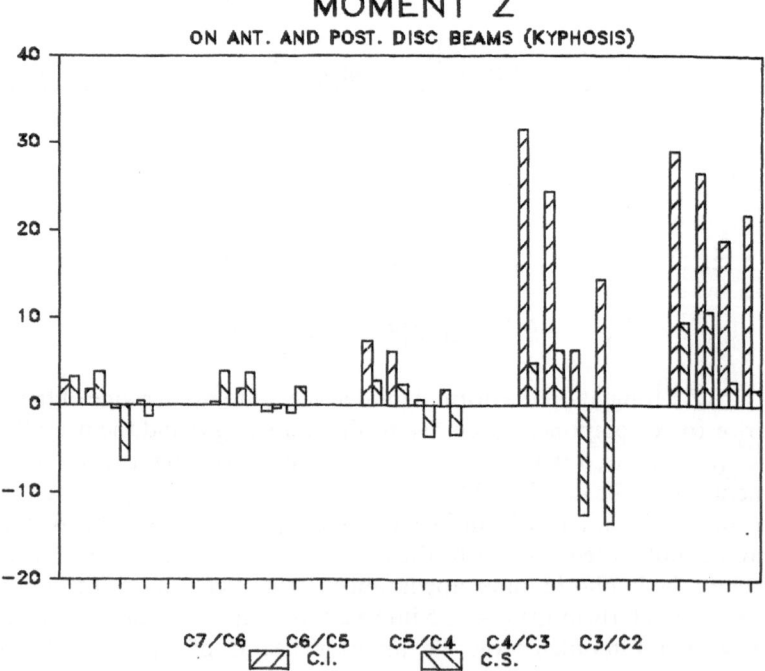

Fig. 7c

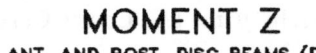

MOMENT Z
ON ANT. AND POST. DISC BEAMS (DISLOC.)

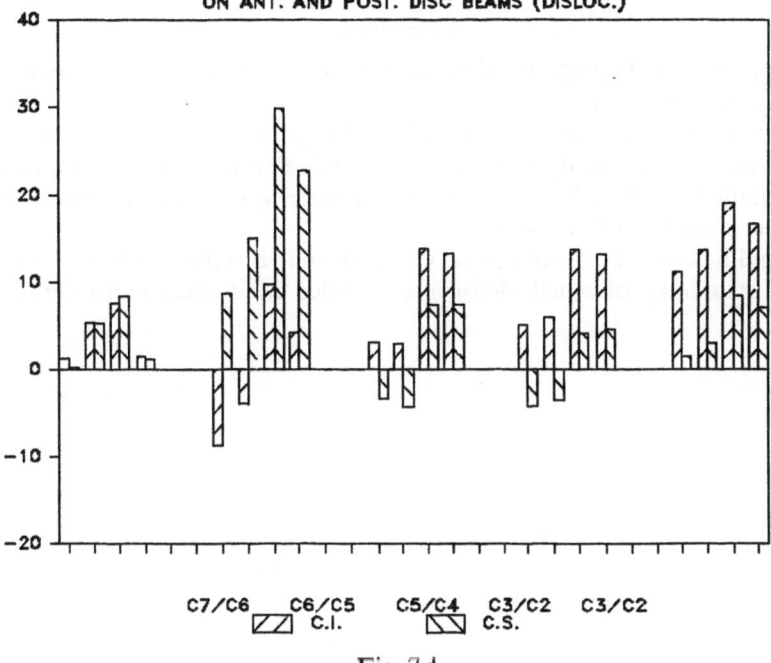

Fig. 7d

SHEAR FORCE Y
ON THREE FUNCTIONAL COLUMNS

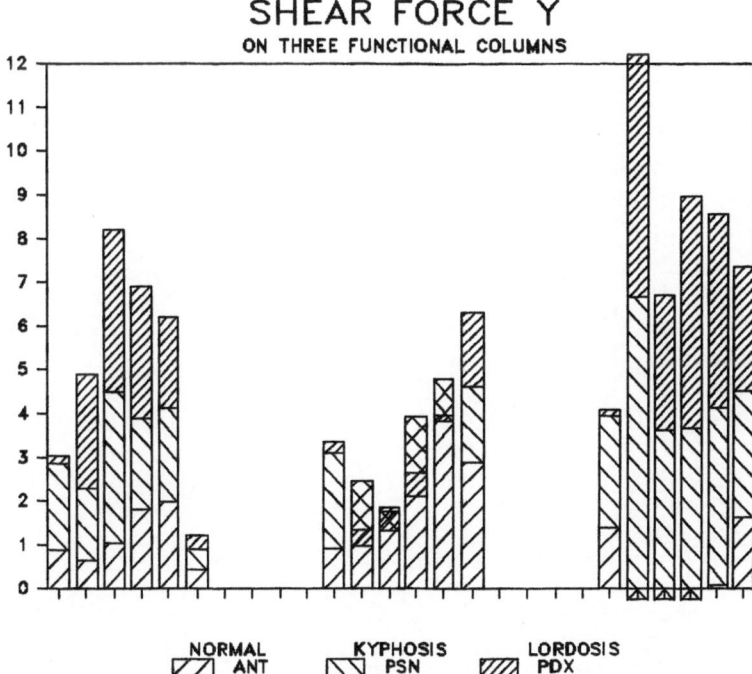

Fig. 8. A representation of loadings according to the three-functional columns theory: an overload on the anterior column in kyphosis and an opposite behavior in lordosis is again shown

References

1. Tranquilli Leali P (1983) Tecniche computerizzate in diagnostica ortopedica I, Jasillo, pp 1–56
2. Tranquilli Leali P, Bartolini F, Merolli A, Sanguinetti C (1984) Videotape "3-D Computer assisted analysis of spine. Videotape section, SICOT 84, London
3. Tranquilli Leali P (1985) Aspetti biomeccanici e clinici dell'osteosintesi vertebrale. Newsletter I, 1: 54–55
4. Tranquilli Leali P, Romagnoli O, Bartolini F (1985) Diagnostica computerizzata interattiva nelle deformita rachidee. Medicina ed informatica I: 13–19

1.7. Cervical Facetectomy and Its Effect on Stability

(Cervical Spine Stability as a Function of the Articular Facet)

R. B. Raynor, J. Pugh, and I. Shapiro, New York, N.Y., U.S.A.

Stability and the factors affecting it are of paramount importance for evaluating therapeutic modalities in the treatment of cervical spine disorders. Measurements have been made on the ligamentous structures singly and as a group. Some measurements have also been made on the facets and their ability to influence or alter normal spine strength [1]. Work to date regarding facets has been done with these structures either intact or absent. Objective criteria regarding stability have therefore been an all or none situation in the experiments performed. When the ligamentous structures are sectioned posteriorly or anteriorly, half of them must be cut before instability results unless the articular facets are removed [2, 3, 7]. Such extensive distinction rarely occurs except in severe trauma [6]. However, clinical situations arise where facet resection is necessary or advantageous. There have been no measurements made concerning the amount of facet that may be removed before instability results. Our objective in these experiments was to determine when this point was reached.

Materials and Methods

Fourteen cervical motion segments were used. These consisted of adjacent vertebral bodies and their connecting ligaments. Three series of tests were run. *Group I* consisted of five fresh frozen cadaver specimens that had been thawed and mounted as will be described. *Group II* contained five specimens that were formalin fixed and had a bilateral facetectomy of 50% or less on each side. The facet resection was performed utilizing a high speed air drill and standard surgical technique [4]. All ligamentous structures were left intact other than the capsular ligaments. A satisfactory facetectomy exposed the nerve root from the axilla distally. The superior and inferior margins of the root were well visualized and free from encompassing bone. Previous work had shown that the clinical estimate of the percent of facetectomy was reasonably accurate. This estimate was checked at the end of the experiment when the motion segment was disarticulated. *Group III* contained four specimens and was similar to Group II except that a 70% facetectomy was performed bilaterally. Into the exposed surface of each vertebral body a 0.028 K wire was inserted and then the K wires and exposed surfaces were fixed to aluminum plates with methylmethacrylate cement. The aluminum plates, which were held parallel to each other, were attached to an MTS electrohydraulic tension-compression testing unit and loaded in shear. A cross-head speed of 0.01 inch per second was used until a load of 80 pounds was achieved. Load deflection curves were recorded for multiple cycles alternately in tension or compression. The specimen was then loaded to failure, again recording load deflection curves. Failure load and mode of failure were noted.

Results

Compression and distraction stiffness (load divided by displacement) were similar in the fixed, facetectomized groups. Group I, which consisted of fresh frozen specimens that had been thawed but had not undergone facetectomy, were less stiff than the fixed specimens. This represented the greater elasticity of the fresh ligamentous structures as compared to the fixed ones, as other investigators have shown. However, our principal interest was in bone strength at moderate to high loads. Once firm contact between the opposing facet joints is established with higher loads, the principal resistance to shear is due to the opposing bone surfaces. Sedlin [5] has shown minimal effects of fixation on the mechanical properties of bone.

A facetectomy of 70% exposed from 8 to 10 mm of nerve root measured from the axilla. When 50% of the joint was removed, from 3 to 5 mm of nerve root could be visualized. The differences in length exposed reflect the variations in the facet configuration from specimen to specimen, a factor noted by others. These anatomical variations also account for the differences noted in the loading curves from specimen to specimen.

There were two principal modes of failure (Table 1). In three of the four specimens where 70% facetectomy had been done, fractures occurred in the remaining facets. One specimen also had fractures in the pedicles and one side of the lamina. The ligamentous structures including the disc were not strong enough to prevent acute dislocation once the fractures occurred.

Four of the five Group II specimens (50% of less facetetomy) failed when one of the vertebral bodies tore loose from the acrylic cementing it to the mounting plate. One specimen failed because of fracture of the facet.

The mean load where fracture was the cause of failure was 159 ± 37 lbs. Fixation failure occurred at 208 ± 26 lbs. The differences are significant at p 0.05, a confidence of greater than 95% (Table 2). Only two of the fresh whole specimens were loaded to failure. In one, the fixation broke while in the second, the facets dislocated at 235 lbs resulting in disruption of the ligaments and disc.

Table 1. *Failure Load (lbs) and Mode of Failure*

Type of specimen	No.	Mode	Load
Fresh	1	dislocation	235
	1	fixation	195
Fixed 50%	4	fixation	212
facetectomy	1	fracture	135
Fixed 70%	1	fixation	195
facetectomy	3	fracture	167

Table 2. *Mean Load (lbs) of Different Type of Failure*

Type of failure	No.	Load lbs	t	p
Fixation	6	208 ± 26	2,165	$P < 0.05$
Fracture	4	159 ± 38		

Discussion

Many clinical situations require facet removal to greater or lesser degrees. There is general agreement that total removal of a facet produces an unstable situation and leaves the cervical vertebra prone to dislocation at the involved segment.

The facets form the posterior and postero-lateral wall of the canal containing the nerve root as it exits from the bony spine. Previous work has shown that the axilla and up to 5 mm of the root can be exposed by resecting less than 50% of the medial facet joint [4]. This is more than adequate to decompress the root or remove osteophytes at the entrance to the neural canal or in the uncovertebral joint.

Some authors feel that 8 to 10 mm of root should be visualized to decompress a cervical root in its canal. The normal course of the root through its canal is antero-lateral to its foramen of exit. Our measurements indicate that 60 to 70% of the facet must be removed to expose this length of root. This degree of bone removal seriously compromises the strength of the remaining joint and most of our 70% facetectomy specimens failed because of fracture. The ligamentous structures and disc do not have sufficient strength to prevent dislocation of the vertebral bodies.

If less than 50% of the joint was removed, failure occurred because of fracture in only one instance. The remaining specimens suffered fixation failure at 208 lbs and a fracture load could not be established. When more than 50% of the facet is removed bilaterally, the joint will fracture at a mean of 159 lbs when stressed by a shearing force. The difference in these loads is significant.

Panjabi *et al.* have shown that joint strength and stability at light loads is provided by the ligamentous structures [2, 3]. At least half of them must be sectioned for the motion segment to become unstable, unless the entire facet is removed. In these experiments the intact ligaments were unable to prevent dislocation if half of the joint was removed and fracture of the remaining joint occurred. Based on this, we feel that the integrity of the facet joint is essential for stability. Unless there are compelling reasons, *no more than 50% of the facet should be resected* since the remaining joint will fracture under loads in the physiological range and instability will result. If it is necessary to do a wider resection, other means of stabilization must be considered.

References

1. Johnson RM, Wolf JW (1980) Stability of the cervical spine using a human cadaver model. Ortho Trans, J Bone Joint Surg 4: 46.
2. Panjabi MM, White AA, Johnson RM (1975) Cervical spine mechanics as a function of transection components. J Biomech 8: 327–336
3. Panjabi MM, White AA, Keller D, Southwick WO, Friedlander G (1978) Stability of the cervical spine under tension. J Biomech 11: 189–197
4. Raynor RB (1983) Anterior or posterior approach to the cervical spine: an anatomical and radiographic evaluation and comparison. Neurosurgery 12: 7–13
5. Sedlin ED (1965) A rheologic model for cortical bone: a study of the physical properties of human femoral samples. Acta Orthop Scand [Suppl] 83
6. Stauffer ES, Kelly EG (1977) Fracture-dislocations of the cervical spine: instability and recurrent deformity following treatment by anterior interbody fusion. JBJS 59 A: 45–48
7. White AA, Southwick WO, Panjabi MM (1976) Clinical instability in the lower cervical spine. Spine 1: 15–27

1.8. Forces and Motions Across the Neck in Patients Treated with Halo-vest for Unstable Cervical Spine Fractures

B. LIND, H. SIHLBOM, and A. NORDWALL, Göteborg, Sweden

Introduction

The Halo-vest apparatus is used for stabilizing cervical spine injuries [1–6]. The device is considered to restrict motion in extension/flexion more effectively than other orthoses. Johnson *et al.* [2, 3] found only 4% of normal motion possible. Patients treated with Halo-vest are allowed to be ambulated immediately, and yet the apparatus is as effective in promoting healing of cervical spine injuries as other conservative methods of treatment. However, little is known about motions of the spine and the forces across the neck in different exercises during the Halo-vest treatment [4].

Material and Methods

In this study 31 patients, 13 women and 18 men, were investigated regarding extension/flexion motion of the cervical spine during the Halo-vest treatment. The average age of the patients was 41 years, with the range 13–79 years. Seventeen of the patients were also studied regarding distraction and compression forces across the neck during the treatment. About 50% of the patients had tetraparesis and most of the patients were injured in traffic accidents.

The motion in extension/flexion of the cervical spine was registered by lateral radiograms while the patient performed the following exercises: supine, prone, sitting, weight-lifting in supine and sitting, wheel-chair driving and push up. The angle between occiput and C6 was registered, *i.e.* the flexion/extension of the entire cervical spine, and the sum of the angles between each vertebra (Fig. 1). During the exercises, forces were registered with a strain gauge mounted on the vertical bars of the Halo-vest apparatus. The forces were also measured during a deep breath, with the arms elevated and the shoulders shrugged. We also measured the adjustment of the vest as the distance between the skin surface over the sternal bone and the top of the vest, and the distance between the skin surface over the costal arch and the bottom of the vest. The vertical shifting of the vest between supine and standing positions was also registered.

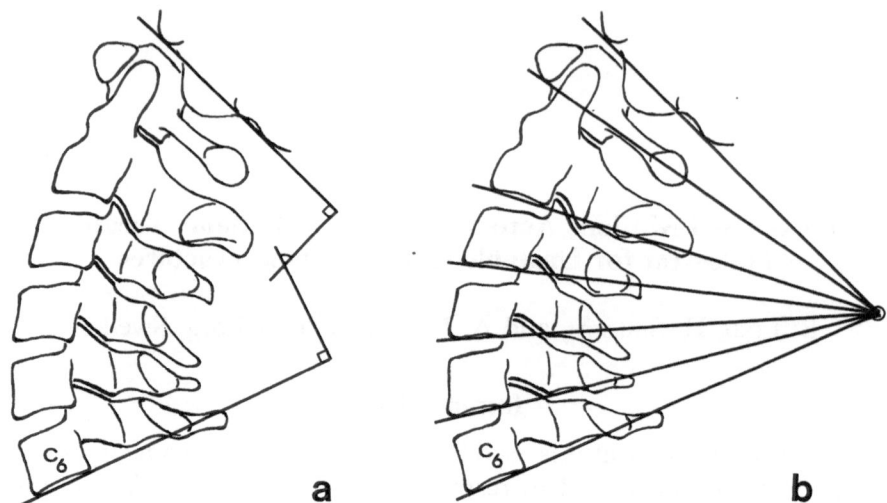

Fig. 1. Method of determination of the angle between occiput and C 6 (a) and of the angles between each vertebra (b)

Results

Between maximum extension and maximum flexion there was an average total motion of 9° between occiput and C 6. However, when movement in each segment was measured, the sum of the motion angles amounted to 51° (Table 1). Compared to normal motion according to White and Panjabi [6], this means that almost 70% of normal motion remains. We found that during the different exercises the cervical spine moves like a snake that is fixed in both ends (Fig. 2). While there is a flexion motion in one segment, there is at the same time an extension motion in the segment above or below. This changes with the position of the body and with the type of exercise.

The forces across the neck varied widely in the patients, depending on the position of body and exercise. All patients had a distraction force in the supine position (Table 2). This force averaged 53 N and it was reduced in sitting to 17 N and in standing to 3 N. In 4 patients, the force changed to compression in standing and in 1 patient the compression was 47 N. This variation of force, depending on the position of the body is probably explained by the fact, that the vest in sitting and standing better adjusts to the upper part of the trunk. This could also be measured by the vertical shifting of the vest in standing, when it sinks an average of 8 mm. The highest forces of distraction were registered during 3 different exercises: deep breath, the arms lifted or the shoulders shrugged. Six patients then had a distraction force of more than 200 N and one patient reached 305 N of distraction.

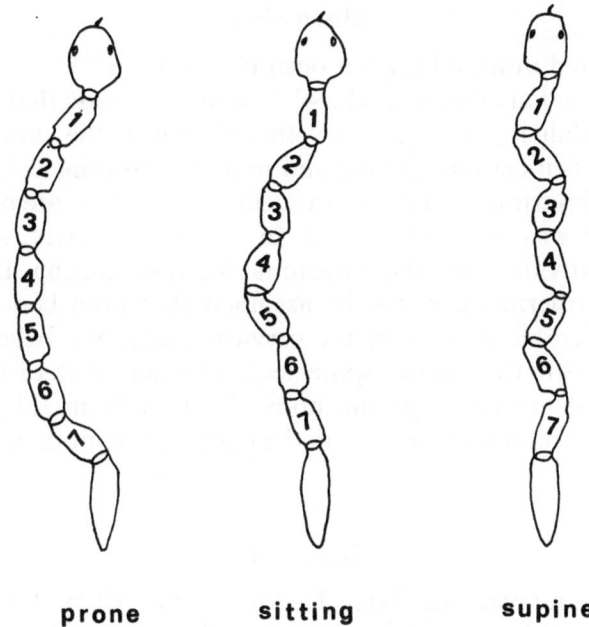

prone   **sitting**   **supine**

Fig. 2. Motion in Halo-vest

Table 1. *Motion in Flexion/Extension*

	Mean	Range
Sum of all segments Occ. –C 6	51°	43°–61°
Normal spine [White-Panjabi (6)]	73°	41°–157°

Table 2. *Forces in Halo-vest*

	Mean	Range
Supine	—53 N	—5 – —110 N
Sitting	—17 N	+ 20 – —56 N
Standing	—3 N	+ 47 – —14 N

— = distraction, + = compression.

Discussion

The measured motion between occiput and C 6 of 9° corresponds well with that reported in other series [2–4], and may indicate that a Halo-vest is effective in stabilizing the cervical spine. However, the sum of segmental motion of 51° is most remarkable and may be alarming as we are dealing with unstable injuries, yet it does not seem to affect the rate of union of the injuries which was more than 90% in the whole series. Probably, the stability is provided by the constant traction during the Halo-vest treatment. Furthermore, it can be assumed that even bed-skull traction implies considerable motion in the cervical spine. We believe that most unstable injuries in the cervical spine need treatment with distraction in the Halo-vest in all positions of the body. Exempt from this rule may be fractures of the odontoid process and major ligamentous injuries.

References

1. Cooper R, Maravilla K, Sklar F, Moody SF, Clark KW (1979) Halo immobilization of cervical spine fractures. J Neurosurg 50: 603–610
2. Johnson RM, Hart DL, Simmons ES, Ramsby GR, Southwick WO (1977) Cervical orthoses. A study compairing their effectiveness in restricting cervical motions in normal subjects. J Bone Joint Surg 59-A: 332–339
3. Johnson RM, Owen JR, Hart DL, Callahan RA (1981) A guide to their selection and use. Clin Orthop Rel Res 154: 34–45
4. Koch R, Nickel V (1978) The Halo-vest: An evaluation of motion and forces across the neck. Spine 3: 103–107
5. Lyddon DW (1974) Experience with the Halo and body vest in the ambulatory treatment of cervical spine fractures. Ill Med J 146: 458–461, 490
6. White AA, Panjabi MM (1978) The basic kinematic of the human spine. A review of past and current knowledge. Spine 3: 12–20
7. Young R, Murphy DJ (1977) Step by step procedure for applying the Halo Vest. Ace Orthopaedic Company Literature

1.9. Stability of the Lower Cervical Spine

H. H. SHERK, Philadelphia, Pennsylvania, U.S.A.

The stability of the cervical spine has been defined as maintenance of normal vertebral alignment under physiologic loads. The ligaments of the cervical spine appear to be responsible for stability under test conditions which usually involve stressing two spinal segments in various directions. These studies for the most part have been carried out on specimens which have been stripped of overlying muscles and subjected to unidirectional forces. Previous work has yielded useful data regarding stability but the testing of two or three isolated vertebrae and their ligaments may place undue emphasis on the passive ligamentous supporting structures. These passive elements do not actively position or support the cervical spine under conditions of normal use.

The purpose of this paper is to reconsider the concept of cervical stability taking into account the effect of cervical musculature on cervical alignment. The questions which arise are: 1. Are the ligaments the only stabilizers? 2. Can cervical musculature maintain stability? 3. How do the cervical ligaments and musculature interact in providing stability to the biomechanical construct of the cervical spine?

The ligamentous anatomy of the neck is familiar to most workers in this area, but a brief review of the anatomy of the cervical musculature would be in order (see Figs. 1–3).

Posteriorly, the extensor muscles of the cervical spine can be divided into three groups, 1. the splenii, 2. the erector spinae and 3. the transversospinalis muscles. The trapezius and levator scapulae muscles, while attached to the cervical spine, are considered muscles of the upper limb.

The deepest muscle layers are the transversospinalis muscles including the interspinalis muscles, multifidi and intertransversarii.

In flexion and extension, the vertebrae move about centers of rotation which are probably in the anterior-inferior part of the vertebral body. The arc of motion is defined by radii from the center of rotation to the arc of the facet joints. The extreme of flexion appears limited by passive tension on the inter-spinous ligament, ligamentum nuchae, facet joint ligaments, posterior longitudinal ligament and the posterior annulus fibrosis.

Under physiologic conditions when the cervical spine and head are in full flexion and the passive restraints under full tension, the effect of contraction of the interspinalis and multifidus muscles can be demonstrated mathematically by shortening the distances between the spinous processes and laminae.

The neck from cervical two to cervical seven is thereby shortened and stiffened. It is converted to a rigid lever arm, the position of which can be further refined by tension generated in the semispinalis cervicis, inserting primarily into the bifurcated spinous processes of C 2–C 7.

The prominence of the spinous processes of cervical two and cervical seven seem significant in this regard. They overhangs the smaller spinous processes of the adjacent vertebrae. This birfucated projection provides for posts on which a large muscular semispinalis cervicis can act advantageously in modulating the degree of extension of the lower cervical spine and positioning the lever arm of cervical two through cervical seven for adjustment of head position.

Fig. 1. The interspinalis muscles are more developed in the cervical spine than in the thoracic and lumbar levels. They arise and insert on the midline of adjacent spinous processes from the axis to the first thoracic vertebra. The multifidi arise from articular processes on each side from the third cervical to the first thoracic vertebra and they insert onto each side of the entire spinous process of the two vertebrae above their origin. The multifidi and the interspinalis muscles, therefore, have a very short excursion spanning one or two segments and they generate tension close to the axis of rotation of each intervertebral joint

Fig. 2. The two semispinalis musles are part of the transversospinalis muscle group but these two muscles operate over many segments and appear to function well away from the axis of rotation of the intervertebral joints. The semispinalis cervicis is the deeper of the two. It arises from the transverse processes of the upper six thoracic vertebra and inserts into each side of the apex of the spinous process from the axis to cervical seven. It will be recalled that the spinous process of the axis is always bifurcated. The right and left halves of the semispinalis cervicis insert on the right and left projection of this bifurcated process

Fig. 3. The semispinalis capitus has an extensive and quite caudal origin from the transverse processes of thoracic one through seven, from the articular process of cervical seven and thoracic one. The very large muscle ascends to insert on a broad area of the base of the skull. This area is between the superior and inferior nuchal lines extending laterally almost half the distance from the foramen magnum to the mastoid process. The geometry and biomechanics of the transversospinalis muscle groups have received little attention

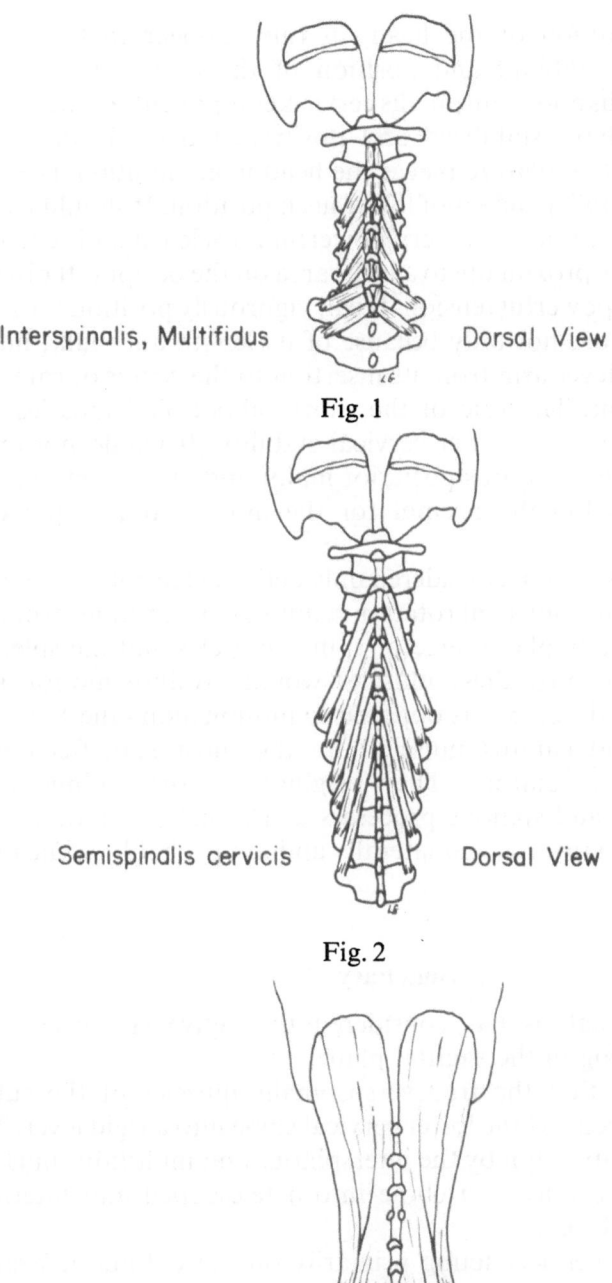

Interspinalis, Multifidus   Dorsal View

Fig. 1

Semispinalis cervicis   Dorsal View

Fig. 2

Semispinalis capitis   Dorsal View

Fig. 3

Stability and position of the head, in turn, appear to be relatively independent of the stability and position of the neck. Thus once the multifidi, interspinalis and semispinalis cervicis components of the transversospinalis muscles have stabilized and positioned the subaxial cervical spine, the occipital musculature places the head in an additional degree of extension seemingly independent of lower neck position. It should be noted that the semispinalis capitus is a very powerful muscle extending from the mid and lower thorax proximally to a large area on the occiput. It obviously generates extremely powerful tension. It can vigorously position the head in considerable extension, not only because of its length and bulk, but also because of the long lever arm from its insertion to the center of rotation of the atlantoaxial joint. The role of the short suboccipital muscles is not germane to a discussion of lower cervical stability. It would not appear, however, that the rectus capitus posterior major and minor, act over short distances to preposition the occiput for the more major action of the semispinalis capitus.

The foregoing discussion considered only active extension in the sagittal plane. Lateral bending and axial rotation requires contributions from more superficial and laterally placed erector spinae muscles and the splenii.

Acting asymmetrically, these muscles would produce motion in the coronal plane along the Z axis as opposed to motion along the X axis. The splenius cervicis and capitus muscles are the most superficial of the posterior-cervical musculature. They originate in the midline on the ligamentum nuchae and spinous processes as far distally as thoracic six. They pass obliquely upwards and laterally and are probably prime movers in axial rotation.

Summary

The foregoing analysis has considered the active stabilizers of the cervical spine working in the sagittal plane.

It has suggested that the transversospinalis muscles of the subaxial portion of the neck convert the lower cervical spine into a rigid lever. This is accomplished by contraction by the interspinous and multifidus muscles to draw the lower six cervical vertebrae into a telescoped and interlocked position (Figs. 4 and 5).

The semispinalis cervicis acting primarily on the C 2 and C 7 spinous processes, powerfully completes and maintains extension. It stabilizes the lower neck because of its bulk and long excursion so that head extension can be adjusted by the semispinalis capitus (Figs. 6–9).

These muscles are active stabilizers of the neck on extension augmenting the passive stability provided by the ligaments. Forces generated by the cervical musculature can be calculated on the basis of cross sectional

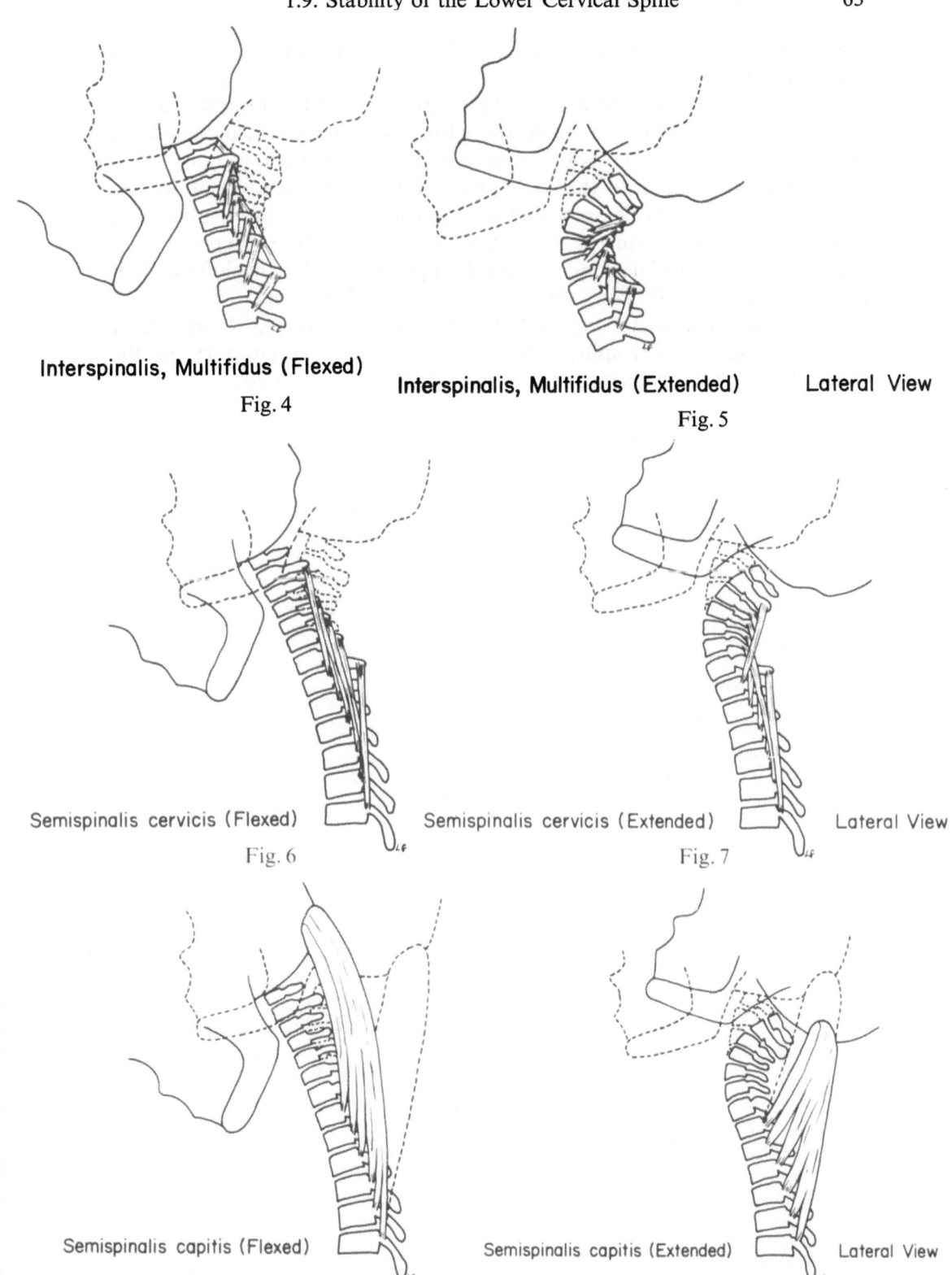

Interspinalis, Multifidus (Flexed)

Fig. 4

Interspinalis, Multifidus (Extended)

Fig. 5

Lateral View

Semispinalis cervicis (Flexed)

Fig. 6

Semispinalis cervicis (Extended)

Fig. 7

Lateral View

Semispinalis capitis (Flexed)

Fig. 8

Semispinalis capitis (Extended)

Fig. 9

Lateral View

diameter of the muscles length of excursion of the muscles and velocity of contractions.

The torque or moment created by contraction of the muscles can be calculated and compared to the maximal force to failure of the ligaments. A normal physiologic load is considered to be 25% of the body weight, which is 2½ times the weight of the body above the first thoracic vertebra. The musculature of the neck operating in extension in the sagittal plane can probably generate torque in this range. The musculature, therefore, can stabilize the head and neck against loads approaching the physiologic limit and augment the stabilizing effect of the cervical ligaments.

It is concluded, therefore, that the cervical musculature is capable of stabilizing the cervical spine. The passive ligamentous supports of the cervical spine become critical when these loads are exceeded.

1.10. Comparative Stability of Anterior or Posterior Cervical Spine Fixation—*in vitro* Investigation

Chr. Ulrich, O. Woersdoerfer, L. Claes, Ulm, Federal Republic of Germany,
and F. Magerl, St. Gallen, Switzerland

The stability of a cervical spine motion segment is guaranteed by intact disco-ligamentous structures [3]. If these have been destroyed, only bony fusion of the affected unit can prevent impending instability or ensure long-term stability. Operative treatment involves the application of anterior and posterior spondylodesis procedures to obtain immobilization of the motion segment. However, controversy still exists concerning the primary stability of these procedures [1]. The purpose of this comparative experimental study is, therefore, to examine *in vitro* the primary stabilizing effect of posterior and anterior internal fixation procedures under differing conditions of instability.

Materials and Methods

Ten fresh deep-frozen cervical spines were detached from their muscles. The motion segment C 5/6 was removed, and C 6 was embedded in methacrylate. A tensile force was applied in a vertical direction to the base of the spinous process of C 5, so that a flexion-bending load could be introduced into the unit. This was registered with a vertical electrical displacement transducer at the posterior edge of the end-plate (Fig. 1). The tilting angle α was calculated on the basis of the measuring sections a, b, c, Δx and the pertinent tangent (Fig. 2). The vertical tension was applied in five steps (2, 4, 6, 8, 10 N) from 1 mm/min to Fmax = 10 N; each step was repeated five times. Based on the average values of the individual steps, the load-displacement curves characteristic of each individual testing condition were created. The stability of the various spondylodesis procedures was then tested under standardized instability conditions. Firstly only severance of posterior ligamentous structures was performed, then anterior fixation with H-plate, posterior fixation with hook-plate as introduced by Magerl, posterior fixation with sublaminar wiring, and combined anterior and posterior fixation with H-plate/hook-plate and H-plate/sublaminar wiring were tested. After that, all disco-ligamentous structures were severed and stability was again tested in the above-mentioned sequence. In all posterior fixations a small interspinous osseous block was used as abutment.

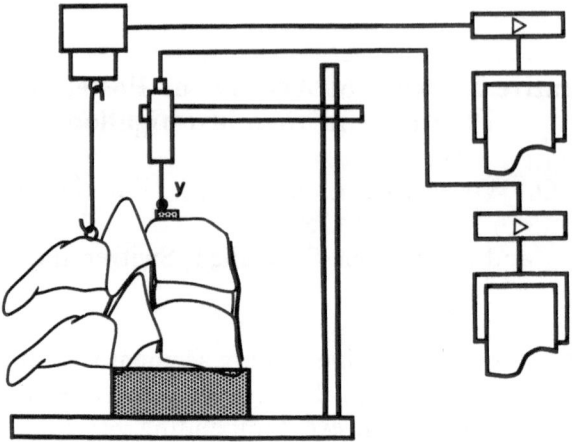

Fig. 1. Test fixture

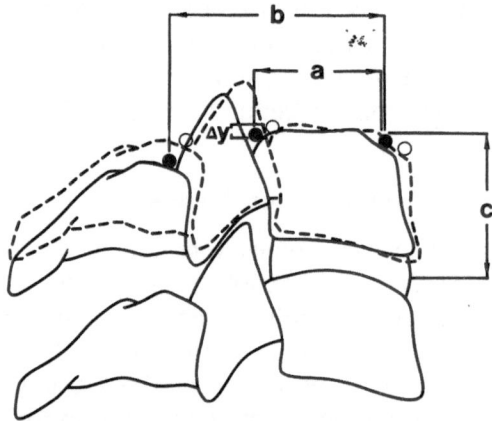

Fig. 2. Measured length used to determine the tilting angle α of the functional spine unit

Results

With F max = 10 N after posterior ligamentous severance the tilting angle was α = 0.415 + 0.041 with a curve characteristic of unstable situations. Anterior H-plate stabilization resulted in a narrowing of the tilting angle (α = 0.415° + 0.092) with a comparable curve (Fig. 3). Stabilization with posterior hook-plate (α = 0.014° + 0.002) achieved the smallest tilting angle with the linear course of the curve in the measuring range; additional anterior H-plate fixation showed identical tilting angles. The value for α was

0.03° + 0.016 after sublaminar wiring; in combination with the anterior H-plate it was possible to lower this value to 0.015° + 0.005 (Fig. 3). Complete disco-ligamentous severance of the specimens resulted in the lowest value of

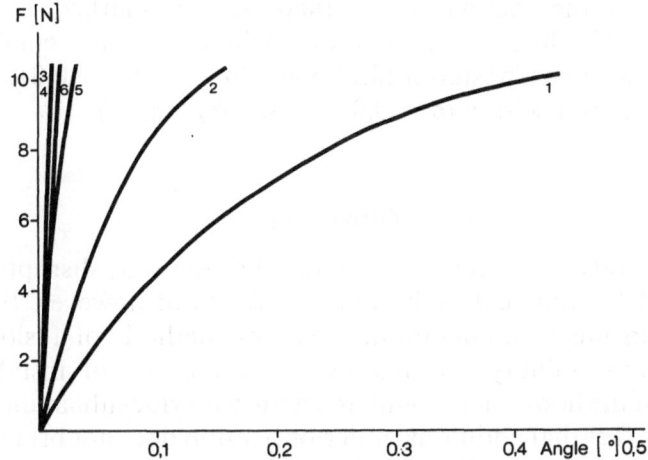

Fig. 3. Load-displacement curves for posterior ligamentous disrupture. *1* Without stabilization, *2* anterior H-plate, *3* posterior hook-plate, *4* anterior H-plate plus posterior hook-plate, *5* posterior sublaminar wiring, *6* anterior H-plate plus posterior sublaminar wiring

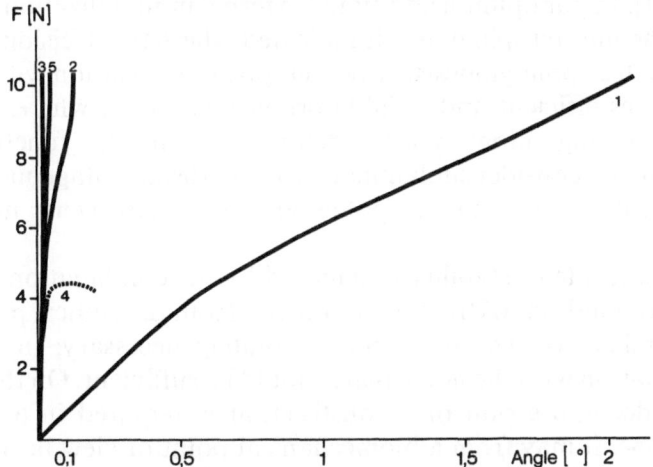

Fig. 4. Load-displacement curves for complete disco-ligamentous instability. *1* Anterior plate fixation, *2* posterior hook-plate, *3* anterior H-plate plus posterior hook-plate, *4* posterior sublaminar wiring, *5* anterior H-plate plus posterior sublaminar wiring

stability ($\alpha = 2.01° + 0.74$) for the exclusive H-plate-fusion and a curve characteristic of a state of instability. Posterior fixation with the hook-plate produced a maximal tilting angle of 0.111° + 0.089; with a short nonlinear deformation the curve corresponds with a stable situation. After exclusive posterior wiring fixation and as soon as 4 N were applied, the specimen did not resume its initial condition because of plastic deformation and cutting of the wires into the lamina. Also, there was a marked tendency for retrolisthesis. The highest stability was achieved by the combined procedures anterior plate/posterior hook-plate ($\alpha = 0.012° + 0.013$) and anterior plate/posterior wiring ($\alpha = 0.023° + 0.008$) (Fig. 4).

Discussion

The instability produced by posterior ligamentous disruption can be compensated to some extent by anterior fixation; however, the curve is typical for an unstable condition. Posterior methods of fusion produce higher primary stability, for fixation is at the site of instability. The superiority of the hook-plate compared with posterior sublaminar wiring, is shown by the fact that additional anterior fixation does not bring about any measurable gain in stability. Under experimental conditions, exclusive anterior plate-spondylodesis does not seem to bring about satisfactory results in complete disco-ligamentous instability; clinically this corresponds with a high number of possible secondary kyphotic processes following this procedure [1]. In our opinion additional external immobilization preventing flexion of the injured spinal unit is indicated where the decision is taken in favour of such a spondylodesis. However, posterior fixation with the hook-plate produces efficient and reliable primary stability, whereas posterior sublaminar wiring allows plastic deformation in the functional unit. Furthermore, we consider sublaminar wiring as disadvantageous because of possible dural lesions and the potential risk of iatrogenic neurological sequelae [2].

The highest rate of stability is achieved by the combination of anterior and posterior methods of fixation. However, from the clinical point of view such comprehensive fixation is not absolutely necessary; in most cases posterior fixation with the hook-plate should be sufficient. On the contrary, if anterior decompression or reconstruction is required in a completely unstable spine, it may from a biomechanical point of view be advisable to add a posterior fixation.

References

1. Capen DA, Garland DE, Waters RL (1985) Surgical stabilization of the cervical spine. A comparative analysis of anterior and posterior spine fusions. Clin Orthop 196: 229–237

2. Mc Afee PC, Bohlman HH, Wilson WL (1985) The triple wire fixation technique for stabilization of acute cervical fracture-dislocation: A biomechanical analysis (abstract). Orthop Trans 9 (1): 142
3. White III AA, Southwick WO, Panjabi MM (1976) Clinical instability of the lower cervical spine. Spine 1: 15–27

Cervical Spine I
© by Springer-Verlag 1987

1.11. The Part of the Macromolecules of the Extracellular Matrix in the Biomechanics of the Lower Cervical Spine

M. Misasi, C. Piergentili, and Gf. Tajana, Napoli, Italy

Introduction

The molecular characteristics of the matrices have mostly been studied through the use of sophisticated methods which require an advanced technology and which can very often be carried out on animals only. The aim of our work was to set up a fast and practical technique of analysis of matrices based on relatively simple tools, and adequate to be applied also to routinary histological preparations (paraffine inclusions).

These requirements led us to improve the technique of examination by polarized light after treatment with suitable "amplifier probes" which allow to observe simultaneously both the fibrillar and matrix components.

The knowledge of the location of the molecular components of the normal and pathological human intervertebral disc may be useful in order to relate biomechanical problems to the molecular composition of the extracellular matrix of the disc. With the use of antibodies against some glycoproteins of the matrix (fibronectine and laminine), and against the different kinds of collagen, it is presently possible to localize some basic components of matrices. Furthermore by the use of monoclonal antibodies against the link-protein it is possible to detect specific loci of the proteoglycanic molecules. However, the identification of proteoglycans, particularly of hyaluronic acid—whose biomechanical role represents the clue for the understanding of molecular control mechanisms of the vertebral statics—is still difficult. In fact, so far there is no existing method allowing the direct detection of hyaluronate by the optical or electronic microscope. The localization of hyaluronic acid may be, however, managed by evaluating the intensity of the staining with Alcian Blue on different preparations, or the autoradiographical distribution of H-glucosamine grains before and after treatments with hyaluronidase. A further trouble rises from the difficulties in collecting and fixing the intervertebral disc. Recently a technical expedient aiming at reducing such fixation artefact utilizes tannic acid or piridin ethil chloride which decreases GAG leakage. However, even this step proves to be highly aspecific for the different GAGs and for the hyaluronic acid itself; this latter being possibly extracted or transferred in nontypical tissular loci.

Sirius Red (F3 BA) is a polyazoic stainer with molecular weight 1,373 characterized by 4 —N=N azoic group and by 6 —SO$_3$Na sulphonic group, about 46 A long.

This molecule can increase the birefringence of collagen in histological sections. When Sirius Red is used as specific stainer for collagen it is prepared in picric acid-saturated water solution of 1 mg/ml. This solution has a pH of 1.8–2. In these conditions the stainer binds prevalently the collagen and at polarized light the specificity is absolute. The reaction occurs at low pH between Sirius Red —SO$_3$ groups and tissue cationic groups. The binding is prevented by the increase of pH and of ionic strength. Other factors which can decrease or prevent the binding of the stainer are the deamination of amino groups by treatments with nitrose acid, the block of amino and guanidinic groups by acetilation and the chloration of amino groups [1]. On the basis of the above consideration the binding should be formed between —SO$_3$ groups and basic groups.

At working pH each free ionizable amino group of the protein can bind one azoic stainer. The staining specificity of the picric acid-Sirius Red solution depend on the competition of the stainer and picric acid for the tissular cationic groups. Junqueira [1] calculated that a single molecule of collagen (MW 300,000) is able to bind about 120 molecules of stainer. Under this condition when using a polarizing microscope, it is possible to see bands of interferences in the spectrum of red, while in the conventional sections, bands of interference corresponding to orange, yellow, and green are observed. These variations are related to the degree of packaging of collagen and particularly to the presence on it of the glycoprotein and proteoglycanic macromolecules [2]. Therefore from the variations of the sections observed at polarized light, after treatment with specific enzymes for collagen it is possible to assess approximately the amount of proteoglycanic molecules associated with collagen inside the human intervertebral disc. Furthermore it should be possible to detect structural differences at different levels of the spine and to relate them to the extent and the kind of regional biomechanical activity.

Materials and Methods

Intervertebral discs taken from cervical and lumbar spine have been used. The discs have been taken from corpses of subjects not older than 30 years, or during surgical arthrodeses.

The autoptic or surgical material was fixed in a solution of Alcohol/Formol (9 : 1) containing 1% of CPC (cetyl pyridine chlorine) and 0.5% of ammonium sulphide.

The tissue was dehydrated, included in paraffine and sectioned at 5 μm. The analysis of the affinity of Alcian for homologous zones in sections treated respectively with buffer (control sections) or with enzyme has been carried out by the method of double wavelength (according to Patten). The preparations have been read by the use of Zeiss photomicroscope with microphotometric head 01 K. The reading was performed on spots of diameter L-25 μm at wavelengths of 650–585. The relative concentration of Alcian in a given zone is expressed as the average of the absorbancy values on five readings. In a parallel study the sections were treated with the same enzymatic solutions containing PMSF (Phenyl Metossil Sulphonil Fluoride) as inhibitor of protease.

Results and Discussion

From these preliminary results it is possible to draw the following considerations:

1. The intervertebral discs of the cervical level are about 2–5 times less rich in hyaluronic acid than the ones of lumbar level.

2. The distribution of chondroitin-4(6)-sulphate is on the contrary completely different showing the highest values at cervical level and the lowest ones at lumbar level.

3. As to dermatic sulphate we have not observed significant differences of its concentration at any level of the spine.

4. In case of discal herniation deep alterations of molecular composition of the matrices are detectable along with changes of the distribution of the different molecular components.

In conclusion, from these preliminary results we might confirm that the histochemical investigation integrated by the use of polarizing microscopy, after treatment with specific subtraction enzymes, may represent a useful system of investigation for the analysis of the molecular components of the intervertebral disc. The asymmetric distribution of the concentration of hyaluronic acid is presumably related to the different biomechanical roles of these two levels. The hyaluronic acid may absorbe or release water from the tissue of the intervertebral disc with relationship to pressure force. The low concentration of hyaluronic acid at cervical level, where shear stresses prevail, and the high concentration at lumbar level, where compression forces prevail, seems to correlated the molecular findings with the biomechanical ones.

The meaning of the distribution of the other GAGs is at present under study.

References

1. Junqueira LCU, Bignolas G, Brentani RR (1979) Picrosirius staining plus polarizing microscopy a specific method for collagen detection in tissue sections. Histochem J 11: 447
2. Dziedzic-Goclawaska A, Rozycka M, Czyba T, Moutier R, Lenczowski U, Ostrowski K (1982) Polarizing microscopy of Picrosirius stained bone sections as method for analysis of spatial distribution of collagen fibers by optical diffractometry. Basic Appl Histochem 26: 227–229

1.12. Chronic Atlanto-axial Instability in the Down Syndrome*

St. W. Burke, H. Graeme French, Th. S. Whitecloud, III, and J. Ollie Edmunds, Jr., New Orleans, Louisiana, U.S.A.

Introduction

The atlanto-axial segments of the cervical spine in children with the Down Syndrome have a predilection for the development of localized anomalies which are of particular interest, because of the danger of atlanto-axial dislocation [4, 6, 7, 13, 18, 23, 27, 28, 31]. All previous studies are limited by the fact that they are not longitudinal [17, 18, 26, 29]. They only describe the incidence of the abnormalities in the Down Syndrome in a population and do not attempt to study the natural history of either the anomalies or the C_1–C_2 instability.

In 1983 we studied one hundred forty patients with Down Syndrome at the Pinecrest State School for upper cervical instability. The study was prompted by an acute C_1–C_2 dislocation resulting in quadriplegia that occurred at this institution. Thirty-two of the patients were identified as having been radiographically screened for C_1–C_2 instability approximately thirteen years earlier. These 32 patients are described in the present report.

Methods and Materials

All the 1970 radiography had been obtained as part of a screening program for C_1–C_2 instability. In 1983, each patient had in addition a physical examination in which we recorded the neurologic status, associated physical anomalies, birthdate, sex, race, activity level, and intelligence. The radiographs we made of the upper cervical spine included flexion-extension views.

Each set of 1983 radiographs was classified in one of three categories, based on the C_1–C_2 measurements and stability, and the presence or absence of an ossicle in the atlas was also recorded. If the C_1–C_2 interval measured more than four millimeters in patients under age 15 years, or more than three millimeters in patients over the age of 15 years (see below) it was

---

* The opinions or assertations contained herein are the private opinions of the authors and are not the official views of the Department of The Air Force.

judged abnormal. Excessive motion at the C_1–C_2 level meant instability. The radiographs were therefore classified as either *normal,* or *stable,* or *unstable.* Normal indicated an interval of less than 3 or 4 mm, with no motion on flexion extension lateral cervical radiographs and no ossicle on the atlas. Stable indicated at least one millimeter of atlanto-axial motion and a maximum interval of less than 3 or 4 mm. Unstable meant more than 3 or 4 mm of motion, or a fixed interval of more than 5 mm.

Except for the one patient who died of dislocation of C_1–C_2 all thirty-one remaining patient are still living.

Results

In 1970, in 26 sets of radiographs, the findings were classified as normal, in five as stable, and in one as unstable. The analogous numbers in 1983 were 19, 3, and 7, and two patients who had developed ossicles, had atlanto-dental intervals of 2 mm and 3 mm.

In 1970 seven of the patients had some motion at the C_1–C_2 level, the mean being 2.78 mm (S.D.—0.95 mm) but only one of these met our criterion for instability (*i.e.,* more than a 4 mm interval under age 15). In seven other patients in 1983 the average motion of C_1–C_2 was 6.93 mm (S.D.—4.04 mm). Evaluation by Student T-test demonstrated that the difference between these two groups was statistically significant at the p less than 0.005. During 1983 four of the patients who had some motion in 1970 had no evidence of motion, including the patient considered unstable on the 1970 X-rays. Of the seven patients who had instability at C_1–C_2 in 1983, 6 had no C_1–C_2 motion in 1970. There was one who had less than 3 mm interval in 1970, and 19 other patients who were normal in 1970 remained unchanged (stable). The three patients who developed accessory ossicles on the atlas between 1970 and 1983 did not have associated motion at C_1–C_2, but one patient had a fixed interval of 6 mm. The initial average age of the group that improved was 9.25 years and it was 18.16 years in the group that deteriorated (p less than 0.05). The one patient, case 4, that was unstable in 1970 was radiographically normal in 1983.

Discussion

Instability

Our criteria for atlanto-axial instability, based on several reports in normal individuals [11, 12, 15, 17, 30], prescribes the normal adult C_1–C_2 interval as less than 3 mm and that of children between the ages of one month and sixteen years as less than 4 mm. Based on these criteria we have demonstrated only one instance of instability in the original X-rays of our 32 patients but a 22% (seven instances) incidence at follow-up after 13 years. These data agree with those of other reported series [5, 17]. In the present series, the magnitude of the atlanto-axial subluxation increased with age. This represents a reversal of the trend in normal individuals toward increased stability (*i.e.* narrowing of the C_1–C_2 interval) with maturation. Evaluation by age of those patients who showed increasing instability indicated that they usually were older than ten at the time of initial evaluation. Those patients less than age 10 years at first evaluation were more likely to improve (p less than 0.05). This probably reflects the fact that the younger patients have more physiological motion at C_1–C_2.

Ossicles

The three patients in our series who had accessory ossicles in 1983 did not show them on the 1970 X-rays, implying that these ossicles may develop late in childhood.

All three of our patients who developed an ossicle in the atlas by 1983 clearly had a normal apophysis of the upper dens in 1970. Therefore, any congenital accessory ossicle should have been visible when each patient had the initial X-ray [11]. The 1983 films in the three patients with ossicles all show a dens of normal length with an ossicle superior to its tip; therefore, the presence of an ossicle above the dens suggests that there had been an avulsion fracture of the upper end of the dens. This implies that there may have been instability of the atlanto-axial level at some time, despite the fact that no C_1–C_2 motion was evident in 1983 in any of the three patients. It appears that the degree of instability in C_1–C_2 in patients with Down Syndrome increases with age as shown in our cases 1–3, 5–8, and that the ossicles may be associated with instability of transient character.

The etiology of the upper cervical instability in Down's Syndrome is most likely a defect in collagen that is manifested by generalized ligamentous laxity. The weak connective tissue is susceptible to injury and stretching. The combination of an increasing mechanical disadvantage at a joint because of lengthened fibrous structure leads to progressively increasing instability of the joint with minor trauma. The collagen of the structures supporting the dens may be susceptible to an avulsion fracture. There also may be decreased tensile strength in the growth plate during the adolescent growth spurt, that may lead to such an injury at that time of life.

The chronic subluxation at the level of instability may explain the sudden postoperative respiratory arrest that occasionally is associated with reduction and fusion of C_1–C_2 [7, 13, 18, 23, 27] because impingement of the spinal canal may occur because the reparative scar tissue narrows the spinal canal. Even minor cord compression at this level is likely to result in respiratory arrest as previously noted by Nordt [23].

Because of the predisposition of patients with Down Syndrome to instability of the cervical spine and because our data indicate that it is progressive, presumably the result of repetitive trauma to constitutionally lax ligaments, and most importantly because the instability can cause a catastrophe, we recommend that all patients with the syndrome whether stable or unstable be restricted from all high risk activities. Patients with potential or actual instability can be identified. They have either more than four millimeters of atlanto-axial subluxation when over 10 years of age, or an accessory ossicle at C_1-C_2, or a fixed C_1-C_2 interval of more than 4 mm and they should be treated with stringent restriction of activity and close observation. We further recommend that C_1-C_2 fusion should be considered in all healthy patients with instability whose activity cannot be restricted.

References

1. Bailey DK (1952) The normal cervical spine in infants and children. Radiology 59: 712–719
2. Cattel HS, Feltzer DL (1965) Pseudosubluxation and other normal variations in the cervical spine in children. JBJS 47 A: 1295–1307
3. Clark AM, Clarke ADB (1973) Mental deficiency, the changing outlook, third edn. The Free Press, New York
4. Curtro BII, Blank S, Fisher RL (1968) Atlanto-axial dislocation in Down's Syndrome. JAMA 205 (6): 212–213
5. Diamond LS, Lyne D, Sigman B (1981) Orthopaedic disorders in patients with Down's syndrome. Orthop Clin North Am 12 (1): 57–71
6. Dzentis AJ (1966) Spontaneous atlanto-axial dislocation in a mongoloid child with spinal cord compression. J Neurosurg 25: 458–460
7. Finerman GAM, Sakai D, Weingarth S (1976) Atlanto-axial dislocation with spinal cord compression in a mongoloid child. JBJS 58 A: 408–409
8. Gladstone RJ, Wakeley CPG (1924) Variations of the occipito-atlantal joint in relation to the metameric structure of the craniovertebral region. J Anat 59: 195–216
9. Halley L (1948) Atlanto-occipital fusion, ossiculum terminale and occipital vertebra as related to basilar invagination with neurologic symptoms. Am J Roen 59: 511–524
10. Hawkins RJ, Fielding J, Thompson W (1976) Os odontoideum: congenital or acquired. JBJS 58A: 413–414
11. Hefke HW (1940) Roentgenologic study of anomalies of the hands in one hundred cases of mongolism. Am J Dis Child, Dec: 1319–1323
12. Hinke VC, Hopkins CE (1960) Measurement of the atlanto-dental interval in the adult. Am J Roen 84: 945–951
13. Hreidarsson St, Magram G, Singer H (1982) Symptomatic atlanto-axial dislocation in Down's syndrome. Pediatrics 69 (5): 568–571
14. Juhl JH, Miller SN, Roberts GW (1962) Roentgenographic variations in the normal cervical spine. Radiology 78: 591–597
15. Locke GR, Gardener JI, VanEpps EF (1966) Atlas-dens interval (ADI) in children. Am J Roen 97: 135–140

16. Lombardi G (1961) The occipital vertebra. Am J Roen 86: 260–269
17. Martel W, Tishler JM (1966) Observations on the spine in mongolism. Am J Roen 97: 630–638
18. Martel W, Uyham R, Stevenson C (1969) Subluxation of the atlas causing spinal cord compression in a case of Down's syndrome with manifestations of an occipital vertebra. Radiology 93: 839–840
19. Mauntner H, Barnes A, Curtis G (1950) Abnormal findings on the spine in mongoloids. Am J Mental Def 55: 105–107
20. McCrae D (1960) The significance of abnormalities of the cervical spine. Am J Roen 84: 3–25
21. McCrae D (1954) Bony abnormalities in the region of the foramen magnum: correlation of the anatomic and neurologic findings. Acta Radiologica 40: 335–348
22. Nicholson JT, Sherk HH (1968) Anomalies of the occipitocervical articulation. JBJS 50 A: 295–304
23. Nordt JC, Stauffer ES (1981) Sequellae of atlanto-axial stabilization in two patients with Down's syndrome. Spine 6 (5): 437–440
24. Plautt HF (1937) Fracture of the atlas or developmental abnormality. Radiology 29: 227–231
25. Ricciardi JE, Daufer H, Louis D (1976) Acquired os-odontiodeum following acute ligament injury. JBJS 58 A: 410–412
26. Semine AA, Ertel AN, Goldberg MJ, Bull MJ (1978) Cervical spine instability in children with Down's syndrome (Timsomy 21). JBJS 60 A: 649–652
27. Sherk HH, Nicholson J (1969) Rotatory atlanto-axial dislocation associated with ossiculum terminale and mongolism. JBJS 51 A: 957–964
28. Sherk HH, Pasquarsello PS, Watters WC (1982) Multiple dislocations of the cervical spine in a patient with juvenile rheumatoid arthritis and Down's syndrome. Clin Orthop 162: 37–40
29. Tishler J, Marte W (1965) Dislocation of the atlas in mongolism. Radiology 84: 904–906
30. von Torklus D, Gehle W (1972) The upper cervical spine. Grune and Stratton, New York
31. Whaley WJ, Gray WD (1980) Atlanto-axial dislocation and Down's syndrome. Can Med Assoc J 123: 35–37

2. Diagnostic Evaluation

Cervical Spine I
© by Springer-Verlag 1987

2.1. Initial Sensory Examination as a Predictor of Neurologic Recovery Following Anterior Spinal Cord Injury

B. E. Northrup, D. Ball, and J. L. Osterholm,
Philadelphia, Pennsylvania, U.S.A.

Introduction

Sensory incomplete spinal cord injuries frequently recover a variable degree of motor function. We wished to ask the question: Does the pattern of retained sensation enable one to predict the extent of motor recovery?

Population

Over a five year period five hundred and twenty-nine patients with spinal cord injuries were admitted to the Delaware Valley Spinal Cord Injury Center at Thomas Jefferson University Hospital. Of these patients, thirty were judged to have on admission complete paralysis and partially preserved sensation (sensory incomplete injury).

The thirty patients varied with respect to type of bony pathology: Five had dislocations of the cervical spine, eighteen had flexion compression injuries, and six had spondylosis. One patient received a paravertebral gundhot wound. The average age of the spondylosis group was 54.4 years, of the dislocation group, 34.2 years, and the flexion compression group, 26.8 years. The etiology of the injuries were varied (vehicle accidents 13, diving 11, falls 5, gunshot wound 1). Two thirds of the patients were operated upon, and one third were treated with halo vest immobilization only.

Method

Assessment and treatment in the spinal cord injury center was accomplished by a team consisting of orthopedists, neurosurgeons and physiatrists. The patients were graded retrospectively on the basis of the admission sensory findings according to the following scale:

1. Appreciation of pin prick sensation in the lower extremities.

2. Proprioception and/or touch in the lower extremities, but without pin prick appreciation.

3. Irregular or patchy distribution of sensation in the lower extremities, no appreciation of pin prick.

4. Sacral sparing.

The patients were subsequently graded by the physiatrists at the time of discharge, and at one, three, six months, and one year intervals. The patients were rated retrospectively on their motor abilities on the anniversary of the spinal injury according to the following scale:

1. Independent walking.
2. Walking with assistive device.
3. Weak movements only.
4. No improvement.

Results

The patients were found to have a wide spectrum of severity of neurologic injury. One fourth were found to have preserved pin prick in the lower extremities, slightly over one half had a preservation of touch and/or proprioception in the lower extremities, and one fifth had sensation restricted to sacral segments only.

Long tract recovery. Seventy percent of patients retaining pin prick regained the ability to ambulant independently, as compared to ambulation in one third of patients who retained only touch and/or proprioception in the lower extremities. Independent ambulation did not occur with five patients who were found to have irregular sensation or sacral sparing only.

Zone of injury recovery. Two thirds improved one level or more. This was noted in sixty percent of nine immobilized patients. In patients operated upon seventy-two percent improved one or more levels. Two patients with spondylosis improved more than one level: Three levels and two levels respectively. One patient with a flexion compression injury improved two levels. Three patients with good to excellent recovery of distal cord function retained significant impairment at the level of injury.

Mortality. In this group of patients there was a seven percent mortality at three months and ten percent mortality one year following injuries. The cause of the last death is unknown, but suicide is suspected.

Type of bony injury. In the five patients with cervical dislocation sensory function was relatively good initially. Four of the five subsequently regained the ability to walk independently. In the six patients with spondylosis, only sacral sparing was present in five of the six. The one patient retaining sensation in the lower extremities was able to walk independently. In the flexion compression group, all patients with retention of pin prick were able to walk without braces. In those who retained touch and/or proprioception of the lower extremities, but had lost the ability to perceive pin prick, one third were able to walk. None of the patients with meager patchy sensory retention or those with sacral sparing only regained the ability to walk.

Type of bony treatment. The patients received a variety of treatments, dependent largely on the type of bony injury (dislocation, spondylosis or flexion-compression injuries). Patients with dislocation were reduced (one case required operative reduction) and a posterior cervical fusion performed. An anterior fusion was undertaken in one patient in order to provide better decompression of the root of the level of injury. Patients with spondylosis were evaluated myelographically, and decompressed where significant cord impingement occurred. In one patient a corpectomy was performed. This patient who had retained pin in the lower extremities, was able to ambulate independently at one year. A wide spectrum of bony injury was seen in the patients with flexion compression injury. When the canal could not be restored to anatomic position, and myelographs did not indicate cord compression, immobilization was carried out, followed by flexion—extension radiographs at three months. In patients with significant neural impingement corpectomy was done followed by fusion. When bony deformity did not intrude into the canal, but ligamentous injury was judged to be significant, a posterior fusion was done.

Discussion

The degree of recovery is in nearly all patients a reflection of the neurologic deficit on admission. Patients with a greater degree of sensory preservation tend to improve motor performance more. When pin prick sensation is preserved, the likelihood of significant motor recovery is quite good.

The anterior cord syndrome includes patients with preservation of posterior column function: Touch, vibration, and position sense. Since the spinothalamic tracts are located in the anterior portion of the cord, pain and pin prick are not appreciated below the level of the lesion. Seven of the twenty-seven survivors were found to have pin prick sensation in the lower extremities; these patients regained the ability to ambulate.

The outcome of the recovery process is influenced greatly by population composition. The current study is limited by sample size. Variability of treatments once that patient reached the center tends to compromise the results further. A retrospective analysis is made difficult by systematic errors, such as the exclusive of certain patients (older, more severely injured, etc.) from surgical groups.

Because of this variability it is not possible to conclude as to whether any particular treatment was more effective in restoring neural function.

Cervical Spine I
© by Springer-Verlag 1987

2.2. Sectorization of the Axial Image of Cervical Vertebrae, a Heuristic Approach for Automatic Analysis in Artificial Intelligence

A. WACKENHEIM, Strasbourg, France

Three cervical vertebrae are very similar: C 3, C 4, and C 5. They build a morphological unit which is perceived globally because it is formed by three proximal and identical vertebrae.

In practice, the rules we found out for the heuristic analysis are the same for each of these three vertebrae so that we have to consider only one pattern. It comprises three anatomical levels which are demonstrated in this paper.

In Fig. 1 these three levels are localized schematically. Each of them, A, B, and C is divided into nine image-sectors. These sectors have a heuristic value because they are very closely linked to the medical thinking and to the pathological processes. Sector 1 and 3 are connected with the vertebral artery and its pathology. Sector 2 concerns the vertebral body and its pathology (traumatic, metabolic, tumoral, ...). Sector 4 and 6 are connected with rheumatic diseases. Sector 5 is linked to the neurological pathology. Sector 7 and 9 are silent and sector 8 is very poorly informative.

Let us describe the three cuts:

Cut A (Fig. 2): It is very easy to identify this cut with respect to the two others. Indeed its characteristic is the presence in sector 1 and 3 of the section of the rounded canal of the vertebral artery, the foramen transversarium. The automatic analysis of shape recognition identifies this structure and by this mean recognizes the level A. The cut A is concerned by a very rich pathology which is indicated above and especially by the relations between rheumatic pathology (sector 4 and 6) and compression of the vertebral artery (sector 1 and 3). It is for example very easy to suspect a constitutional aplasia of one vertebral artery when one foramen transversarium is too small.

Cut B (Fig. 3): This cut is characterized by the density of the vertebral body, *i.e.* ⩾ 300 UH. Indeed, this density distinguishes cut B from cut C. The absence of foramen transversarium distinguishes cut B from cut A. The most informative sectors of cut B are 4 and 6 because they contain the articular interspace of the posterior articular processes. At the level of this

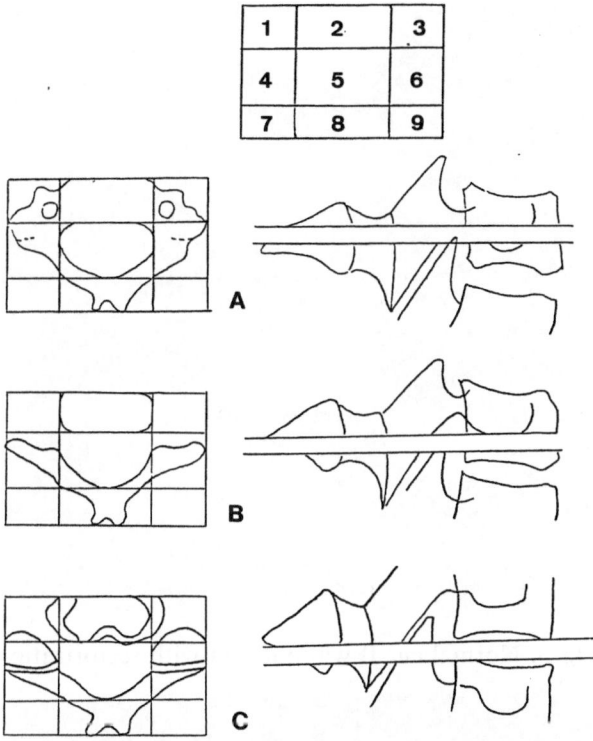

Fig. 1. Schematic representation of the sectorization in three levels of clinical CT
axial cuts

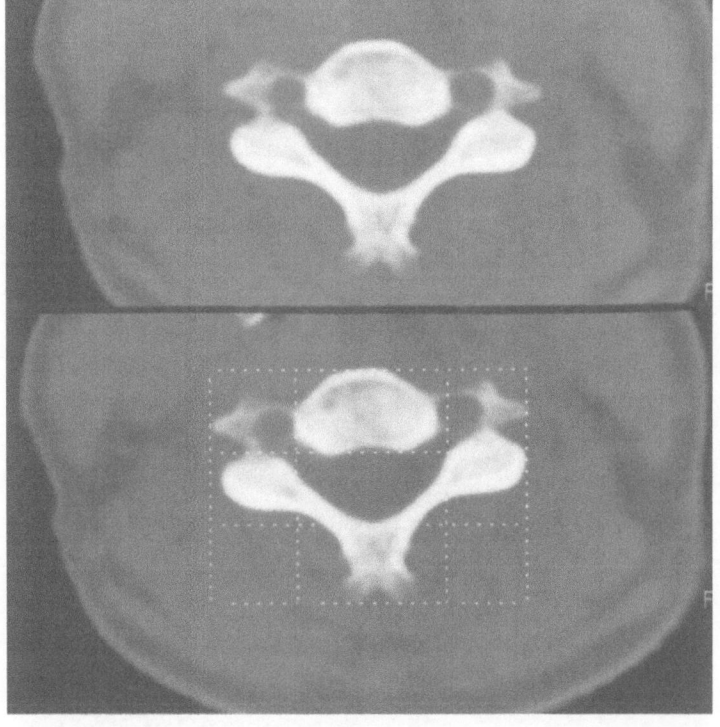

Fig. 2. Normal cut A without and with sectorization

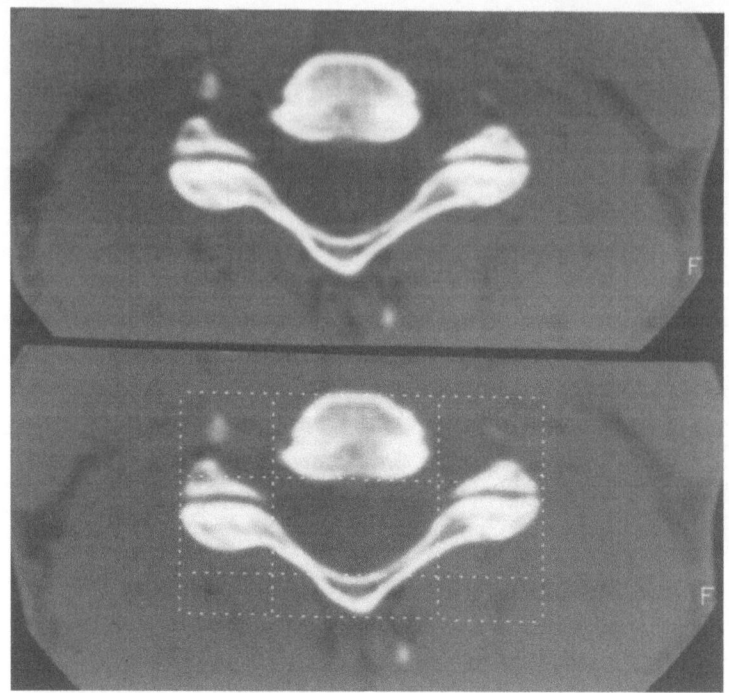

Fig. 3. Normal cut B without and with sectorization

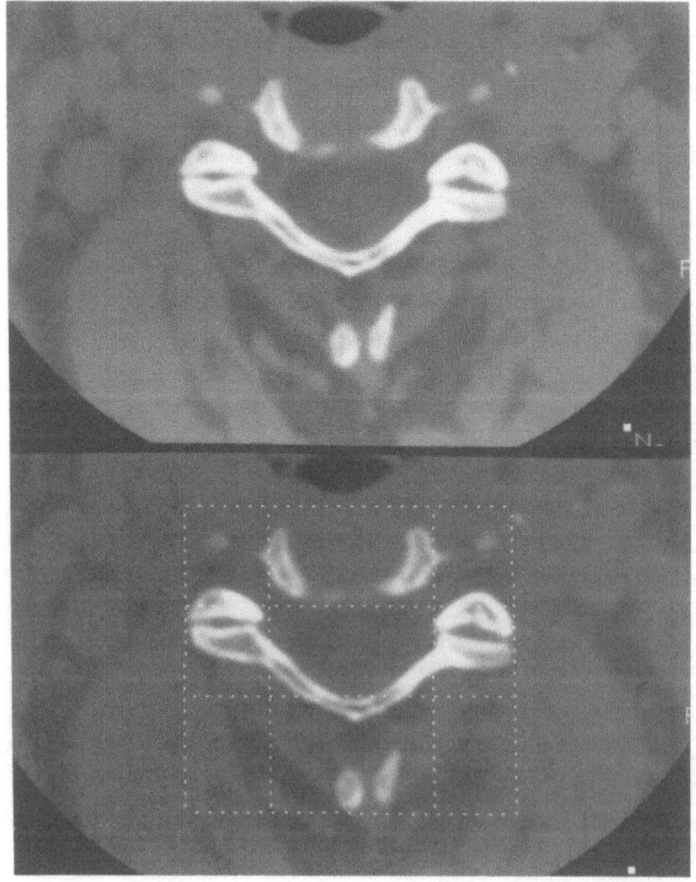

Fig. 4. Normal cut C without and with sectorization

cut, we have to invent specific rules for the expert system concerning the pathology of degenerative and inflammatory rheumatics.

Cut C (Fig. 4): It is the specific level of the intervertebral disc. It is characterized by the density of sector 2 which is $\leqslant$ 200 UH. The value of the density distinguishes cut C from cut B. The absence of the foramen transversarium distinguishes the cut C from the cut A. In this image, the rules concern the intervertebral foramen in its basal part, *i.e.* the most pathogenic one because it shelters the corresponding cervical root. Thus the rules we have to determine concern on one hand the pathology of the disc (soft and hard hernias) and on the other hand the hypertrophy as well of the uncus as of the superior articular process of the underlying vertebra which are responsible for narrowness of the intervertebral canal.

Summary

The author describes the method of a heuristic approach of automatic analysis in the axial views of three very similar vertebrae: C 3, C 4, and C 5. He demonstrates a method of sectorization and traces the general lines concerning the rules which are to be elaborated for an expert system in artificial intelligence.

Cervical Spine I
© by Springer-Verlag 1987

2.3. Unstable Cervical Trauma and Traumatic Conditions Inducing Neurological Complications as Investigated by CT-Scanning

P. Capesius and M. C. Kaiser, Luxembourg, Grand-Duchy of Luxembourg

Introduction

One of the main advantages of CT-scanning in traumatic conditions of the cervical spine resides in the fact that CT investigations may easily be carried out during the acute stage of the trauma as only minimal patient movement is necessary, soft tissue and bone structures being equally well shown during one visit to the Radiology Department only [1, 6, 8]. As a general rule CT-scanning is performed as a complementary investigation after careful appreciation of conventional X-rays. In most of the cases CT obviates the need for myelography at this stage, intrathecal contrast injection should only be performed whenever avulsion of the brachial plexus is suspected in a view to perform CT myelography [2]. In those cases the injection of contrast may be performed using the latero-cervical approach between C 1 and C 2, the patient remaining in a supine position.

1. Diagnosis of Cervical Instability

Traumatic instability of the cervical spine is due to fractures of the posterior arch which are in general much better outlined by CT than by conventional radiography. This is mainly true in the study of the posterior articular facets where CT may easily delineate fractures and luxations causing vertebral instability. In cases where bilateral interarticular fractures or luxations are present, traumatic spondylolisthesis may be shown by CT. If on one CT slice a band of disc material is enclosed by the upper and lower vertebral end plates, this CT feature may be considered as being pathognomonic for spondylolisthesis. In cases of unilateral fracture or luxation of the posterior facets a unilateral antelisthesis may be observed which is objectivated by vertebral rotation with the spinous process moving towards the affected side [3, 7]. In our serie we encountered 7 patients presenting this type of unilateral dislocation fracture of the posterior facets (Fig. 1). Electronically generated reconstructions in the sagittal plane permit a more accurate evaluation of global or unilateral vertebral displacement (Figs. 2

and 3) and as well of the luxation within the posterior facets. This is even more true in cases where good quality standard films and complex motion tomography are not available.

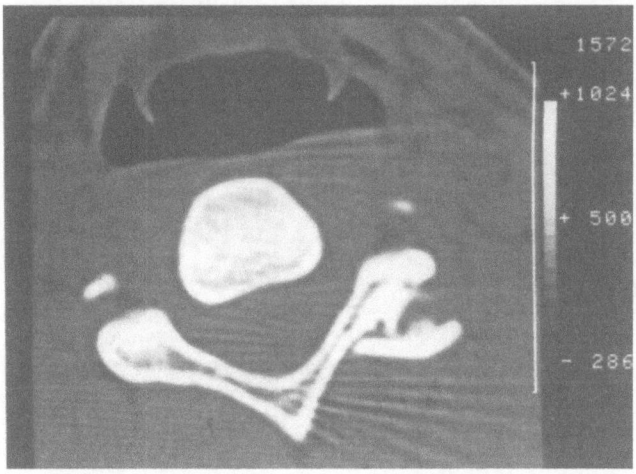

Fig. 1. Unilateral dislocation fracture of posterior facets with lateralized spondylo-listhesis due to vertebral rotation

2. Neurological Complications

Apart from instability other traumatic lesions capable to induce serious neurological complications may be delineated by CT.

a) Vertebral Fractures with Interruption of the Posterior Wall

CT easily shows prolongation of a vertebral fracture into the posterior wall with eventual avulsion and protrusion of a bone fragment inside the neural canal. A particular type of fracture, the tear-drop fracture, is almost constantly associated with posttraumatic paraplegia. The CT features in this type of fracture are quite characteristic: sagittal and coronal fracture lines isolating an antero-inferior bone fragment (tear-drop) and posterior widening of the sagittal fracture line which appears to open into the neural canal. This fracture causes narrowing of a A–P diameter of the vertebral canal due to protrusion of the posterior wall. Also bilateral fractures of the posterior arch are constantly encountered (Fig. 4).

b) Intracanalar Herniation and Protrusion of Disc Material

To establish a diagnosis of cervical hernia by conventional radiography is not possible, even with myelography the diagnosis may remain difficult and uncertain. CT may show cervical hernias causing posttraumatic

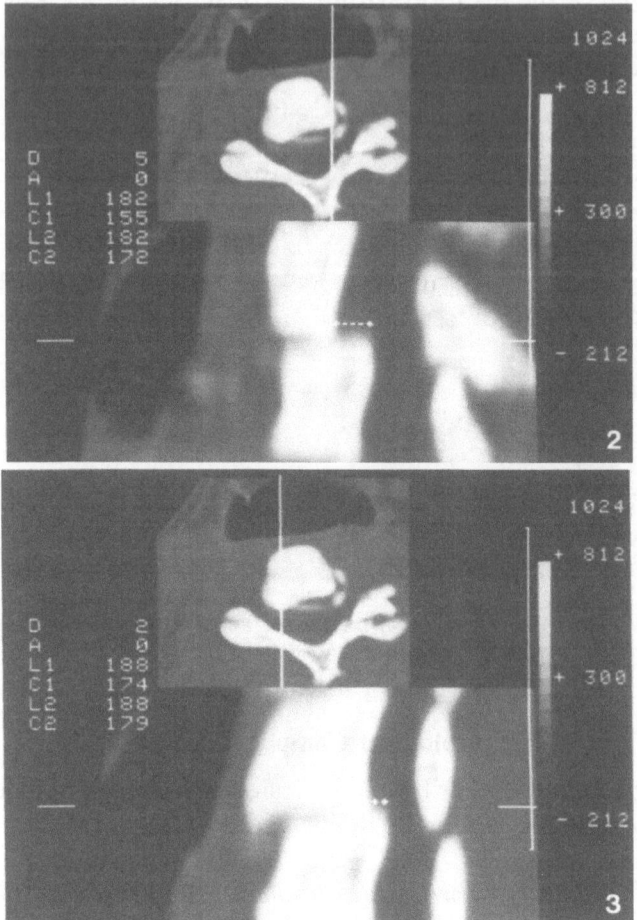

Figs. 2 and 3. Electronically generated reconstructions in a sagittal direction demonstrate vertebral displacement of 5 mm on the side of the posterior dislocation fracture while on the opposite side the antelisthesis measures only 2 mm. Notice some degree of vertebral rotation

neuralgia or paraplegia. The herniated disc is seen as a relatively hyperdense structure protruding out of the intervertebral disc space inside the neural canal. The hernia may be in the midline or more laterally. In some instances massive disc herniations may fill up almost all the intracanalar space facing the affected disc space.

c) Hematomas and Medullary Contusions

Their diagnosis is very difficult on CT images. They are mainly recognized as hyperdense areas of relatively irregular delineation within a diffusely enlarged cord.

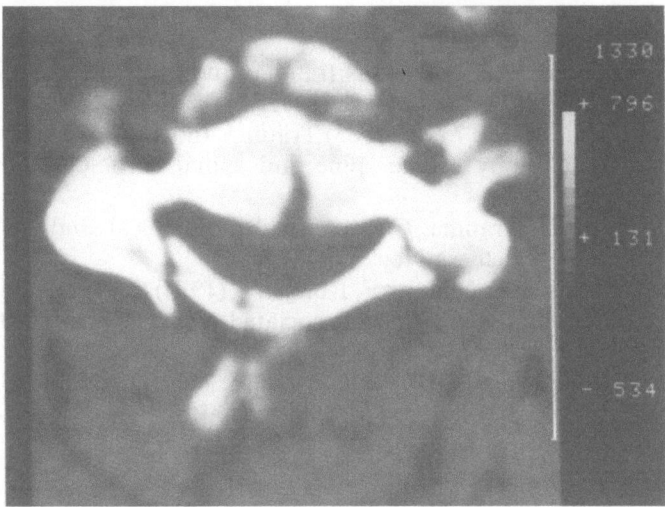

Fig. 4. Axial cut. Tear-drop fracture of cervical vertebra. A sagittal and coronal fracture line are seen separating an antero-inferior bone fragment. Notice bilateral fractures of the posterior arch and canal narrowing due to protrusion of the posterior vertebral wall

d) Perimedullary Hematomas

Epidural and subdural hematomas have only exceptionally been diagnosed by CT [4, 9]. A hyperdense perimedullary area is seen on one side of the neural canal with contralateral deviation of the cord. This aspect confirms the compressive nature of the process which represents a neurosurgical emergency.

e) Avulsion of the Brachial Plexus

The diagnosis of nerve root avulsion may be established in the acute posttraumatic period by injecting watersoluble contrast intrathecally to perform CT myelography. At the site of avulsion a pseudo-diverticular pouch may be seen at the tearing point of the nerve sheath. This pouch or pseudo-meningocele may progressively increase in size and may even expand into the axilla or into the pulmonary apex [5].

Conclusion

With the advent of CT-scanning the acute posttraumatic investigation of the cervical spine has been greatly facilitated. By using CT it is possible to establish early and precise diagnosis of anatomical lesions and to detect physiopathological mechanisms explaining vertebral instability or neurological complications. This allows adequate and rapid adjustment of the therapeutic management of the lesions and early prognostic evaluation is possible.

References

1. Babin E, Babin SR (1981) Lésions traumatiques du rachis cervical moyen et inférieur. Radiologie J CEPUR 1: 111–122
2. Brant-Zawadzki M, Post MJD (1983) Trauma. In: Newton TH, Potts DG (eds) Computed tomography of the spine and spinal cord. Clavadel Press, San Anselmo, pp 149–186
3. Dosch J CL (1985) Trauma. Conventional radiological study in spine injury. Springer, Berlin Heidelberg New York Tokyo
4. Kaiser MC, Capesius P, Ohanna F, Roilgen A (1984) Computed tomography of acute spinal epidural hematoma associated with cervical root avulsion. J Comput Assist Tomogr 8: 322–323
5. Kaiser MC, Capesius P, Petti M (1983) Thoracic inlet mass due to cervical root avulsion diagnosed by CT-scanning. Fortschr Röntgenstr 4: 505–506
6. McInerney DP, Sage MR (1979) Computer assisted tomography in the assessment of cervical spine trauma. Clin Radiol 30: 203–206
7. O'Callaghan JP, Ullrich CG, Yuan HA, Kieffer SA (1980) CT of facet distraction in flexion injuries of the thoracolumbar spine: the naked facet. AJNR 1: 97–102
8. Petti M, Roilgen A, Kaiser M, Capesius P (1982) Exploration scanographique des traumatismes du rachis cervical. J Radiol 63: 141–143
9. Post MJD, Seminer DS, Quencer RM (1982) CT diagnosis of spinal epidural hematoma. AJNR 3: 180–192

2.4. CT Diagnosis of Cervical Hernias

M. C. Kaiser and P. Capesius, Luxembourg, Grand-Duchy of Luxembourg

General Considerations

With the advent of high-resolution CT-scanners the diagnosis of cervical disc herniation can easily be made without intrathecal injection of contrast. A localizing CT "Scoutview" or "Topogram" is at first obtained for proper siting of the CT slices to the cervical region of interest. In the study of cervical pathology the use of thin slices (2 or 4 mm) is necessary and the images obtained should be electronically enlarged to permit adequate delineation of pathology. The examination should not be limited to the intervertebral disc space only, but should also be extended upwards and downwards as migration of hernias is known to occur in both directions. In order to obtain optimal hard copies of CT images a narrow window with a low center level should be used for optimal visualization of relatively low density disc fragments. In some instances CT demonstration of a hernia may be improved by utilizing a high-lighting computer program. As a matter of fact the CT density of hernias varies according to its structural components: disc material, calcifications, associated bone avulsions or degenerative changes including necrosis and gas formation [1–5].

In the presence of midline herniation it may be important to obtain sagittal reconstructions for better appreciation of eventual antero-posterior narrowing of the neural canal or compression of the cord. The main diagnostic problem is not to confirm or exclude the presence of disc herniation, but to determine the degree of compression to nervous structures due to the hernia. For this purpose differentiation between midline or lateral disc herniation should be made [6, 7].

1. Midline Herniations

This type of disc herniations has only pathological significance in those cases where they cause antero-posterior narrowing of the neural canal. Compression of the cervical cord may induce symptoms consistent with cervical myelopathy.

The degree of canal narrowing in the cervical region may be assessed

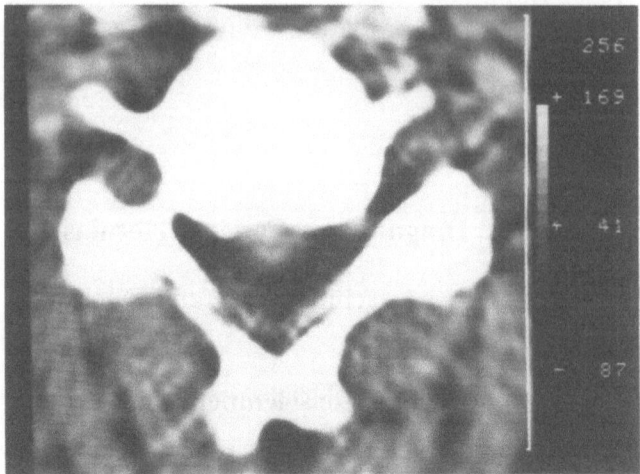

Fig. 1. Plain CT, cervical region. Midline hernia obviously shown. Cervical cord not visualized and cord compression can not be evaluated

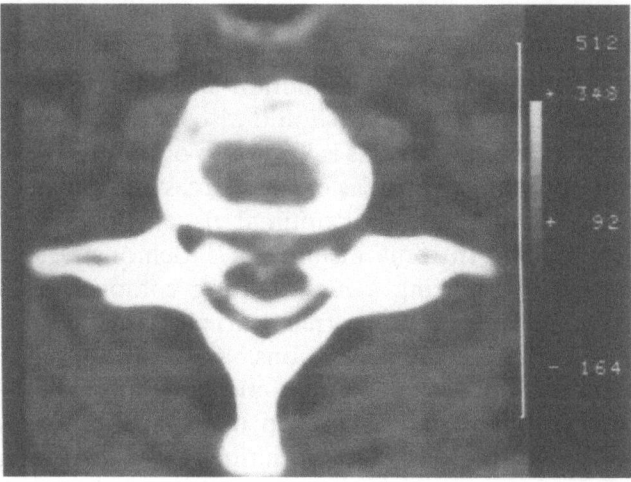

Fig. 2. CT myelography. Obvious midline hernia shown compressing cervical cord

with difficulty and measurements may sometimes be more accurate and informative on sagittal reconstructions than on axial images. The cervical cord may even not be clearly shown on plain CT-scanning and intrathecal injection of contrast material is required to demonstrate the cord and its compression due to midline herniation of disc material (Figs. 1 and 2).

2. Lateral Cervical Hernias

These hernias may obstruct the intervertebral foramen. Nerve roots may not be visualized in the cervical region without injection of intrathecal

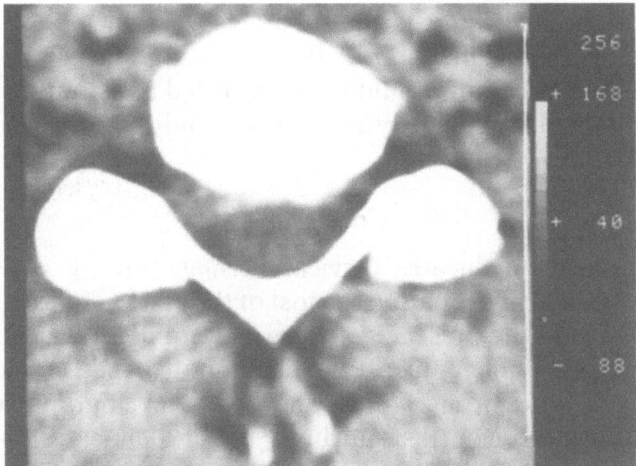

Fig. 3. Plain axial CT scan. Lateralized disc hernia shown obstructing left foramen

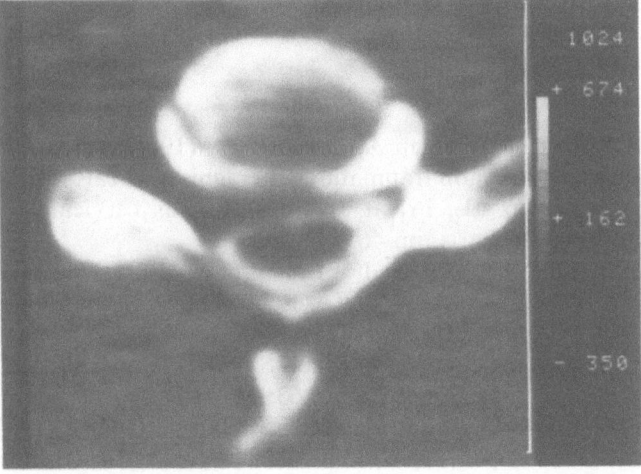

Fig. 4. CT myelography, different patient as in Fig. 3. Nerve root seen on the right, root compression seen on the left by lateral hernia

contrast medium [2–5]. Nevertheless nerve root compression at this level may be confirmed with a high degree of accuracy by plain CT scans in most of the cases by their topography and size. If a large hernia sites in the vicinity of the traject of the nerve roots, compression may definitely be asserted (Fig. 3).

A highlighting computer program may advantageously show the epidural fat which encloses the nerve roots. In cases of increased intraspinal pressure the epidural fat line disappears and this may be considered as a sign of nerve root compression inducing cervico-brachial neuralgia. In some cases rapid injection of a high dose of intravenous contrast medium may enhance surrounding ligaments and subarachnoid structures. This phenomenon permits better delineation of the hernia. Nevertheless, intravenous contrast medium injection should be disregarded as a routine technique as the results obtained are unsteady and it should only be performed in selected cases (Fig. 4).

Conclusions

Plain CT easily delineates cervical hernias causing cervico-brachial neuralgia or cervical myelopathy. In most of the cases CT alone is capable to confirm or exclude the presence of a hernia and complementary myelography with watersoluble contrast media should be performed in selected cases only. Sometimes primary or secondary CT myelography may be done as the subarachnoid contrast medium better delineates the cord and emerging nerve roots. Nuclear magnetic resonance imaging (MRI) greatly facilitates the diagnosis of cervical cord compression by disc herniation as it allows for sagittal imaging of the spine.

References

1. Capesius P, Kaiser M, Roilgen A, Tamisier JN (1985) Exploration scanographique de la pathologie non traumatique du rachis cervical: résultats et limites. In: Simon L, Leroux JL, Privat JH (eds) Rachis cervical et médecine de réeducation. Masson, Paris, pp 46–53
2. Capesius P, Meoli S, Petti M, Radice L, Kaiser M (1985) Studio scannografico del rachide cervicale. In: Russo P, Tedeschi A (eds) La patologia del rachide cervicale. Idelson, Napoli, pp 131–138
3. Capesius P, Sandt G, Lemaitre Y, Meoli S (1982) Diagnostic scanographique des hernies molles cervicales. J Radiol 63: 141–143
4. Capesius P, Smaltino F, Kaiser M, Meoli S, Gambardella A (1981) Computed tomography of the cervical spinal canal. J Neurosurg Sci 25: 265–270
5. Coin CG, Coin JT (1981) Computed tomography of cervical disc disease. Technical considerations with representative cases reports. J Comput Assist Tomogr 5: 275–280
6. Miyasaka K, Isu T, Iwasaki Y, Abe S, Takei H, Tsuru M (1983) High resolution computed tomography in the diagnosis of cervical disc disease. Neuroradiology 24: 253–257
7. Williams AL, Haughton VM (1983) Disc herniation and degenerative disc disease. In: Newton TH, Potts DG (eds) Computed tomography of the spine and spinal cord. Clavadel Press, San Anselmo, pp 231–249

2.5. Magnetic Resonance Imaging of the Cervical Spine and Spinal Cord

Ch. G. Ullrich, Charlotte, North Carolina, U.S.A.

This report subjectively summarizes more than 300 magnetic resonance imaging (MRI) examinations of the cervical spine performed with a 0.15 Tesla resistive magnet imaging system (Technicare) installed at the Charlotte Memorial Hospital, Charlotte, North Carolina, U.S.A. Since the initial patient study in March, 1983, advances in system design, including a recently available surface coil, have considerably improved image quality. Current applications include:

1. *Cranio-cervical junction lesions:* MRI is excellent for the evaluation of congenital anomalies such as the Chiari malformation and associated lesions of syringohydromyelia (Fig. 1) and tethered spinal cord. Spinal cord compression due to a foramen magnum mass or cervical instability is well visualized. Structural bone abnormalities may be detected by MRI, but are often better evaluated by conventional or computed tomographic (CT) techniques.

2. *Intrinsic (intra-axial) spinal cord lesions:* The exceptional tissue contrast resolution of MRI makes it a superior noninvasive method for the detection and surveillance of spinal cord tumor, syrinx (Fig. 1) and atrophy. MRI has detected several intra-axial lesions not demonstrated by X-ray imaging techniques. MRI failed to detect a small cervical syrinx and several cases of subtle spinal cord atrophy which were demonstrated by CT myelography. Other workers have used intraoperative ultrasound to detect spinal cord cysts which have not been correctly identified by either MRI or CT. The spinal cord lesions of multiple sclerosis and amyotrophic lateral sclerosis have not been consistently demonstrated by any imaging technique, but spinal cord compression clinically mimicking these diseases can be effectively excluded by MRI.

3. *Cervical myelopathy and extra-axial lesions:* MRI is excellent for demonstrating spinal cord compression due to tumor, abscess and large central disc herniation (Fig. 2). Osteophytes and other densely calcified lesions provide a very low MR signal (Figs. 2 and 3) and are primarily detected as a "negative shadow" deforming the margin of the high intensity

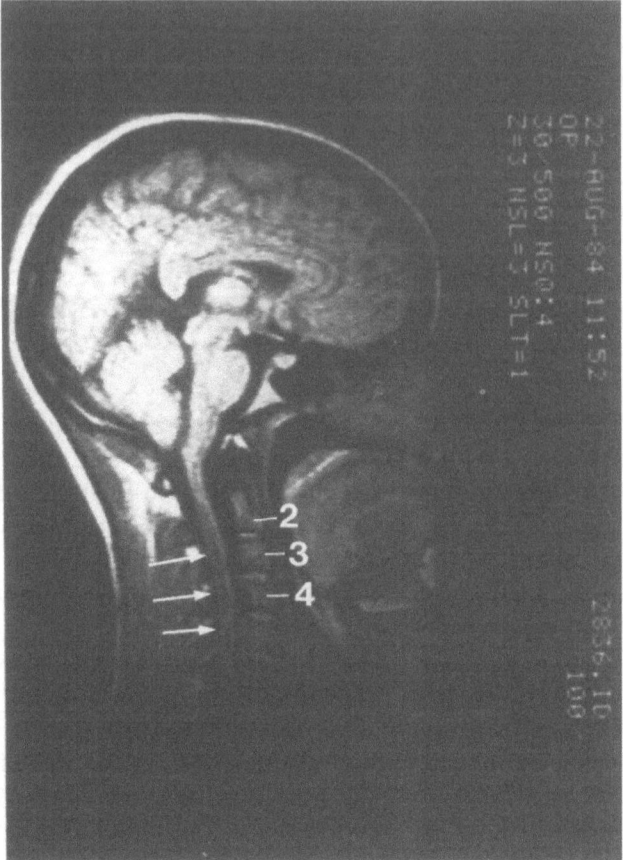

Fig. 1. A Chiari I malformation with associated cervical syringohydromyelia (→) is easily recognized (Spin-echo technique, TR: 500 msec, TE: 30 msec, sagittal projection, obtained with "head" imaging coil)

thecal sac in a T 2 weighted MR image (Fig. 2 c). MRI is very sensitive to tumor or infection involving the spinal column. In the absence of a bone or disc space abnormality, it may be extremely difficult to distinguish an intradural from an extradural lesion by MRI. Screening MRI examination of the cervical spine is usually performed in the sagittal projection. This technique has allowed small epidural lesions including a lymphoma and a neurofibroma to go undetected by MRI. Cervical disc herniations producing only radiculopathy have been very difficult to reliably detect by MRI. CT and/or myelography remain the imaging procedures of choice in such cases.

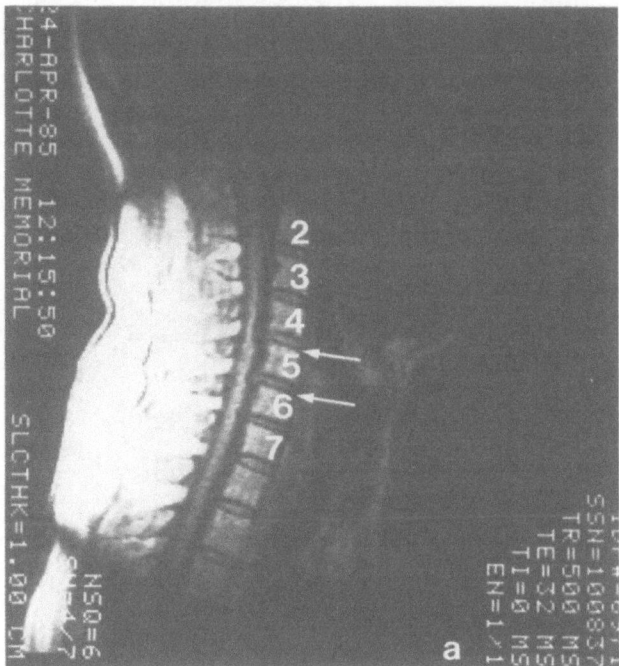

Fig. 2. a) Cervical spinal cord compression due to a large central C 4–5 disc herniation (→) and a smaller C 5–6 disc herniation (→) in a 42-year-old dentist with clinical symptoms of myelopathy. Note the deformity of the spinal cord (Spin-echo technique, TR: 500 msec, TE: 30 msec, sagittal projection, obtained with surface coil). b) A magnified image showing the disc herniations (→) and spinal cord compression to better advantage. c) T 2 weighted image turns the spinal cord and cerebro-spinal fluid white, producing a "pseudomyelogram". The herniated cervical discs (→) are producing anterior extra-dural defects at C 4–5, and C 5–6 (Spin-echo technique, TR: 1,800 msec, TE: 120 msec, sagittal projection, obtained with surface coil)

4. *Traumatic lesions:* Bony fractures are poorly demonstrated by MRI because of the low signal intensity derived from the cortical bone. Spinal cord contusion, hematoma, and compression should be detectable by MRI, but I have no experience evaluating acute spinal cord injury patients by MRI. The use of steel tongs for traction may preclude MRI. At present, evaluation by CT without or with intrathecal contrast material is a better choice for most of these patients.

MRI is already making valuable contributions to cervical spine and spinal cord diagnosis and treatment. This technology promises to grow in importance in the years ahead as further refinements in equipment and technique develop.

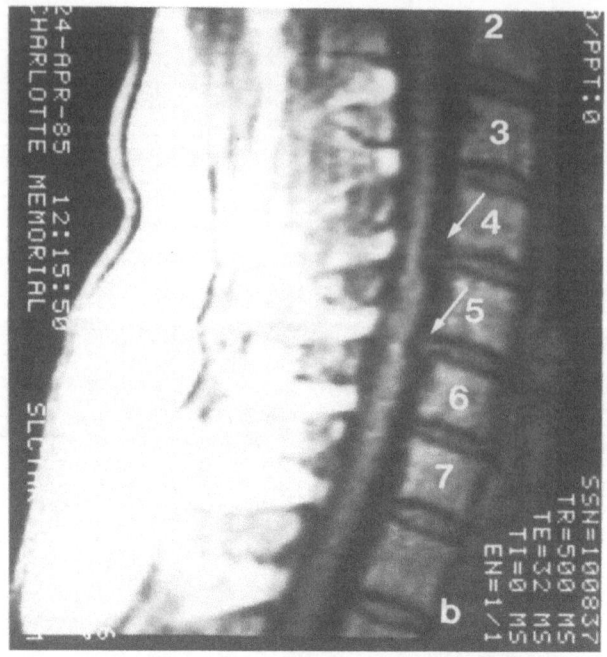

Fig. 2 b

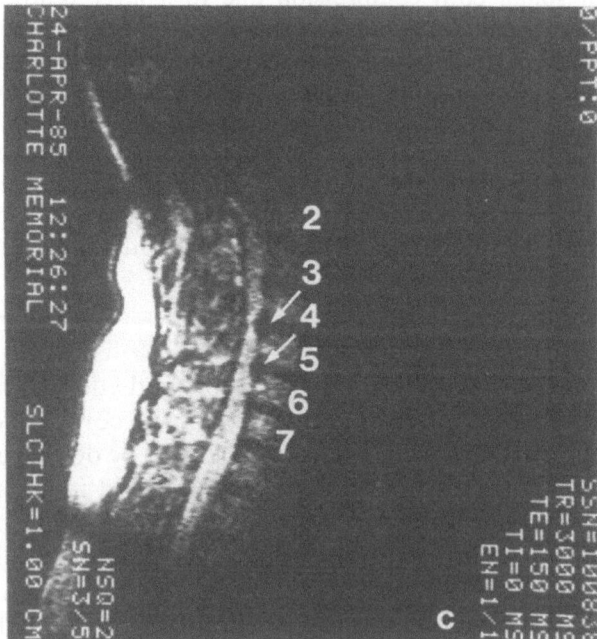

Fig. 2 c

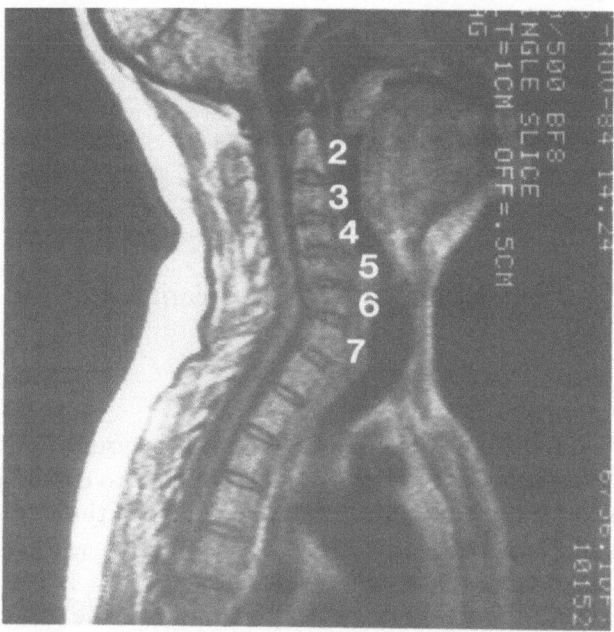

Fig. 3. Cervical cord compression due to cervical spondylosis between lower C 4 and mid C 6. Note the deformity of the spinal cord. The "black line" between the posterior vertebral body and the spinal cord is due to cortical bone and osteophyte, not cerebrospinal fluid (Spin-echo technique, TR: 500 msec, TE: 30 msec, sagittal projection, obtained with "body" imaging coil)

2.6. Osteo-vascular Correlations on Cervical Spine Diseases

A. Solini and G. Orsini, Torino, Italy

Introduction

It is our opinion that selective angiography should be included in the study of cervical spine pathology. In fact, in order to obtain diagnosis, it is quite often necessary to have a topographic image of the cervical cord blood supply [1, 3]. As a matter of fact, many congenital vascular malformations in this region are symptomatic (Figs. 1 and 2).

Many cervical spine tumors, as well as tumors of the cervical cord, cause deviations of the vascular axes so typical as to allow a precise diagnosis (Figs. 3 and 4). Certain impairments of the "carrefour unco-artéro-radiculaire" cause very typical modifications in the course of vertebral arteries. Angiography has been employed by us mainly in pediatric pathology of malformations or neoplastic diseases, as well as in adults to investigate extrinsic compressions of the vertebral artery caused by unco-arthrosis or of posttraumatic origin (anneau fibrotique), according to Jung and Kehr [4, 5]. In this complex pathology we believe the study of an angiography is an important tool to clarify the diagnosis. We make use of bilateral percutaneous brachial injection for reasons that will be explained in the discussion. Nevertheless femoral artery catheterism (as described by Seldinger) is still used by many authors.

Technique

One hour before the start of our study, we inject (intramuscularly) 10 mg of Diazepam. Then we perform xilocaine local anesthesia in the cubital fossa. The contrast media is Iopamidolo (Iopamiro) 300, and the needles used are 18 G 2 or 18 G 4 type by Becton & Dickinson. Different quantities of contrast media are employed, whether the study is carried out on right or left side. On the right side the maximum permissible dose is 35 to 40 cm^3, while on the left it is 30 to 35 cm^3.

The injection time is about 12 cm^3 per sec; this is the same on both sides. With the patient lying on his back, we carry out oblique X-rays, both on right and left side. The time gap needed before starting X-ray is of 1 to

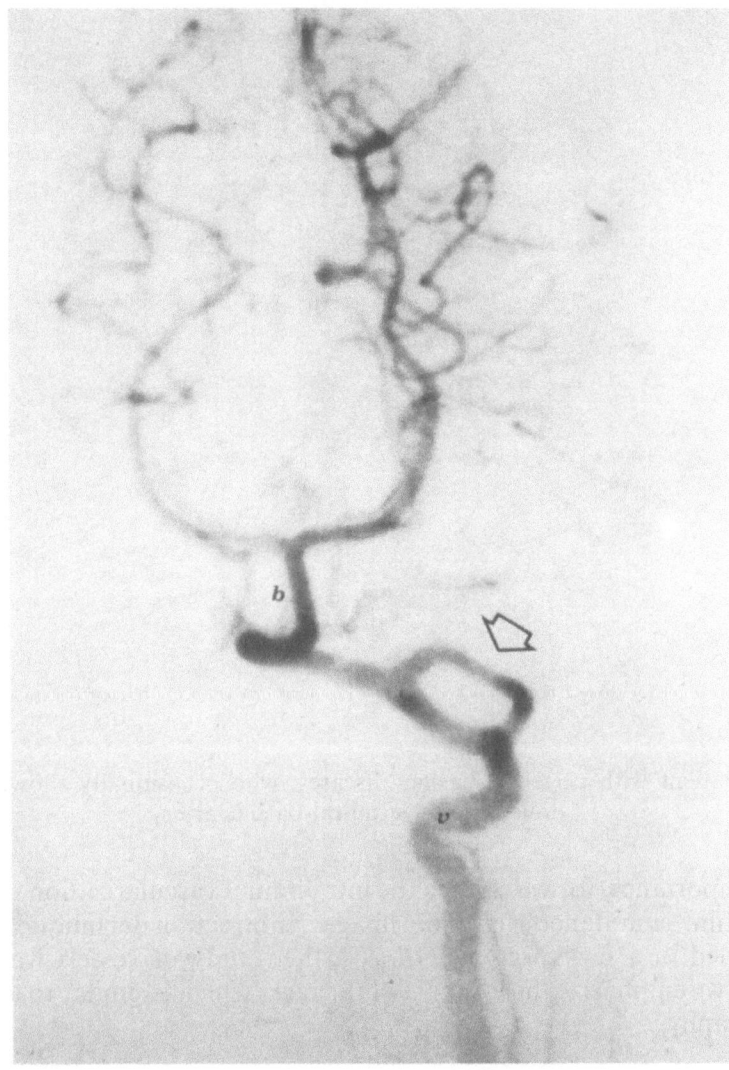

Fig. 1. Child with fenestration of the left vertebral artery at the level of the atlas

1.5 sec on the right side, and 0.6 to 1 sec on the left side. We use 10 X-ray films each projection (therefore using 20 X-ray films in all); exposure planning is 3 X-ray films per sec, plus 1 X-ray film for testing. If X-rays show vascular stenosis, due to "ring-shaped" extravasal compression, we perform a new study by turning the patient's head beyond a right angle and by injecting a new contrast media dose. The whole study needs 20 to 30 minutes.

It is our opinion that angiography performed by Schonander 35 are of

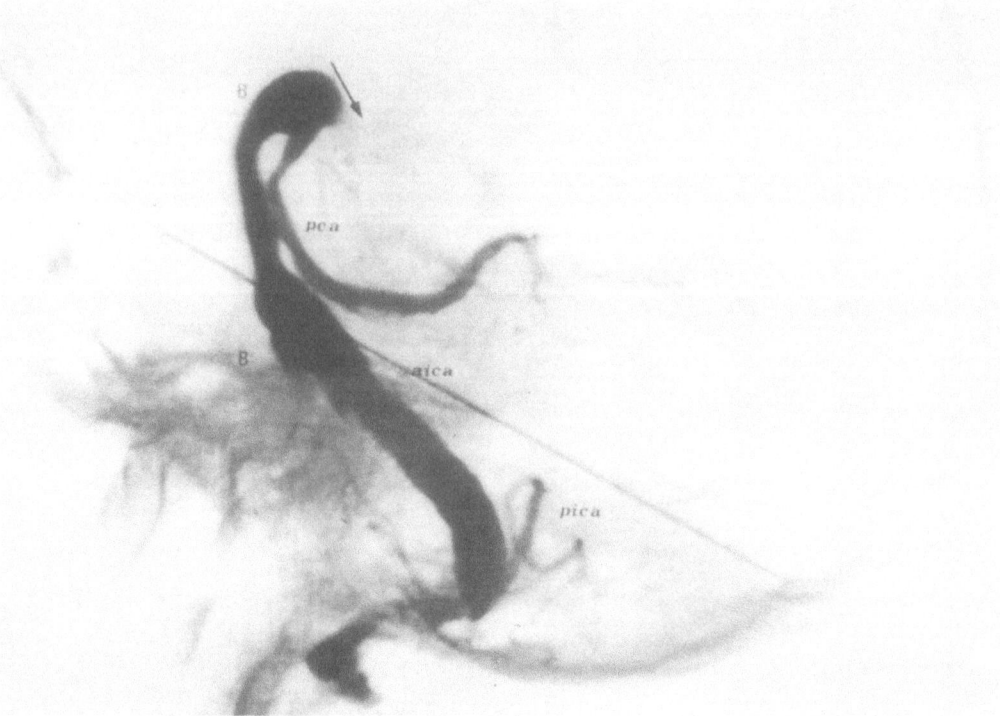

Fig. 2. Patient with vertebral-basilar diseases, who occasionally showed a large dolico-mega vertebral-basilar artery

great importance, for we can see the intracranial vascularization on a single X-ray film simultaneously. The images subtraction technique has been performed in a few cases, where a further study of vessels was needed. Finally we emphasize the low cost of the task, which is similar to a standard tomography.

Discussion

The complexity of the various anatomical structures of th cervical spine level, makes it quite often necessary to use angiography. In fact, with this examination, we are able to acquire new information that will confirm, or sometimes deny, our diagnostic hypothesis.

This examination is particularly important in this research of tumors, both benign and malignant, skeletal or extraskeletal. For this type of pathology, angiography will supply us data on the extent, dimensions and site of the neoplasm and also if it is benign or not. Biopsy, which should in any case be carried out, will then confirm this data. The typical angiographic images of tumoral lesions show vascularization impairments which normally are increased in the malignant neoplasia and, *vice versa,* decreased in the benign ones.

The development of the vascular network is due to the presence of newformed vessels that depart from a main trunk at a sharp angle (characteristic of tumor vessels) and irregularly distribute themselves around the tumor; they show malformations both in the shape and structure (aneurysms, etc.) and cause a change in the circulation time inside the tumor. This explains the phenomena of the persisting opacity, relatively homogeneous, beyond the venous phase.

Furthermore, angiography is suitable in the investigation of those arterial diseases, such as atherosclerosis, which, by reducing the spinal cord blood supply, may explain the vascular etiology of certain neurological damages.

Last, but not least, this examination should be carried out in all cases of suspected arterio-venous malformations, when this suspicion is based on informations obtained by routine tests. In these cases the angiogram shows either vasal coilings, or arterio-venous plexus-like interlacements, or, normally in children, large arterio-venous malformations of the extra-dural vascularization (Type1, 2, 3, according to Di Chiro *et al.* [2].

In conclusion we think that the possibility to visually identify the relation between vascular and bony images in the cervical region is an important tool to guide the surgeon. The exact lesion site, its topographic dimensions, its major or minor vascularization are essential elements for a correct surgical approach. Quite often the patients are children, polytraumatized or old aged subjects with possible generalized vascular disorders. In these conditions it is essential to carry out a very simple and quick examination, nontraumatic for the patient. At the same time this type of investigation must offer the greatest amount of information, both at the cervical and intracranial level. We believe it is very important to have all the vertebro-basilar and posterior cerebral circulation visible in one view.

Many syndroms of vertebro-basilar insufficiency, clinically quite similar, show different angiographic images (Fig. 2). Many intracranial vascular disorders (hemangiomas, arterio-venous shunts, aneurysms, etc.) show, in particular moments of their course, clinical features similar to that of extrinsic compressions on vertebral artery in its second (transversarial-intratransverse) stage (V 2) or in its third stage (V 3). The certainty given by a real anatomical picture can exclude congenital and acquired malformations, surgically non interesting. Many times in fact, vertebro-basilar insufficiency may be due to various diseases and may not be surgically approached. The brachial arteriography is, mainly for this pathology, extremely important. This technique supplies information about syndromes not always well known to the surgeon, helping him to avoid therapeutic misleadings.

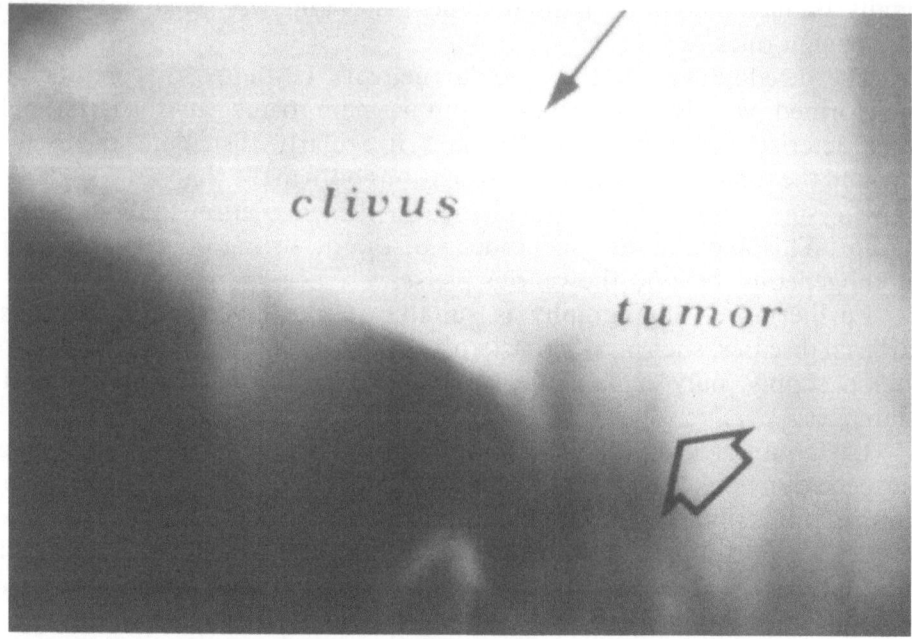

Figs. 3 and 4. Patient with cervicalgia and initial hemiatrophy of the tongue. Tomography of the skull base shows wide osteolysis of the hinder part of the clivus (Fig. 3). Angiography of the left vertebral artery demonstrates a dislocation of the vertebral-basilar arch (Fig. 4). Diagnosis of chordoma was confirmed by biopsy. High-level localization of this type of tumor is uncommon in grown-up people

References

1. Di Chiro G, Fisher RL (1964) Contrast radiography of the spinal cord. Arch Neurol 11: 125
2. Di Chiro G, Doppman JL, Ommaya AK (1971) Radiology of spinal cord arterio-venous malformations. Prog Neurol Surg 4: 329
3. Djindjian R, Hurth M, Houdart R (1970) L'angiographie de la moelle épinière. Masson, Paris
4. Jung A, Kehr P (1972) Pathologie de l'artère vertébrale et des racines nerveuses. Masson, Paris
5. Kehr P (1981) Les traitements chirurgicaux des syndromes cervicocéphaliques et des syndromes cervicobrachialgiques. Rev Therap XXXVIII, pp 660–667

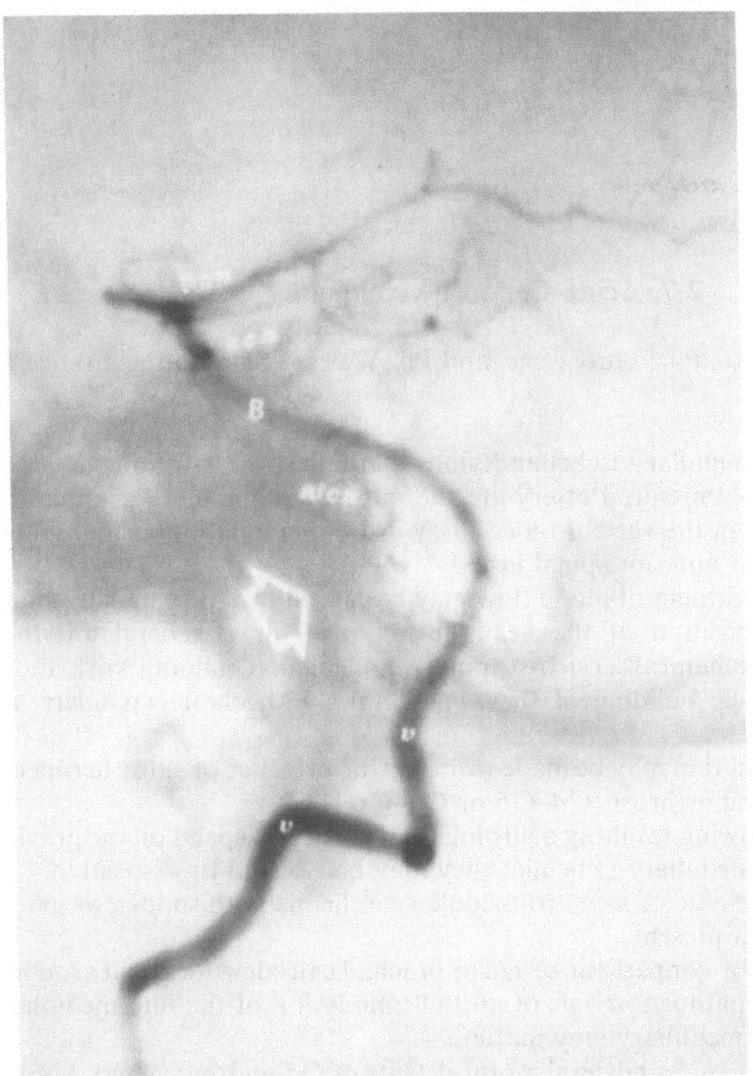

Fig. 4

2.7. Acute Cervical Myelopathy C 5–C 6

M. Jesel, Ph. Vautravers, and Ph. Wasser, Strasbourg, France

Centro-medullary ischemic lesions at the level C 5–C 6 in the area of the sulco-commissurial artery are the most frequent. They are due to an impairment in the vertebro-medullary arterial circulation at the radiculo-medullary or anterior spinal level.

The impairment of blood flow may be caused by a trauma, a prolonged unnatural position of the head during sleep or a general anesthesia, excessive mechanical cervico-scapulary movements (building work, moving house, muscle building of the upper limbs with chest expanders, cast-fishing).

This condition may be made worse by the presence of a disc hernia or an intervertebral arthrosis C 4–C 5 or C 5–C 6 [1, 4].

The following resulting neurological disorders, depend on the gravity of the centro-medullary ischemia; they may be isolated or associated:

— in the case of a centro-medullary ischemia with sudden onset, neck pain is often present,

— pain of sympathetic origin or brachial causalgia localized around the shoulder is pathognomonic of an ischemic lesion of the intermediolateral area of the medullary grey matter,

— unilateral or bilateral motor deficits of C 5 and/or C 6 are symptomatic of an ischemic lesion of the anterior horncells. The deficiency may be severe, with serious atrophy of the paralysed muscles, or slight, but at the same time accompanied by a reduction of the deep tendon reflexes C 5–C 6,

— sensory losses, (more often unilateral) at the C 5 and/or C 6 area, are of dissociated type like in syringomyelia and correspond to an ischemic lesion of the anterior grey commissure.

The *clinical course* of the centro-medullary ischemia is variable: There might be a full recovery with disappearance of pain and improvement of the neurological disorders within 3 months. When the functional motor recovery is incomplete, the EMG registration of an interference pattern can provide for a complete recovery within one additional month. The prognosis, concerning the motor recovery, is favorable when, after a period of 3 to 4 weeks, no spontaneous fibrillation potentials appear in the paralysed muscles.

In the contrary after 3 months, sensory deficit which has not regressed will be permanent, and motor deficit with EMG patterns of chronic neurogenic muscle atrophy (the decrease of the number of the motor unit action potentials) may also be permanent. Even with a complete functional recovery in this case, muscles may remain hypotrophic and less efficient.

In case of surgery, it is useful to look for an obstacle hindering the medullary arterial circulation (disc hernia, bony spurs due to spinal arthrosis). The aim of the surgical procedure (removal of the disc alone or combined with an intersomatic arthrodesis) is to decompress as soon as possible the radiculo-medullary artery. It can be performed later in order to prevent any risks of recurrence. These risks exist. In case of recurrence, the motor deficit may be very severe.

This acute C 5–C 6 myelopathy was described by Turner [5] first. Yet the author did not believe in the medullary origin of the neurological troubles [4].

In spite of the characteristic clinical findings and course, the acute C 5–C 6 myelopathy was not well known, and was classified into the heterogeneous group of neuralgic amyotrophies around the shoulder girdle, known as the shoulder girdle syndrome or Parsonage and Turner [2, 6] syndrome.

Summary

The authors analyse clinical characteristics and clinical course of the acute C 5–C 6 myelopathies, firstly described by Turner in 1944 (acute brachial neuritis). They present the clinical aspects and the EMG of an acute C 5–C 6 ischemia in a 26 years old female. Full recovery occurred within three months (Fig. 1).

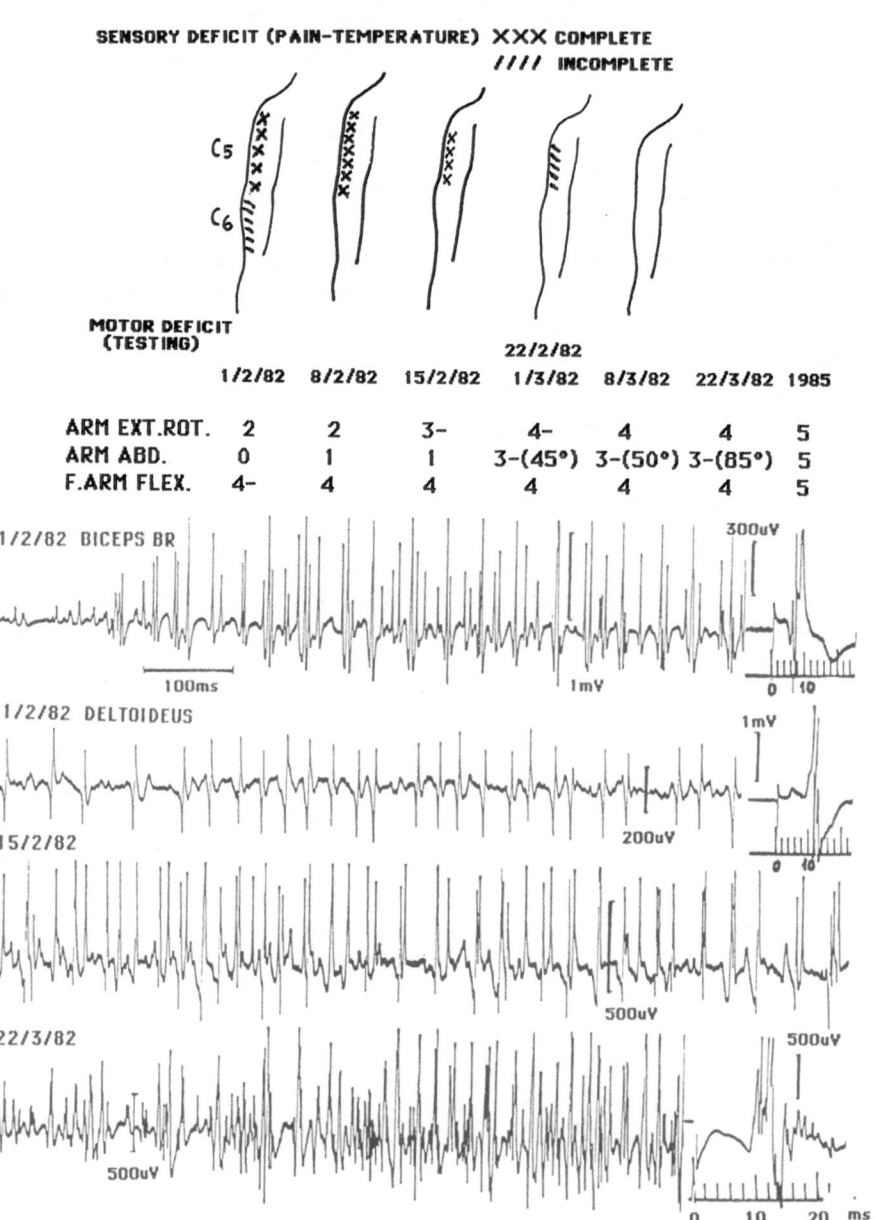

OBS. EMG. 234/82   Mrs M.....M.-FRANCOISE, 26 y.

26/01/82: ACUTE CERVICAL RACHIALGIA
27/01/82: RIGHT SHOULDER CAUSALGIA
28/01/82: ACUTE RIGHT C5–C6 MOTOR AND SENSORY DEFICIT

SENSORY DEFICIT (PAIN-TEMPERATURE) XXX COMPLETE
//// INCOMPLETE

	1/2/82	8/2/82	15/2/82	22/2/82 1/3/82	8/3/82	22/3/82	1985
ARM EXT.ROT.	2	2	3–	4–	4	4	5
ARM ABD.	0	1	1	3-(45°)	3-(50°)	3-(85°)	5
F.ARM FLEX.	4–	4	4	4	4	4	5

Fig. 1

References

1. Jesel M, Vautravers Ph (1985) Myélopathies cervicales aigues et subaigues par accident ischémique médullaire. Collection de pathologie loco-motrice n° 10, Masson, Paris, pp 376–381
2. Parsonage MJ, Turner JW (1948) Neuralgic amyotrophy; The shoulder-girdle syndrome. The Lancet 26 Juin, pp 973–978
3. Ruh D, Boyer P, Jesel M (1980) Apport de l'électromyographie au diagnostic des paralysies aigues radiculaires ou médullaires cervicales d'origine discale. Rev Electroencéphalogr Neurophysiol Clin 10, 1: 33–46
4. Ruh D, Malibary H, Jesel M, Isch F (1981) Le syndrome de Parsonage et Turner: entité nosologique? Compte rendu des deuxièmes journées languedociennes d'électromyographie t. II. Euromed Ed., Montpellier, pp 437–451
5. Turner JW (1944) Acute brachial radiculitis. Br Med J 2: 592–594
6. Turner JW, Parsonage MJ (1957) Neuralgic amyotrophy (paralytic brachial neuritis) with special reference to prognosis. The Lancet 2: 209–212

Fig. 1. Case no. 234/82 of acute C 5–C 6 ischemic myelopathy concerning Mrs. M. M. Françoise, 26 year old. Acute C 5–C 6 myelopathy starting with an acute neck pain (January 26, 1982) and a right shoulder causalgia (January 27, 1982). The cervical myelopathy was characterized by C 5–C 6 motor and sensory deficits: Sensory deficit on the right arm and forearm with loss of pain and temperature sensibility C 5 (complete loss) and C 6 (incomplete loss on the upper part of the C 6 area). Evolution: spontaneous complete recovery of the C 5–C 6 pain and temperature sensibility after 36 days.—Motor deficit C 5–C 6 concerning, on the right side, the external rotation (testing: 2) and the abduction (testing; 0) of the arm and less severely, the flexion (testing: 4) of the forearm. First EMG assessment: January 1, 1982. Biceps brachii: intermediate activity with potentials of 1 to 2 mV (millivolt) with high frequencies. ERB's point stimulation: normal, direct response; motor latency: 4 ms (milliseconds). Deltoideus: single motor unit pattern with 0.4 mV potential, reaching high frequencies. ERB's point stimulation: reflex response; motor latency: 8 ms. *Follow-up: February 15, 1982.* Deltoideus: spontaneous denervation activity; increasing of the number of motor unit action potentials and of their amplitude. *March 22, 1982.* Deltoideus: recovery of an interference pattern of 2 mV. ERB's point stimulation: reflex response; motor latency: 8 ms. At this date, arm abduction strength is still reduced, possible against gravity with an amplitude of 85°. *In 1985:* complete motor and sensory recovery

2.8. Magnetic Resonance Imaging of Cervical Spinal Stenosis

R. A. Hyman, J. A. Epstein, R. Carras, and N. E. Epstein, Manhasset, N.Y.,
U.S.A.

We have had the opportunity to examine the cervical spines of 121 patients utilizing a 0.6 Tesla magnetic resonance (MR) imaging unit manufactured by Technicare Corporation, Solon, Ohio. Thirty-one patients demonstrated degenerative changes in the cervical spine without cord compression, while 19 patients with myelopathy, demonstrated evidence of cervical spinal stenosis. Fourteen of the latter underwent myelography, 13 of which confirmed the evidence of narrowing of the spinal canal causing resultant compressive changes in the spinal cord. One false positive MR study was encountered. Seventeen of seventeen patients who had plain radiographs demonstrated abnormalities, however, in only 6 cases could one make the definitive diagnosis of cervical spinal stenosis from the plain films alone.

The pulse sequences utilized included relatively T 1 weighted spin-echo series (TR = 500 ms, TE = 30 ms) as well as predominantly T 2 weighted multislice and multi-echo series in both sagittal and transverse projections (TR = 2,240 ms, TE = 30 to 240 ms).

The plain radiographs demonstrating degenerative changes and retrolisthesis at C 5–6 of a 69 year old man are shown in Fig. 1 a. The T 1 weighted series demonstrates marked spinal cord compression at C 5–6 (Fig. 1 b). The T 2 weighted images show marked extradural defects at multiple levels in addition to the single level of cord compression (Fig. 1 c). A second series of films in an additional patient shows in the plain radiographs spinal stenosis with overlapping of the articular facets. The T 1 weighted MR image shows compression of the cord at C 4–C 5. The T 2 weighted image demonstrates compression of the subarachnoid space from C 3 to C 5. The transverse MR demonstrates marked flattening of the spinal cord confirmed by the frontal myelogram. These studies also rule out the question of a cystic tumor or mass lesion of the spinal cord. T 1 weighted images optimally show the cervical spinal cord in contrast to the low signal (black) CSF and are excellent for the identificaton of cord compression. Late echoes of the T 2 weighted image show the CSF as a high signal region

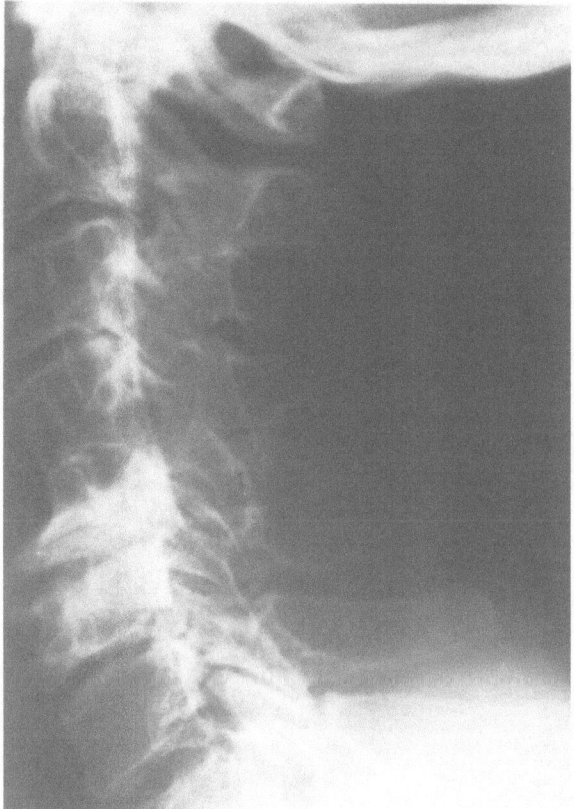

Fig. 1. a) Plain radiograph shows degenerative changes and retrolisthesis at C 5–6 but direct information about the spinal cord is not provided. b) A T 1 weighted spin echo series shows marked cord compression at C 5–6, with the cord appearing white and the CSF black. TR = 500 ms, TE = 30 ms. c) A T 2 weighted spin echo series, utilizing a late echo with the CSF now white, shows multiple extradural defects both dorsally and ventrally although the cord was seen to be compressed at only one level in 1 b. TR = 2,240 ms, TE = 50 ms. (Reproduced with permission of the publisher from Hyman *et al.*: 0.6 T MR imaging of the cervical spine. AJNR 6: 229–236, 1985)

(white) which is particularly helpful in identifying and characterizing extradural processes.

In another patient, a swan-neck deformity is demonstrated in the plain films. The T 1 weighted image demonstrates angulation of the spinal cord at the C 3–C 4 level well above the gibbus deformity with evidence of anterior and posterior compression of the cord and subarachnoid space that is particularly well demonstrated on the T 2 weighted image series (Figs. 2 a and b). This is confirmed in the subsequent myelogram where thickening of

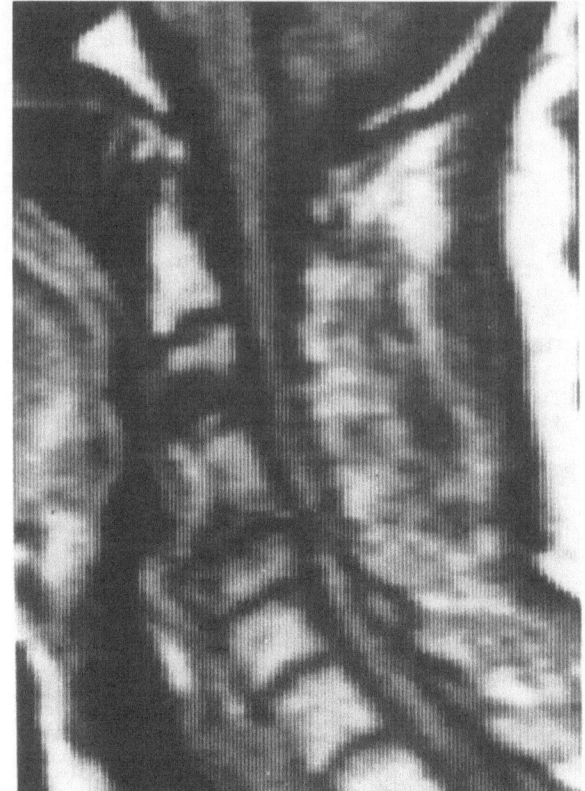

Fig. 1 b

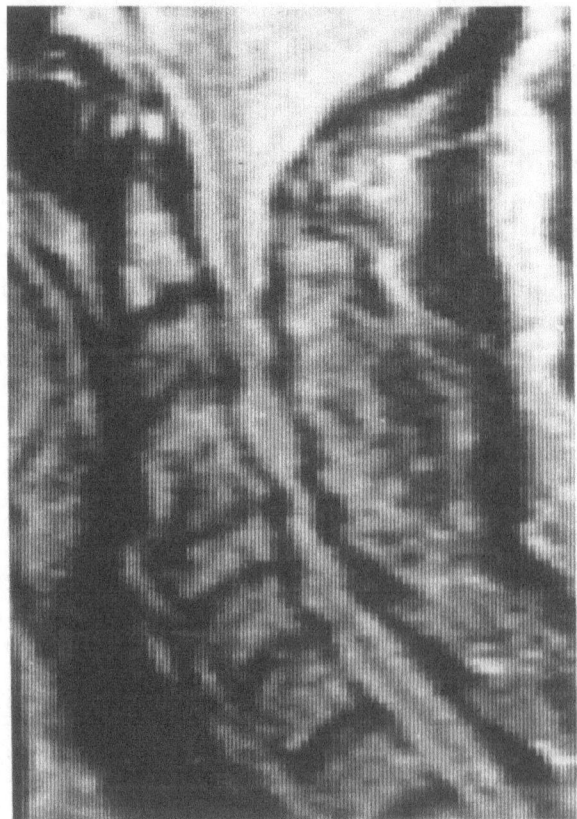

Fig. 1 c

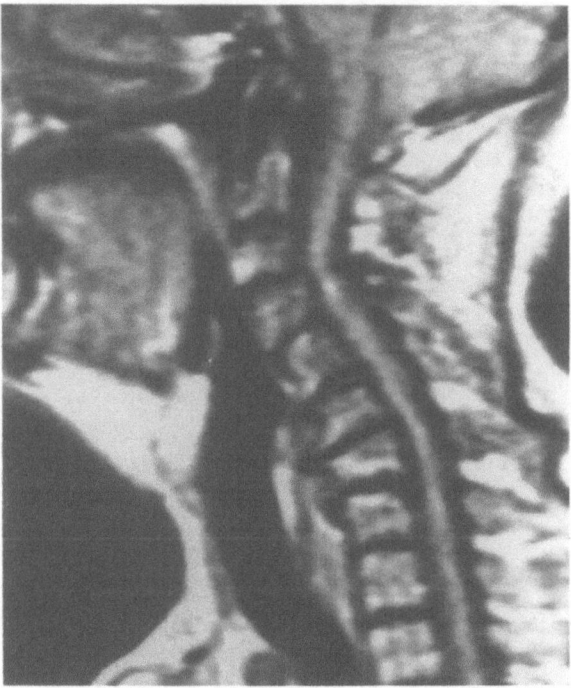

Fig. 2. a) A T 1 weighted image shows angulation and compression of the spinal cord at C 3–4 with degenerative changes inferiorly. TR = 500 ms, TE = 30 ms. b) A T 2 weighted image demonstrates a significant posterior component to the subarachnoid space compression and shows the cord as black against the high signal (white) CSF. TR = 2,240 ms, TE = 120 ms. c) Postoperatively, a T 1 weighted series demonstrates the cord compression and angulation to be corrected (compare to 2 a). TR = 500 ms, TE = 30 ms. d) The T 2 weighted postoperative series confirms the lack of compression and demonstrates posterior out-pouching of CSF where the preoperative compression was seen. TR = 2,240 ms, TE = 180 ms

the yellow ligament is seen posteriorly at C 3–C 4 and C 4–C 5, contributing to the compressive state. In this same patient, a postoperative study demonstrates improvement of the angulation of the cord in the upper cervical levels and absence of anterior and posterior spinal cord compression (Fig. 2 c). The T 2 weighted image series demonstrates posterior outpouching of the CSF where a previously demonstrated extradural defect was apparent preoperatively (Fig. 2 d).

In this study, magnetic resonance imaging of the cervical spine reliably demonstrated the degree and extent of spinal cord compression when T 1 weighted sagittal images were obtained. The ability to diagnose the presence of lateral recess stenosis and encroachment upon exiting nerve roots, however, was limited by the relatively poor quality of the transverse MR

R. A. Hyman *et al.*:

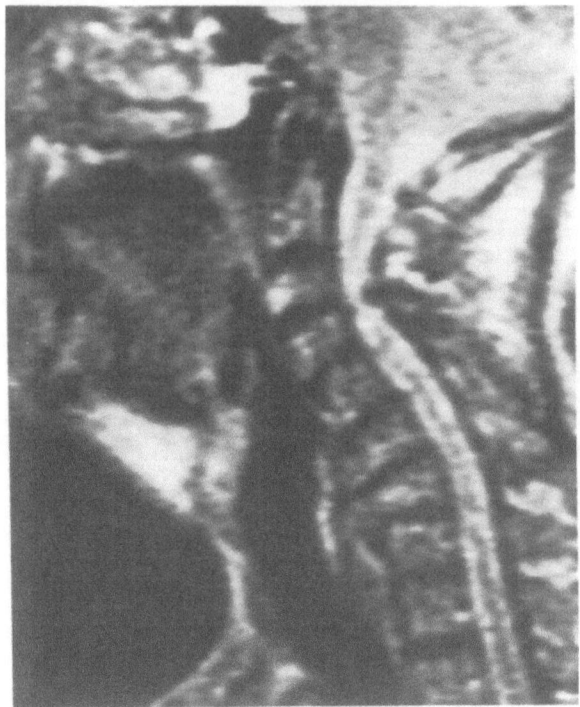

Fig. 2b

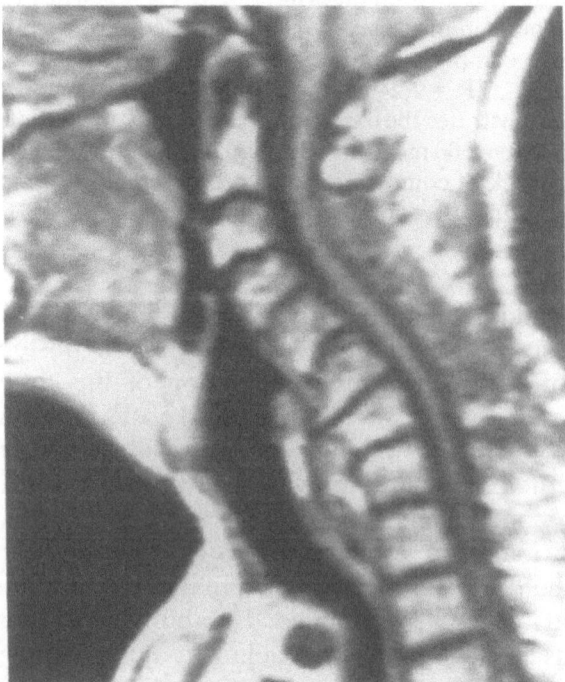

Fig. 2c

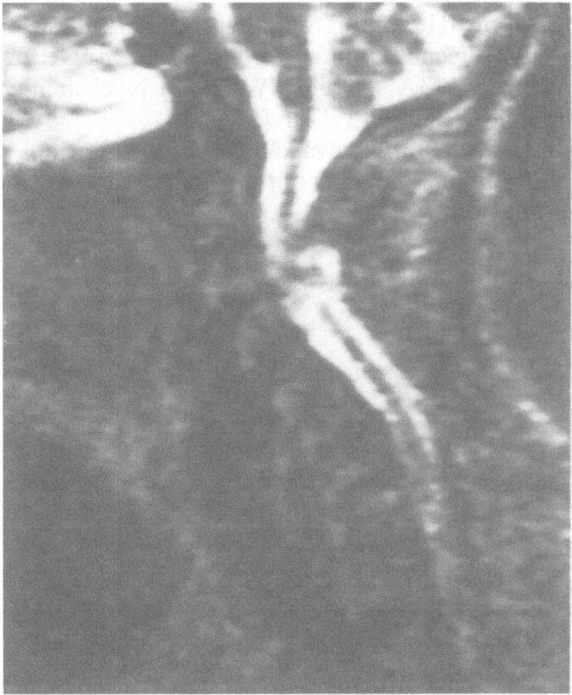

Fig. 2 d

images. Computed tomography both without and with metrizamide consistently outlined bony encroachment on the lateral recess more accurately than MR. T 2 weighted sagittal MR studies, particularly when multi-echo techniques were utilized, imaged well the encroachment of osteophytes and adjacent structures on the subarachnoid space. T 2 weighted images were limited in the ability to perform similarly in the transverse plane.

Routine cervical spine radiographs remain most appropriate for the initial evaluation of patients with suspected cervical spinal stenosis.

When further evaluation is warranted, MR appears to be the imaging modality of choice because of its ability to directly image the cervical spinal cord in the sagittal plane [1–5]. When surgical intervention is appropriate, myelography remains indicated for the most complete evaluation of cervical spinal stenosis.

References

1. Han JS, Kaufman B, El Youset SJ (1983) NMR imaging of the spine. AJNR 4: 1151–1159
2. Hyman RA, Edwards JE, Merten CW, Naidich JB, Vacirca ST, Stein HL (1984) Evaluation of degenerative disease of the spine with MR imaging. Radiology 153 (P): 204

3. Hyman, RA, Edwards JH, Vacirca ST, Stein HL (1985) 0.6 T MR imaging of the cervical spine: multislice and multiecho techniques. AJNR 6: 229–236
4. Modic MT, Weinstein MA, Pavlicek W (1983) Nuclear magnetic resonance imaging of the spine. Radiology 148: 757–762
5. Norman D, Mills CM, Brant-Zawadzki M, Yeates A, Cook LE, Kaufman L (1984) Magnetic resonance imaging of the spinal cord and canal: potentials and limitations. AJNR 5: 9–14

2.9. Developments in the Diagnosis of Cervical Hernias Using the Scanner

D. Krause, F. Buchheit, P. Boyer, D. Maitrot, and
J. Tongio, Strasbourg, France

The authors report their findings in the examination of a homogeneous series of twenty-six patients suffering from typical cervical radiculopathy. By virtue of the scanner, the quality and resolution of the resulting images allowed neurosurgical intervention on twenty-one patients where symptomatology alone was not sufficiently informative to allow successful medical treatment.

Very few publications are dedicated to cervical disc herniation, in particular those of the soft type. At the level of the cervical spine the almost total absence of epidural fat together with the small size of the spinal canal make examination and subsequent interpretations rather difficult. The remarkable advantage in using the scanner is its ability to perform sections with a millimetric precision in the plane of the disc and above in the neural foramen. The aim of this work was to demonstrate the excellent correlation which exists between the images obtained using the scanner and the lesions found after a microsurgical intervention.

Materials and Methods

Examinations of our group of twenty-six patients exhibiting cervical radiculopathy which were not amenable to medical treatment, should have shown the existence of twenty-six cervical soft disc herniations at the lower cervical spine ($20 \times$ C 6–C 7; $5 \times$ C 5–C 6; $1 \times$ C 7–D 1). The patients were young, average age 41 years, and the group consisted of fifteen women and eleven men.

The routine photographs provided little information (loss of the cervical curve, compression of the isolated disc). To investigate the anomalies of the disc, we carried out, like many investigators, millimetric sections using the Scanner CGR CE 10000 (field 130 mm matrix 512), at its maximum performance. Two levels are examined for each patient (C 5–C 6; C 6–C 7) marking their location after a profile view scan.

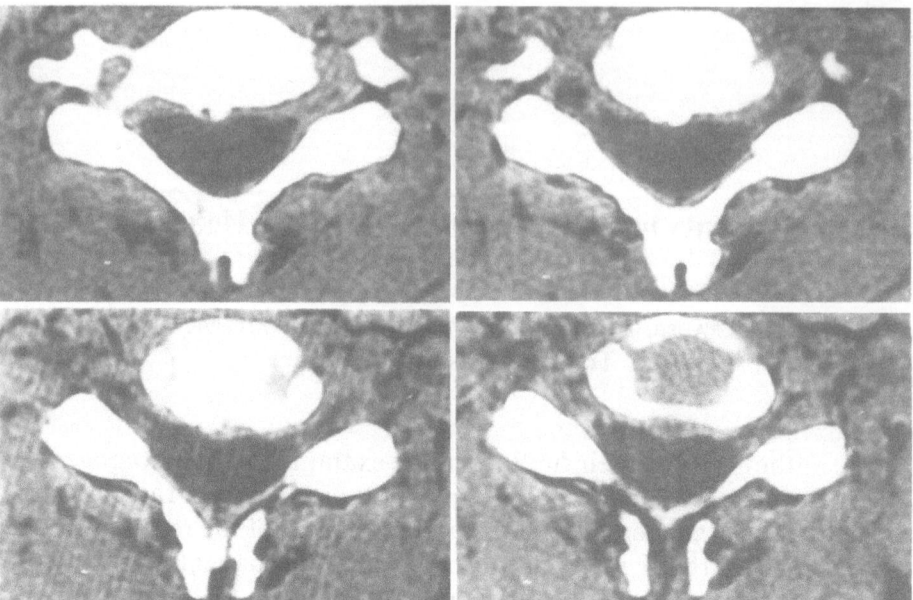

Fig. 1. Normal aspects (after intravenous injection). In the neural foramina the veins are voluminous, the root is visible in the form of a hypodense line. The posterior edge of the disc is reached four millimeters lower. The cord is identified easily with regard to the subarachnoid space

Results

The intravenous injection of a contrast indicator shows up the foraminal veins and the anterior epidural space. The precision level of the study begins with the foramen where the veins are voluminous and exhibit good contrast from one section to another. Here the root is visible in the form of a hypodense line but this time in an intermittent fashion from one section to another. The sections follow on lower down. The foraminal veins are still visible laterally, and mingle progressively with anterior epidural structures towards the front (very fine structures; 1–2 mm thick). Finally the edge posterior to the disc is reached, easily visible with the anterior subarachnoid space; back from this the cord is easily identified. In summary, at the level of the cervical spine the roots exit within the neural foramen above the disc, thus above the level clinically incriminated (Fig. 1).

Soft disc herniation: Taking into account the previously described structures, the anomalies at the examined area appear, for the most part, above the disc. The veins anterior to the neural foramen are abnormally in evidence because of the compression of the adjacent hernia, which develops laterally, towards the foramen. The herniation itself, a few millimeters lower, is always in evidence; we have noticed several types of images (Figs. 2–4):

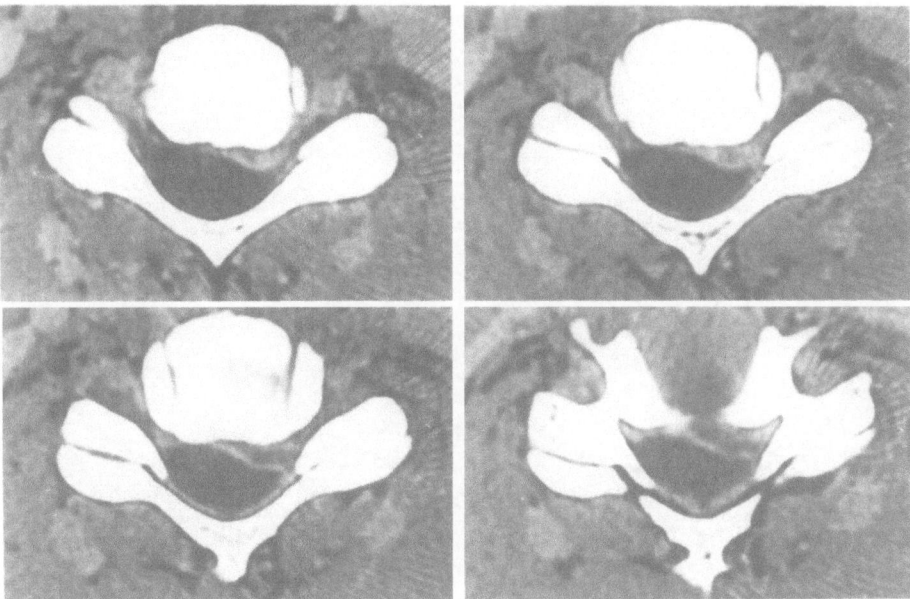

Fig. 2. Radiculopathy C 6–C 7. The veins anterior to the neural foramen are abnormally in evidence; the herniation itself, a few millimeters lower is very well in evidence with hypodense structure (density 30–40 UH). Surgical findings: extruded nucleus and perforation of the posterior ligament

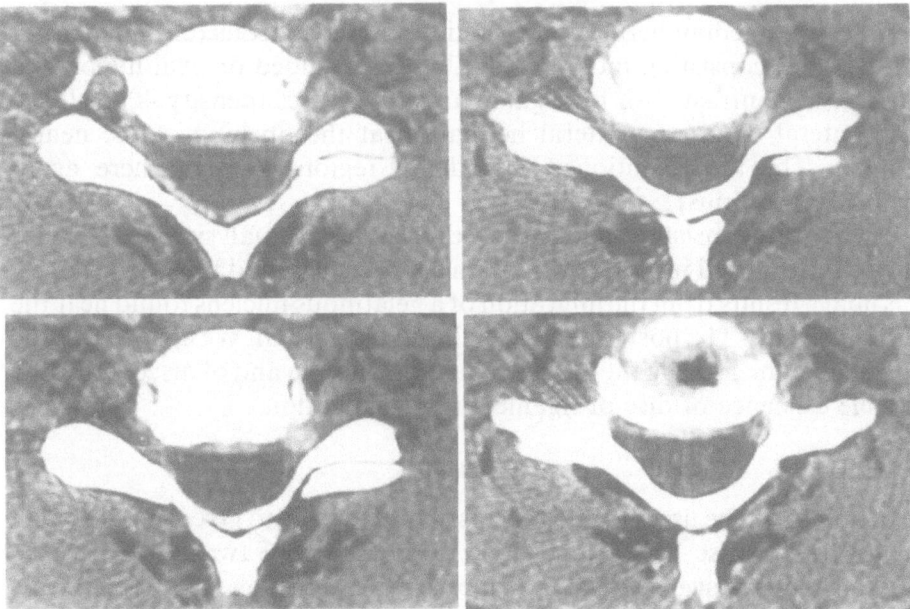

Fig. 3. Unilateral radiculopathy C 5–C 6. A hyperdense structure is localized in the neural foramen, beside the uncus. The posterior edge of the disc is normal. Microsurgical findings: migration of the gelatinous nucleus between the foraminal veins, far from the disc

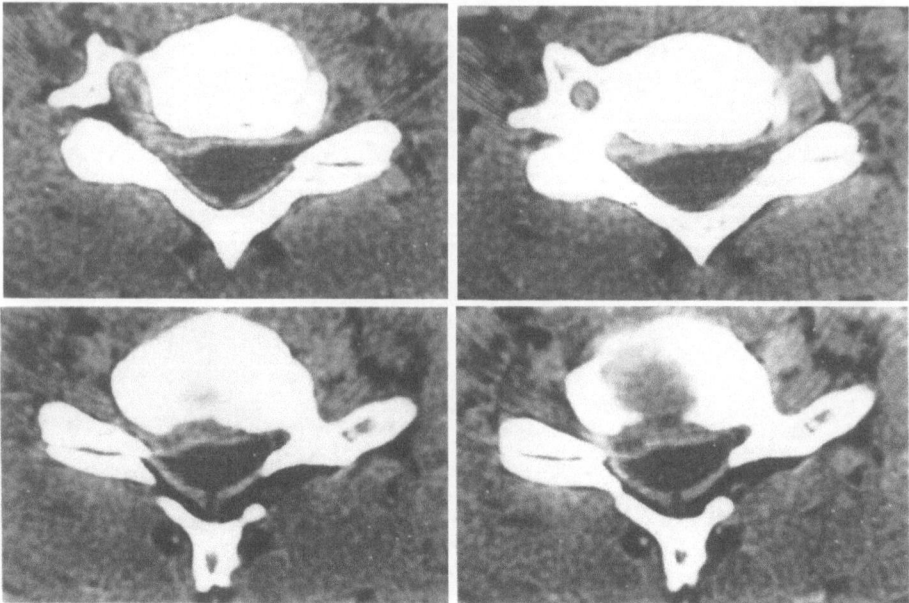

Fig. 4. Radiculopathy C 6–C 7. First the veins are abnormally in evidence in the foramen. The herniation itself is evident 5 millimeters lower. Hypodense structure in the herniation: extruded nucleus and tear of the posterior ligament found at surgery

1. Postero-median herniation sometimes homogeneous (of high density 100–120 UH) consisting most frequently of a rounded or oval hypodense structure in contrast with the ligamentary structures (density 40–50 UH).

2. Lateral or postero-lateral herniation at the opening of the neural foramen. The aforementioned hypodense region is found here again (millimetric sections).

3. This type consists of a hyperdense structure of small size independent of the disc localized in the neural foramen and positioned beside the uncus. This image results from the migration of a gelatinous nucleus found near the foraminal veins. The posterior edge of the disc is normal. We again stress the possibility of measuring the exact height of the hernia and of discovering the possible existence of disc or ligamentary calcifications.

Discussion

In this study the use of the scanner is demonstrated to give images of high quality of soft disc herniation in the examination of twenty-six patients suffering from typical cervical radiculopathy. Twenty-one of these patients were operable uniquely by virtue of the scanner images because intense recurring nocturnal pain which would normally prevent medical treatment during an average of two to six weeks.

We have never performed a complementary cervical myelography. Considering the radiological symptomatology which we have studied very often, a lateral hypodense region is noticed at the center of the image of the hernia. These images indicate the existence of extruded material. By the term "extruded material", we mean the presence of a fragment of gelatinous nucleus at the pre- or intraligamentary level. The discectomy is performed by anterior approach, under microsurgical conditions; the affected disc is lifted out, the neurosurgeon sees the common posterior vertebral ligament perfectly and the gelatinous herniation stuck within. This of course leads to the perforation of the common posterior vertebral ligament. In nineteen out of twenty-one patients operated on, extruded material (nucleus) was found. This underlines the importance of the resolution of the millimetric sections seen on the scanner images. A hypodense structure at the center of this image signifies the existence of an extraligamentary gelatinous nucleus having already migrated towards the foramen. This has to be looked for and found by the surgeon. The level C 6–C 7 is the most common incriminated: Nineteen out of twenty-six patients, sixteen out of twenty-one patients operated on. All patients operated on experienced regression of radicular pain within twenty-four hours and were considered healed.

Conclusions

The examination of patients suffering from typical cervical radiculopathy (but not presenting arthrosis) benefits enormously from the combined use of the scanner and the intravenously injection of contrast medium which improves the compartmentalization of the epidural space and the identification of the root at the center of the foraminal veins in the neural foramen. The millimetric sections permit an extremely precise radiological symptomatology capable not only to give an exact diagnosis in all cases dealt with but also to prove the existence of the extruded material (nucleus) in nineteen out of twenty-one operated on patients. In five cases, surgical intervention was not justified because of the spontaneous regression of the symptoms. In all cases studied the coherence between the observed images and neurosurgical findings was remarkable. It seems therefore that, at least for a young patient suffering from cervical radiculopathy, the scanner provides the only neuroradiological examination to be performed before surgery.

2.10. CT Evaluation of the Multiple Subtotal Somatectomy Results

M. Boni, L. di Guglielmo, V. Denaro, and G. Vadala, Pavia, Italy

In the stenosis of the cervical canal, either constitutional or acquired, the goal of elective surgical treatment is to obtain a "real" enlargement of the spinal canal. The decompression of the cord by anterior approach is indicated if the spinal cord compression is due to the protrusion of the anterior wall of the cervical canal (osteophytosis, herniated disc, bulging annulus, posttraumatic deformity). If the spinal cord compression involves more levels, the surgical procedure of choice is the multiple subtotal somatectomy (MSS) that has been conceived and perfected at the Orthopedics Clinic of the University of Pavia since 1969 [2–4].

The operation consists of a somatectomy, which is the removal of the entire central portion of the vertebral body in its entire depth together with the posterior wall on a width of approximately 15 mm; moreover it is subtotal because it keeps the lateral wall of the vertebral body with the transverse process; finally it is multiple since it involves several vertebral bodies. Therefore it is possible to obtain the spinal cord decompression at more levels and a "real" enlargement of the spinal canal.

The principal steps of the operation are shown in Figs. 1–4.

In the past we have evaluated the results obtained by the MSS either clinically or radiologically [2–4].

At present computed tomography (CT) allows a more precise presurgical study of the spinal canal and of the causes of stenosis [1, 5], and then it shows the effective increase in diameter of the spinal canal in postsurgery.

In this paper we evaluate the results obtained with MSS using CT.

Figs. 1–4. Drawing of MSS technique. Fig. 1. Excision of the three cortical surfaces autograft from the iliac wing. Fig. 2. A) After discectomy the tunnels are performed with the Cloward technique; B) removal of the thin bone bridges between the tunnels; C) insertion of the two arms of the upper and lower bodies; the transplant is shown on the right; D) ready insertion of the autoplastic bone graft in diastasis. Fig. 3. It is very important: the removal of the posterior wall of the vertebral bodies (A) and of the uncus (B). Fig. 4. Lateral view of the graft, inserted in the trench. Its extremities are swallowtail shaped to avoid mobilization

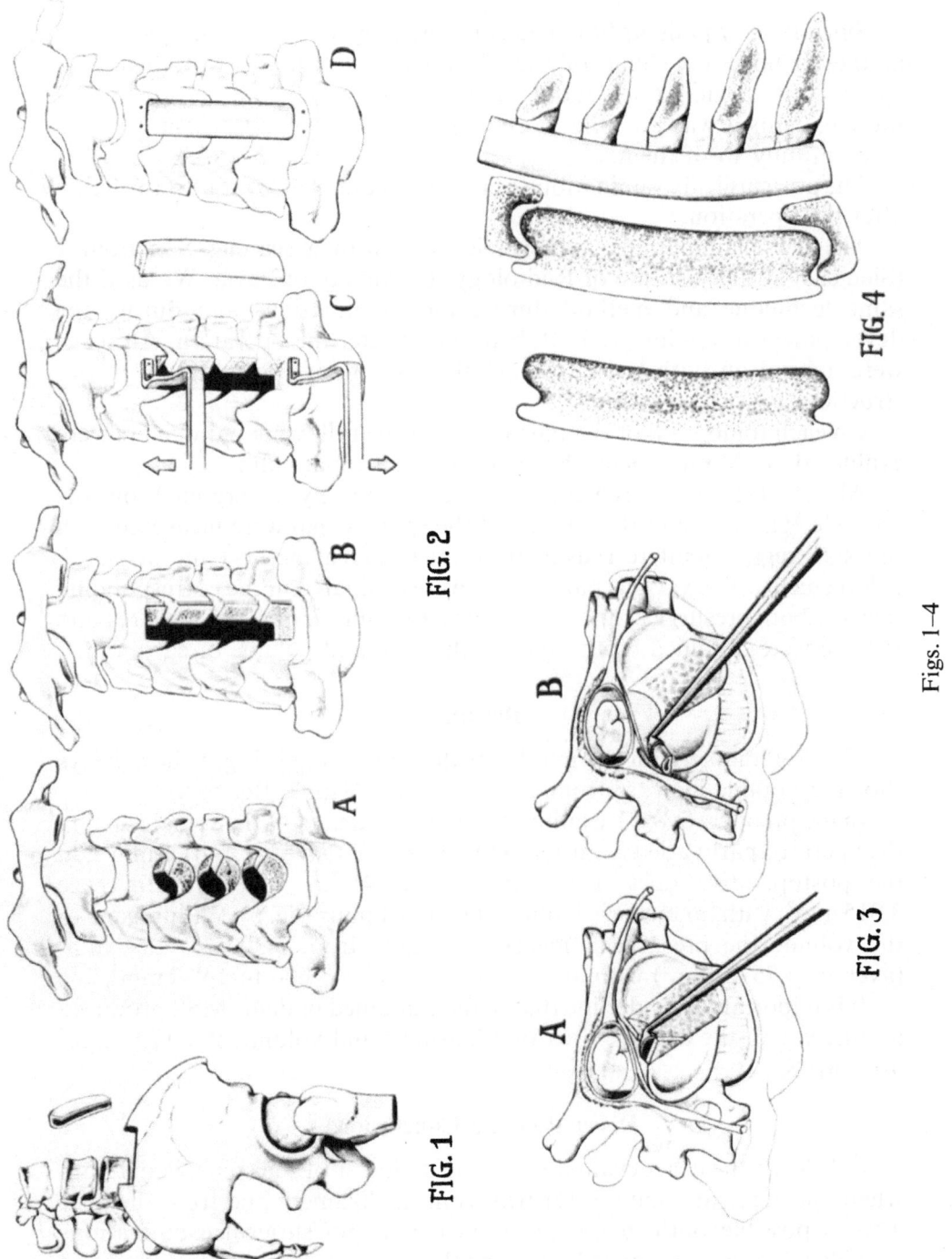

FIG. 1

FIG. 2

FIG. 3

FIG. 4

Figs. 1–4

Material and Method

Since 1969 57 patients have been operated on with this technique (MSS) at the Orthopedics Clinic of the University of Pavia: 42 of them had spondylotic myelopathies and 15 posttraumatic deformities. Among all these patients it was possible to do a systematic pre- and postsurgery CT study in only 15 of them.

The postsurgical examinations were carried out from 6 months to 3 years after the operation.

The CT examinations were carried out with a scanner Somatom 2 (Siemens) at the Institute of Radiology, University of Pavia. We used the same technique and method during the examinations and during the development of the images both before and after the operation. All scans were imaged on both bone and soft tissues windows and sagittal reconstructions were always done.

On each tomogram of the part operated the following parameters were evaluated: a) A–P diameter; b) area; c) spinal canal volume.

All of these measurements were electronically determined on the consolle. The area and the volume of the spinal canal were measured with the ROI (region of interest) using the same technical factors (window, level, enlargement). The various parameters were evaluated in the corresponding scans of both presurgical and postsurgical examinations. The total area and volume were obtained by the sum of the area and volume of each scan.

Results

The A–P diameter in the middle of the spinal canal (Fig. 5) has always shown a notable increase from 2–9 mm to 12–28 mm after surgery.

In the preoperative CT examinations the total area of the spinal canal in the operated part varied from 1,140 to 2,946 mm^2 (average 2,441.8 mm^2); in the postoperative ones it varied from 2,641 to 3,249 mm^2 (average 3,015 mm^2) with an increase from 210 to 1,101 mm^2 Fig. 6). With regard to the volume the presurgical measures ranged from 3,300 to 5,892 mm^3 (average 4,757.5 mm^3) with an increase of between 606 to 1,982 mm^3.

It is important to underline that in the examined patients MSS produced an increase in the average area of 573.6 mm^2 and volume of 1,179.5 mm^3 after MSS.

Discussion and Conclusions

CT allows the exact evaluation of the diameter of the spinal canal both where the edges are bony or formed from the ligament and from the disc. This is possible both in the presurgical and postsurgical examinations provided that they are carried out using the same technique and method and that the diameters are evaluated in the same way.

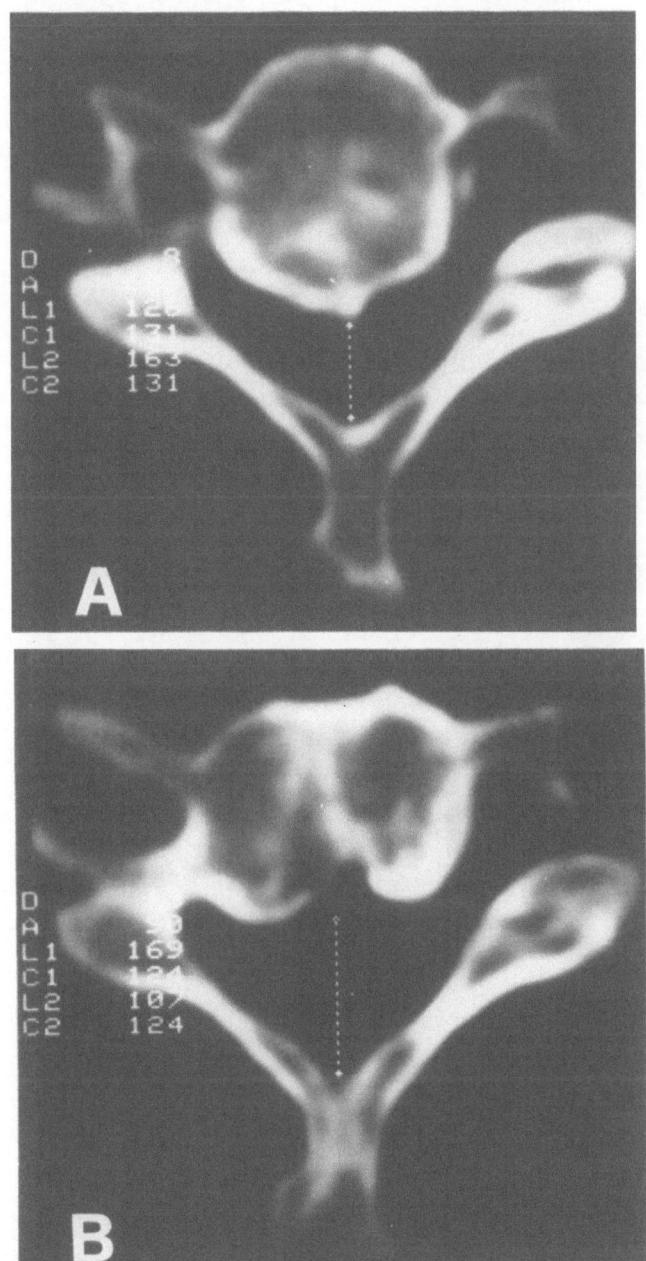

Fig. 5. Measuring of A–P diameter in the same vertebra both before (A) and after (B) MSS

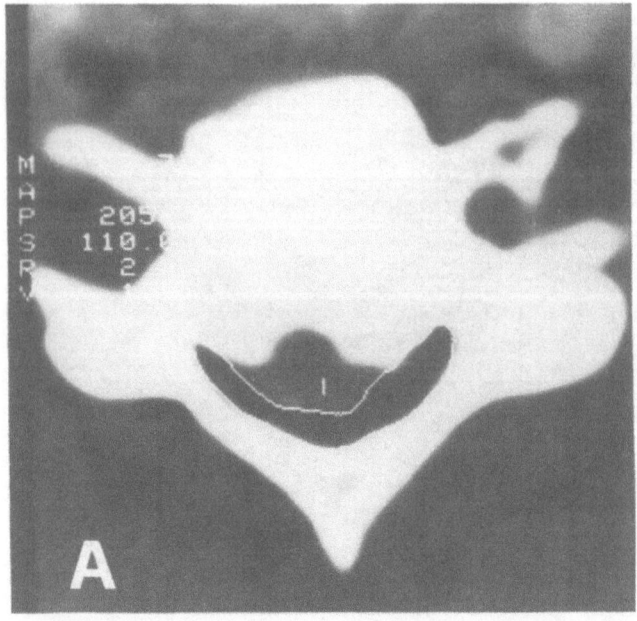

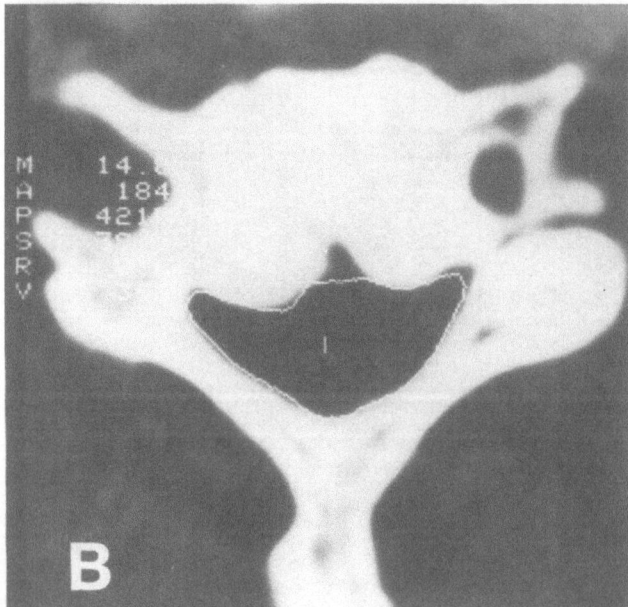

Fig. 6. Evaluation of the area and volume of the spinal canal in a scan showing a large bulging annulus both before (A) and after (B) MSS; the scan having a thickness of 2 mm, the volume value is the double of the area

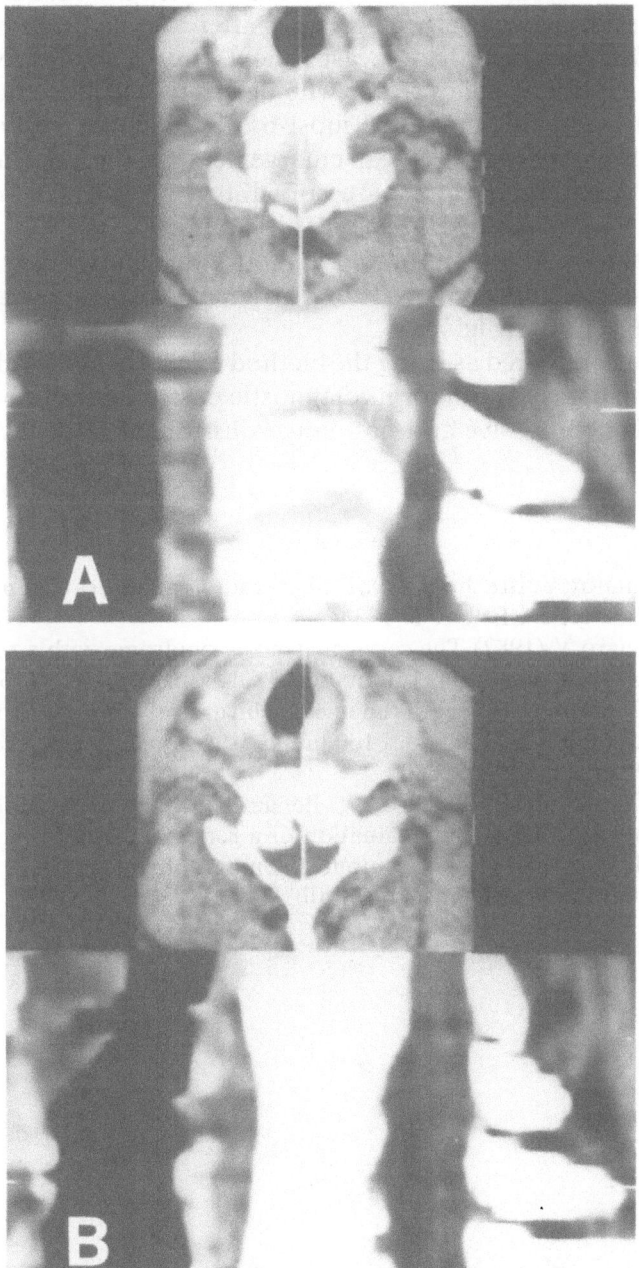

Fig. 7. Same patient as in Fig. 6. Medial sagittal reconstructions photographed with soft tissue window both before (A) and after (B) MSS. Notable enlargement of the spinal canal and decompression of the cord

It is the first time that the area and volume of the spinal canal have been determined electronically both before and after an operation of enlargement with MSS. Although these measurements are approximative because of the variability due to the operator who determines the limits of the area for evaluation, they are among the most precise possible today.

CT has always shown the real enlargement of the antero-posterior diameter of the spinal canal and unquestionably the removal of bone, fibro-cartilaginous tissues and disc in spondylotic narrow canal.

The sagittal reconstructions of the scans appeared particularly useful in a more immediate comprehensive view of the narrow canal and of its longitudinal extension (Fig. 7).

CT must be considered as being the method of choice in the follow-up of the operated on patients both for its diagnostic possibilities and because the examination is noninvasive and not dangerous for the patient.

References

1. Babin E, Lemaitre Y, Bruch JM (1981) Signe radiologique des canaux cervicaux étroits. Radiologie J CEPUR 1: 133
2. Boni M, Denaro V (1982) The cervical stenosis syndrome with a review of 87 patients treated by operation. International Orthopaedics 185: 195
3. Boni M, Denaro V (1982) Traitement chirurgical des cervico-arthroses. Révision à distance (2–13 ans) des 100 premiers cas opérés par voie antérieure. Rev Chir Orthopéd 68: 269–280
4. Boni M, Cherubino P, Denaro V, Benazzo F (1984) Multiple subtotal somatectomy. Technique and evaluation of a series of 39 cases. Spine 9: 358
5. Newton TH, Potts DG (1983) Computed tomography of the spine and spinal cord. Clavadel Press, San Anselmo, Calif., U.S.A.

2.11. Temporal Alterations in Somatosensory Evoked Potentials in Cervical Spondylotic Myelopathy*

J. F. Cusick and J. B. Myklebust, Milwaukee, Wisconsin, U.S.A.

Although a large body of literature exists regarding acute spinal cord trauma, few studies have been devoted to the natural course of the "progressive" myelopathies. The majority of such studies concentrate on cervical spondylotic myelopathy (CSM) and direct attention mainly at the diagnostic criteria and effects of surgical intervention [9, 10]. The paucity of information is understandable considering the immense difficulty in designing a chronic animal preparation to mimic the clinical situation with the timing and character of the compression in the laboratory animals. These limitations suggest that longitudinal clinical studies with associated neurophysiologic observations offer a fruitful method to evaluate the natural history of this disease entity.

Somatosensory Evoked Potential Studies

In considering the value of somatosensory evoked potential (SSEP) monitoring in cervical spondylotic myelopathy (CSM), the correlation of the acknowledged dorsal column dependencies of the SSEPs [2] and the frequent participation of the dorsal columns in the cord degeneration of CSM [1, 12] indicates that SSEPs should be a valuable monitor of the functional spinal cord integrity in this disease process. Evoked responses recorded from the spinal cord have been evaluated by surface recordings or by means of intrathecal electrodes [4, 11], but the need for invasive procedures, inherent risk, and technical problems in recording techniques have made such studies unappealing for evaluating neurophysiologic spinal cord alterations, especially for long-term serial studies. A consensus of these studies relating to the progressive myelopathies, however, indicates that SSEP analysis permits a qualitative evaluation of the functional status of the spinal somatosensory system [3]. These conclusions have mainly been based on variations of latency and amplitude of the primary response components

* This research has been supported in part by Veterans Administration Merit Review No. 1655-03P.

as the indicators of the fidelity of impulse conduction in the human spinal cord. The concept of configuration evaluation has been mentioned but not directly approached. The concomitant involvement of the lateral colums which are also frequently a major participants in CSM can be investigated using methods designed to evaluate reflex and motor coordination systems [5, 7, 8].

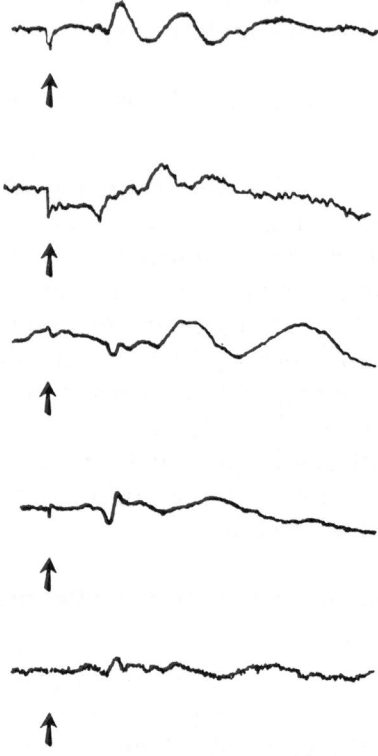

Fig. 1. Serial evoked potential records from a patient diagnosed with cervical spondylotic myelopathy. Recordings were made from scalp electrodes secondary to median nerve stimulation. Top trace was first recording obtained from the patient. Lower traces obtained at 3, 12, 18, and 24 months intervals. Entire trace is 125 ms, stimulus is applied at arrow. Amplitudes and latencies of the components are tabulated in Table 1

Our studies have been directed toward a serial evaluation of patients at risk for or with clinical indications of cervical spondylotic myelopathy. In addition to changes in evoked potential amplitude and latency, waveform alterations are observed as a function of time, and, because of the spinal mobility involved in this disease entity, evoked potentials and muscle activity secondary to tendon of the biceps, triceps, achilles and patella tendons, have been obtained with neck flexion and extension.

Although a certain level of intersubject variability exists, we have found in studies on normal volunteers that there is a stationarity of the primary components (initial 30–45 msec) of the evoked response [6], and no alterations of the SSEPs were observed relative to functional changes of the cervical spine position. In subjects with cervical spondylotic myelopathy, however, serial SSEP recordings over intervals of 3 months to 3 years frequently demonstrate changes in the secondary components of the primary response (Fig. 1). The initial cortical component with onset at 16–20 msec secondary to median nerve stimulation usually remains intact and is not affected until the clinical process is well-advanced (Table 1). The waveform characteristics of the primary response demonstrate a downward shift of the frequency spectrum. These findings are indicative of a temporal

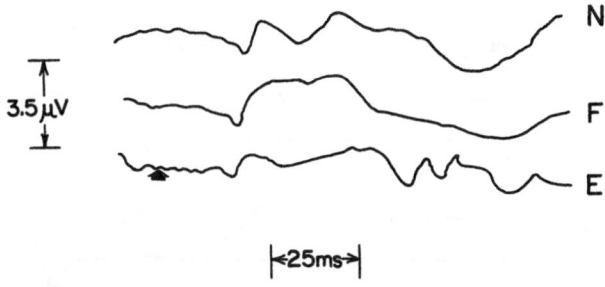

Fig. 2. Evoked responses obtained from a patient with various neck positions. Top recordings were made from scalp electrodes secondary to median nerve stimulation. Trace—neutral, middle trace—flexion, bottom trace—extension. Entire trace is 125 ms, stimulus is applied at arrow

dispersion and suggest that the earlier stages of cervical spondylotic myelopathy are the products of mechanical distortion of the axons with alterations of their conduction capacity. Distortions of SSEP waveform and amplitude variations secondary to changes in neck position are observed in many of these patients (Fig. 2). In these later subjects, flexion may produce little response alteration whereas extension frequently results in amplitude diminution or waveform distortion.

Reflex Pattern Studies

A variety of changes in reflex patterns have been observed with changes in neck position (Fig. 3). Some patients demonstrate coactivation of antagonist muscles while others show amplitude and latency alterations. Correlation of evoked response alterations and abnormalities of reflex testing in these longitudinal studies offers insight into the effects of CSM on long fiber tracts *versus* segmental fibers in the cervical spinal cord.

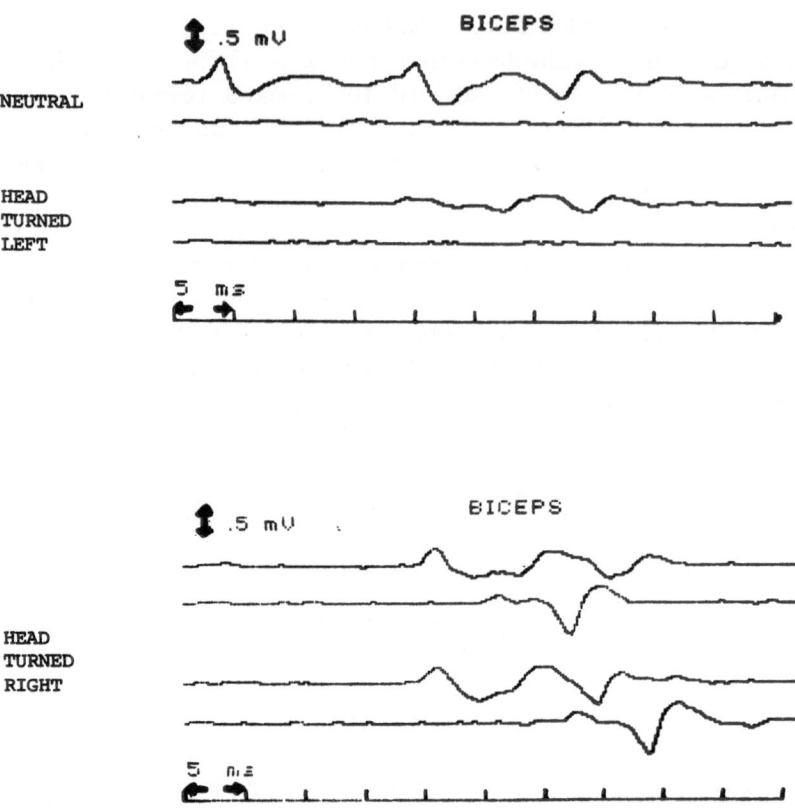

Fig. 3. EMG responses secondary to tap of the biceps tendon. In each pair of traces, the upper one is recorded from the biceps muscle and the lower from the triceps muscle. In the neutral position (top), the response is approximately normal. With the head turned to the left (second pair of traces), the agonist EMG is distorted, but no antagonist activity is present. With the head turned to the right (3rd and 4th pairs of traces) a variable latency response is observed in the antagonist (triceps) muscle

Conclusion

Because cervical spondylotic myelopathy (CSM) is a multifactorial disease process, neurophysiologic monitoring of spinal cord fidelity is an important consideration in defining the natural history of this entity for a specific patient. The predilection for CSM to involve the dorsal and lateral columns indicates the electrophysiologic monitoring of these regions should be of special value. Longitudinal evaluation of somatosensory evoked potentials (SSEPs), especially using configurational analysis and recordings in various functional positions of the cervical spine, have been of assistance in illustrating early changes of dorsal column integrity. The SSEP studies were correlated with tendon tap, joint compliance, and quick stretch measurements designed to offer reproducible quantitative evaluation of lateral column (corticospinal tract) function. The tendon tap examinations using a microprocessor system with an instrumented reflex hammer consistently demonstrated, either singularly or in combination, occasions of amplitude and latency alterations as well as reciprocal excitation at the cervical level. These changes were frequently associated with variations in the functional positions of the cervical spine. It was unusual to find corresponding marked intersubject changes between SSEP and reflex changes suggesting a disassociation between long tract (dorsal column) and short segmental fibers. Reflex changes at the cervical level (biceps and triceps) were more susceptible to positional changes than SSEP recordings.

Table 1 A. *Patient no. 0602. Latencies measured from responses in Fig. 1.* L 1 is the initial deflection from baseline. L 2 is the first (downward) peak. L 3 is the following (upward) peak and L 4 is the next upward peak

Record no.	L 1	L 2	L 3	L 4
1	16.4	18.8	24.4	44.5
2	16.4	18.4	37.5	52.5
3	16.6	19.0	52.2	84.4
4	16.3	18.4	56.2	—
5	16.5	18.5	—	—

Table 1 B. *Patient no. 0602. Amplitudes measured from responses in Fig. 1.* A 1 is amplitude from baseline to the first (downward) peak. A 2–A 4 are the peak-to-peak amplitudes of the following deflections

Record no.	A 1	A 2	A 3	A 4
1	1.5	3.0	3.6	2.4
2	1.5	4.8	2.4	1.2
3	1.6	3.0	3.0	3.0
4	1.6	1.6	—	—
5	1.2	—	—	—

References

1. Bedford PD, Bosanquet FD, Russell WR (1952) Degeneration of the spinal cord associated with cervical spondylosis. Lancet 2: 55–59
2. Cusick JF, Myklebust J, Larson SJ, Sances A, Jr (1978) Spinal evoked potentials in the primate: neural substrates. J Neurosurg 49: 551–557

3. Dorfman LJ, Perkash I, Bosley TM, Cummins KL (1980) Use of cerebral evoked potentials to evaluate spinal somatosensory function in patients with traumatic and surgical myelopathies. J Neurosurg 52: 654–660
4. Ertekin C (1978) Comparison of the human evoked electrospinogram recorded from the intrathecal, epidural and cutaneous levels. Electroencephalogr Clin Neurophysiol 44: 683–690
5. Gottlieb GL, Agarwal GC (1979) Response to sudden torques about ankle in man: myotatic reflex. J Neurophysiol 42: 91–106
6. Myklebust JB, Sances A, Jr., Cusick JF, Friedman RH, Larson SJ, Cohen BA (1984) Stationarity of the somatosensory evoked potential. Med Biol Eng Comput 22: 558–563
7. Myklebust BM, Gottlieb GL, Penn RD, Agarwal GC (1982) Reciprocal excitation of antagonistic muscles as a differentiating feature in spasticity. Ann Neurol 12: 367–374
8. Myklebust BM, Gottlieb GL, Agarwal GC (1984) Effects of body orientation on monosynaptic reflex measurements. Neurosci Lett 48: 223–230
9. Phillips DG (1973) Surgical treatment of myelopathy with cervical spondylosis. J Neurol Neurosurg Psychiatry 36: 879–884
10. Roosen K, Grote W (1980) Late results of operative treatment of cervical myelopathy. In: Grote W, Brock M, Clar HE, Klinger M, Nau HE (eds) Advances in neurosurgery. Springer, Berlin Heidelberg New York, pp 69–77
11. Shimoji K, Matsuki M, Shimizu H (1977) Wave-form characteristics and spatial distribution of evoked spinal electrogram in man. J Neurosurg 46: 304–312
12. Wilkinson M (1960) The morbid anatomy of cervical spondylosis and myelopathy. Brain 83: 589–617

2.12. Calcic Densities in the Cervico-occipital Joint

Y. Dirheimer, J. L. Burguet, and H. Sick, Strasbourg, France

The normal anatomy of the cervico-occipital region of its joints and accessory parts, studied with CT, is now well known [3]; this procedure provides accurate visualization of the bone contours as well as of the soft parts.

During CT investigations carried out for various diseases of the joints, we have detected pathologic calcic opacities; it was however impossible to say whether they were calcifications or ossifications. Only pathologic investigations allow to differentiate amorphous calcic deposits (calcifications) from organized bone tissue (ossifications). Moreover, very often these calcic opacities are not visible on standard radiograms or tomograms.

1. Rheumatoid Arthritis

We have found calcic densities all around the odontoid process, in following locations: atlanto-dental joint, lateral interatlantodental space, syndesmodental joint, transverse and alar ligaments.

As concerns the first of these sites (Fig. 1), we had the impression that there was an ossification filling-up the atlantodental joint space which was widened because of anterior subluxation. The new formed bone seems to be continuous with the anterior arch. In such cases ossification is probably partly responsible for the fact that the subluxation is not reduced by extension during the dynamic test.

When the calcic opacities are located on the lateral aspect of the odontoid, in the interatlantodental space, there are two possibilities: In the first event the bone contours of the lateral masses of the atlas and of the odontoid, and more particularly the transverse tubercles of the atlas, are smooth and perfectly intact (Fig. 1). In the second event there are destructive lesions and the calcic densities could correspond to bony sequesters resulting from destruction of the lateral masses of the atlas and of the odontoid process.

Erosion of the posterior aspect of the odontoid process resulting from syndesmodental arthritis is a classical feature in rheumatoid arthritis [2]. It

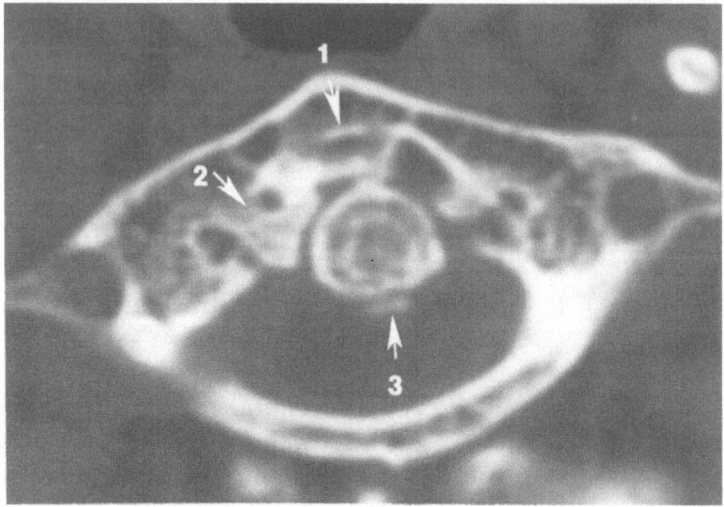

Fig. 1. Anterior atlantodental luxation in a case of seropositive rheumatoid arthritis which has developed over a period of 17 years. The space created by the subluxation is partly filled with new-formed bone tissue developing from the anterior arch of the atlas (*1*) and from the attachment tubercle of the transverse ligament of the atlas on the right side (*2*). There is also a calcic density in the middle part of the transverse ligament, behind the odontoid process (*3*)

may be accompanied by constructive changes with formation of spicules on the posterior aspect of the odontoid process involving also the syndesmo-dental articulation, or by bony sequesters associated with an irregular and partly destroyed dens.

Finally, calcic opacities can also be seen on the ligaments of the cervico-occipital joint, especially on the transverse and alar ligaments [1]. This is mainly seen in cases with anterior atlantodental subluxation (Figs. 1 and 2).

We have also seen a total bone ankylosis in a case of longstanding rheumatoid arthritis, which had caused solidarization of the anterior arch and lateral masses of the atlas, as well as of the odontoid process.

We believe constructive changes at the level of the cervico-occipital joint to be much more frequent than is usually reported; the great number of calcic opacities seen on CT investigations is quite stricking. This fact has also been reported by other authors [2].

2. Ankylosing Spondylarthritis

Chronic inflammatory rheumatism is by definition an ossifying rheumatism comprising ankylosis of the sacroiliac joints and of the posterior interapophyseal joints, intersomatic bridges consisting of syndes-mophytes, and ossification of other intervertebral ligaments (in particular

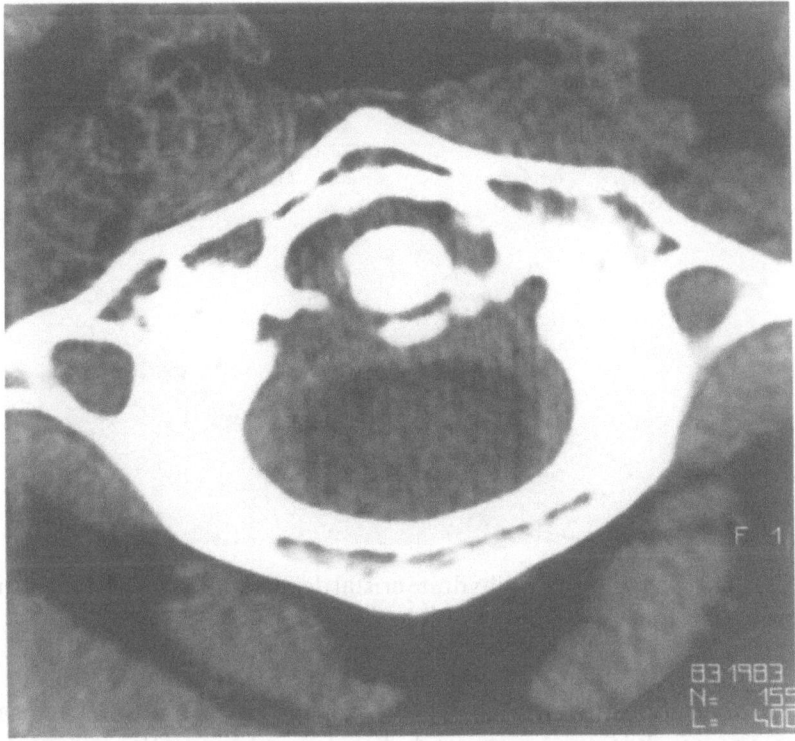

Fig. 2. Moderate anterior atlantodental luxation in a case of seropositive rheumatoid arthritis which has developed over a period of 16 years. The transverse ligament is partly occupied by calcic densities extending from one transverse tubercle to the other

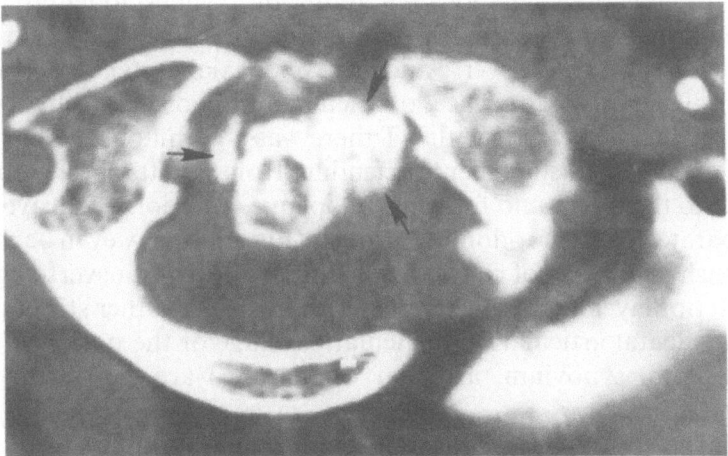

Fig. 3. Severe ankylosing spondylarthritis in a woman aged 59 years. Atlantodental subluxation. Calcic densities in the interatlantodental space (→)

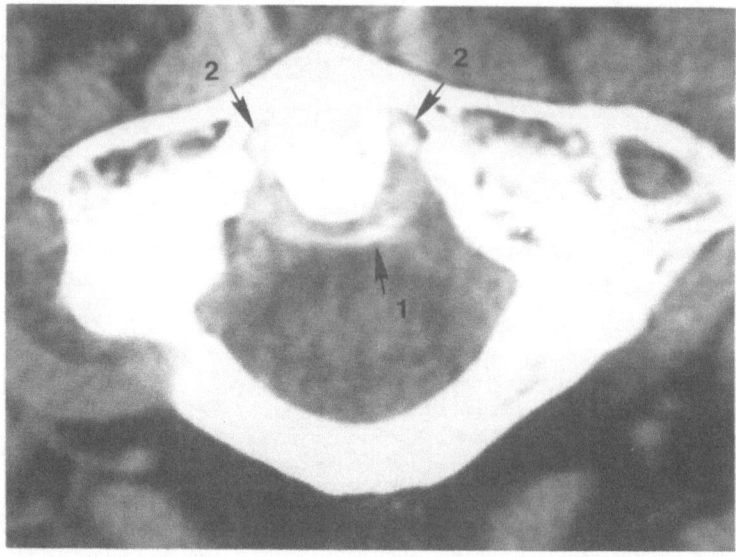

Fig. 4. Calcium pyrophosphate dihydrate cristal deposition disease. Calcification of the transverse ligament (*1*) and of the alar ligaments (*2*)

the interspinous ligaments). Such changes have however only rarely been reported to involve the cervico-occipital joint. CT investigations in a case of ankylosing spondylarthritis showed, besides anterior atlantodental sub-luxation, significant calcic opacities located in the interatlantodental space (Fig. 3).

3. Calcium Pyrophosphate Dihydrate Cristal Deposition Disease

The calcifications are located about the syndesmodental joint and involve following structures: the entire cruciform ligament (the transverse part and the occipitotransverse and transversoaxial parts), as well as the alar ligaments [1, 7]. In the four cases of calcium pyrophosphate dihydrate cristal deposition disease studied with CT there was a granulous, global calcification of the transverse ligament, extending from one transverse tubercle of the atlas to the other, and forming an opaque, anteriorly concave crescent, well separated from the odontoid process (Fig. 4). It may even be possible to distinguish two layers of calcic deposition about the transverse ligament: a thin anterior layer and a thicker posterior layer. The other structures of the syndesmodental articulation (articular cartilage of the posterior aspect of the odontoid, synovium, articular capsule ...) are less readily individualized.

We never saw calcic deposits in the articular cartilage of the atlanto-dental, condyloatlantal and atlantoaxial joints.

In our opinion such transverse ligament lesions could account for the anterior atlantodental luxations described by Resnick [7].

4. Acromegaly

In one case we found a global calcic hyperdensity of the entire transverse ligament, but we do not know whether it was due to an ossification similar to Erdheim spondylosis as it is described in other spinal segments, or to calcic deposits analoguous to those found in calcium pyrophosphate dihydrate cristal deposition disease.

5. Ossification of the Posterior Longitudinal Ligament

Although the posterior longitudinal ligament is ossified behind the vertebral bodies and the intervertebral discs, sometimes from C 2 to C 7, we have never seen calcic deposits at the level of the cervico-occipital joint. In one case only there was a hyperdensity of the transverse ligament.

Conclusion

In several affections computer tomography proves more accurate than conventional radiography for the detection of calcic deposits about the cervico-occipital region. The list reported here is however certainly not exhaustive.

Although in some cases the involved anatomic structure is easily recognized, it may also sometimes be more difficult to be affirmative.

Finally, it is impossible to differentiate between ossification and calcification. By analogy with the lesions involving the other joints in the different diseases we may make suppositions but positive extrapolations are not allowed.

References

1. Burguet JL, Sick H, Dirheimer Y, Wackenheim A (1985) CT of the main ligaments of the cervico-occipital hinge. Neuroradiology 27: 112–118
2. Castor WR, Miller JDR, Russell AS, Chiu PL, Grace M, Manson J (1983) Computed tomography of the craniocervical junction in rheumatoid arthritis. J Comput Assist Tomogr 7: 31–36
3. Daniels DL, Williams C (1983) Computed tomography of the articulation and ligaments at the occipito-atlanto-axial region. Radiology 146: 709–716
4. Dirheimer Y (1977) The craniovertebral region in chronic inflammatory rheumatic diseases. Springer, Berlin Heidelberg New York
5. Dirheimer Y, Wackenheim C, Dietemann JL (1985) Calcification of the transverse ligament in calcium dihydrate deposition disease (CPPD). Neuroradiology 27: 87
6. Martel W (1961) The occipito-atlanto-axial joints in rheumatoid arthritis and ankylosing spondylitis. Ann J Roentgenol 86: 223–240
7. Resnick D, Pinela C (1984) Vertebral involvement in calcium pyrophosphate dihydrate cristal deposition disease. Radiology 153: 55–60

Cervical Spine I
© by Springer-Verlag 1987

2.13. Importance of CT in Fractures of the Cervical Articular Pillar
Report of Three Delayed Diagnosed Cases

P. Kehr and J. P. Steib, Strasbourg, France

Isolated fractures of the articular pillar in the lower cervical spine are difficult to detect, as it is pointed out by Dosch [1] and by Gehweiler, Osborne and Becker [2], who find them in 8% of their patients with spine traumatisms. We report here three cases with similar anamnesis, same level (C7), same clinical cervico-brachialgic manifestation and same diagnostic difficulties.

Here are the observations first:

Observation no. 1: Mr. WY. R., 37 year-old, was sent to see us in November 1981 for a right cervico-brachialgia C7, with motor deficits C6, mainly C7 but also C8 and Th1, settled since a road accident of September 13th, 1981. The initial diagnosis was "cervical sprain" and first treatment was a simple foam collar. Neurosurgeon colleagues see him afterwards because of a persistent cervico-brachialgia and have made a complete neuroradiological check-up which shows:

— a fracture of the right C7 isthmus of the articular pillar:

— a fracture of the right uncus of C7 protruding in the intervertebral foramen C6/C7;

— a C6/C7 subluxation;

— an amputation of the right C7 root showed by amipaque myelography.

The patient was sent to us for freeing of right C6/C7 intervertebral foramen. This operation was performed on December 4th, 1981, after a normal angiography of the vertebral arteries. The operation consisted in the realization of a right C6/C7 discectomy with Robinson fusion and a six-holes-plate osteosynthesis. It was possible to remove the protruded uncal fragment.

Complete subjective and objective recovery with complete regression of the motor deficits as shown on the postoperative electromyogram. Back to occupational life and sports (skiing, shooting); follow-up: 3 years (Fig. 1).

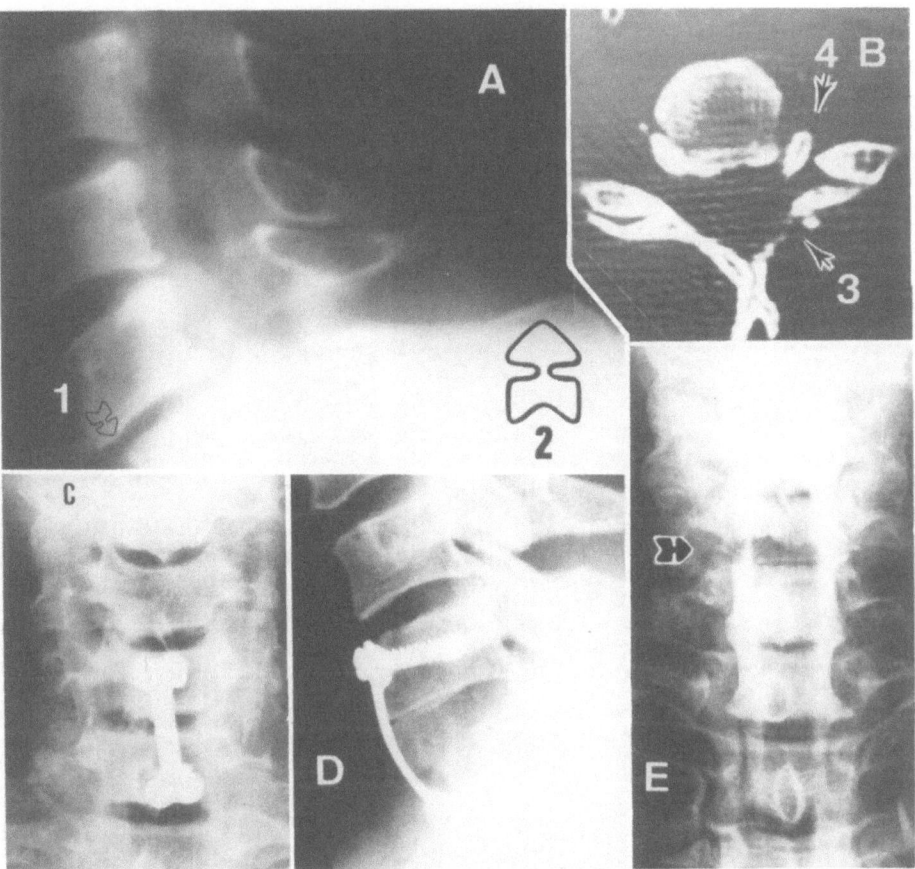

Fig. 1. Mr. WY., 37 years old, ignored separation-fracture of the articular pillar on the right side, resulting from a major road accident which had occurred two month before the first consultation. (A) Lateral tomogram showing the unilateral dislocation of C6/C7 (1), with the interspinous diastasis (2); two very suspect radiological signs of an unstable osteoarticular lesion. (B) Computed tomogram through the superior edge of C7, showing up both fracture lines, one right through the lamine. (3), the other one separating the posterior part of the uncus which finds itself in the intervertebral foramen (4), explaining thus the right C7 cervico-brachialgia. (C) Postoperative A–P roentgenogram showing the osteosynthesis plate. (D) Lateral postoperative roentgenogram on which the intersomatic bone graft C6/C7 is visible. (E) Cervical amipaque myelography demonstrates the nonfilling of the right C7 radicular sheat. Excellent postoperative result; follow-up: 3 years

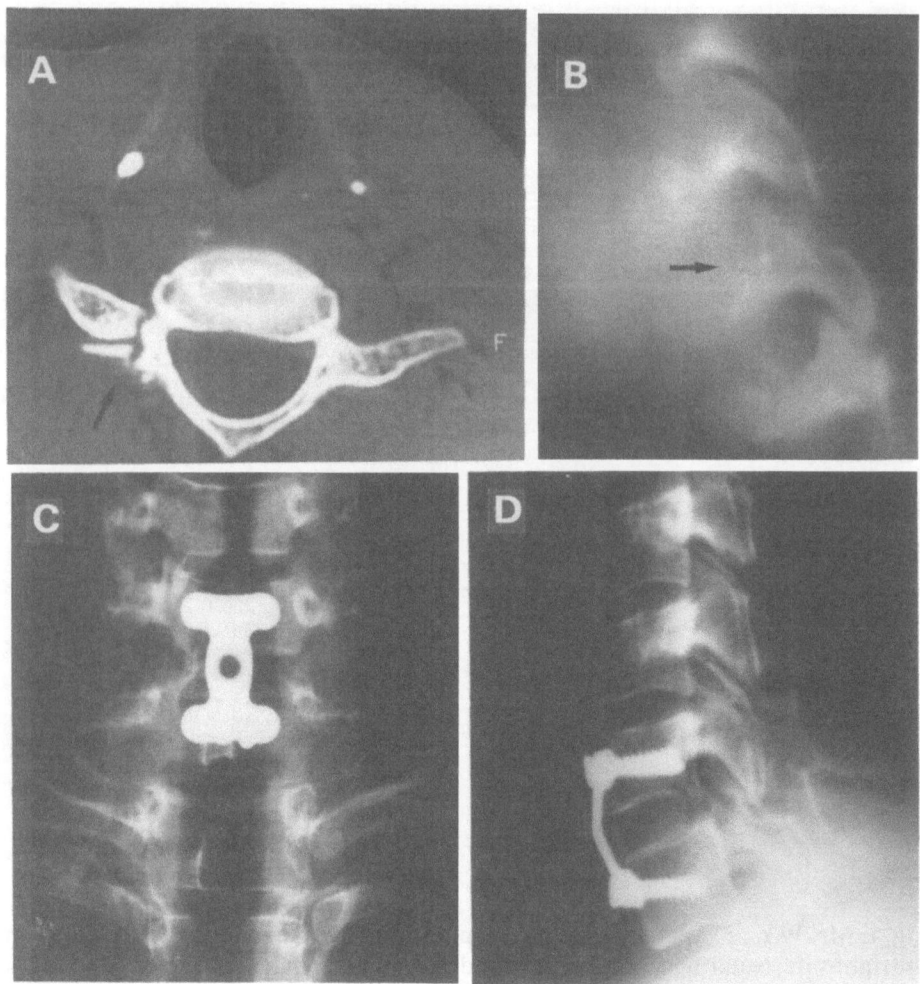

Fig. 2. Mr. PF., 23 years old, consults in May 1984 for a right C7 cervico-brachialgia existing since a skiing accident two month before. The first diagnosis was a "sprain", and vertebral manipulation had even been performed outside! (A) Computed tomogram through C7 showing clearly the fracture of the articular pillar. (B) Lateral tomogram of the right articular pillar of C7; the arrow shows the impaction of this articular part at the front and at the back. (C) Antero-posterior roentgenogram demonstrating the stabilization by using an osteosynthesis plate. (D) Postoperative lateral roentgenogram showing plate and bone graft as well as the excellent realignement of the posterior rachidian wall. Excellent result; follow-up: 1 year

Observation no. 2: Mr. PF. C., 23 years old, consults in May 1984 for a C7 right cervico-brachialgia existing since a ski fall which occurred on March 14th, 1984. The first X-rays made at the ski resort reveal an important C6/C7 functional facet dislocation, which is considered as benign by the doctor at the resort, and treated by foam collar after manipulation!

The neurological check-up made thereafter because of the persisting cervico-brachialgia shows:
— a fracture of the right pillar of C7;
— a fracture of the right uncus of C7;

The electromyogram shows partial signs of denervation in the C7 muscles, particularly at the level of the triceps and the common extensor of the fingers.

Operation on May 15th, 1984: C6/C7 discectomy and Robinson fusion with AO plate osteosynthesis (Fig. 2). The transdiscal C6/C7 foramino-tomy by removal of the posterior part of the uncus succeeds partly because of an important hemorrhage which could be stopped by compression.

Excellent results on a subjective point of view; went back to work; follow-up 1 year.

Observation no. 3: Mrs. LE. J., 51 years old, consults on June 28th, 1984, after a road accident which occurred on June 5th, 1984; she was driving a car, with a seat-belt and a headrest; left lateral shock, dragged along 20 meters.

Treated by a plaster collar brace for 8 days, and then by a Schanz collar because of diagnosis of a severe sprain of C4/C5 as the dynamic X-Rays showed a functional facet dislocation at this level in flexion. Otherwise, pre-existing C5/C6 discal osteoarthritis.

The persistence of neckpain with left C7 cervico-brachialgia (down to the index finger and the middle finger) lead the patient to consult us. The examination reveals an acute pain on the left C6/C7 articular process and a comminuted articular pillar of C7 on the profile X-Ray. A left isthmic fractures of C7 on tomographies (Fig. 3).

Operation on July, 10th, 1984 by posterior osteosynthesis C6/C7/Th1 using Roy-Camille plates on both sides. Excellent early result; immediate improvement of the cervico-brachialgia; unchanged excellent result in May 1985; follwo-up: 1 year.

Comments

1. The lesion is in all three cases an unilateral fracture of the articular pillar of C7 with separation, but in one case the anterior fracture-line does not cross the pedicle but the uncus. The primarily performed X-rays could not establish the diagnosis in any case. In two cases it would have been possible to suspect the lesion because of an interbody subluxation (case 1) or

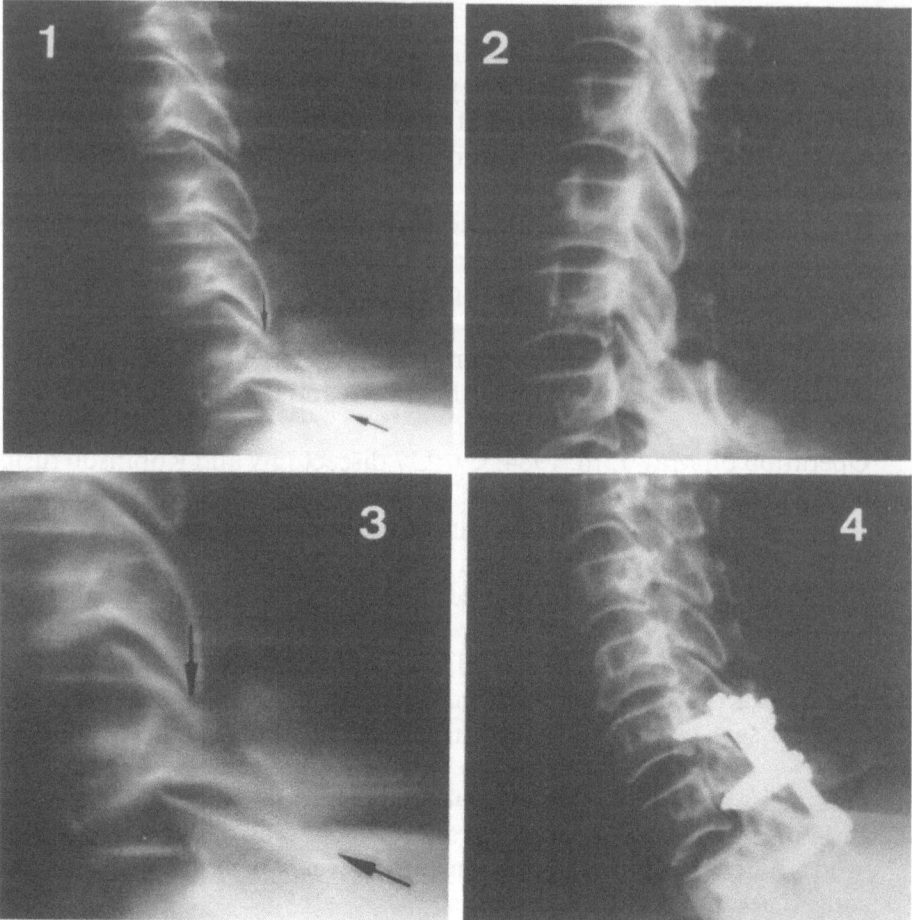

Fig. 3. Mrs. LE., 51 years old, consults three weeks after a road accident which occurred in the beginning of June 1984. The diagnosis of fracture of the left articular pillar of C 7 is seen only on the tomograms. (1) and (3) Lateral tomogram showing the fracture-line passing through the isthmus of the articular pillar. (2) On the standard lateral roentgenogram the abnormal image is the sizeable anterior gasping of the C 6/C 7 disc. (4) Postoperative check-up. Excellent result; follow-up: 1 year

of a functional facet dislocation (case 2). In the third case, the initial X-rays were misleading to the level C 4/C 5; a more careful X-ray study and the correlation to the clinical findings (C 7 cervico-brachialgia and aching point) will lead to C 7.

2. The diagnosis has been confirmed in the three cases by detailed X-rays examinations, tomograms and/or CT scanning.

It might have been possible to see the fracture line in the classical X-rays views (A–P of C 1/C 2, mouth opened—A–P of the lower cervical spine— lateral incidences in neutral position, in flexion, in extension—at an angle of

45° obliquely, right and left incidences—right and left incidences at an angle of 20°—postero-anterior incidence of the posterior arches—right and left posterior oblique incidences of the posterior arches—semiaxial view of the atlas), but these views are difficult to get at the first X-rays examination and dynamic X-ray studies should not be performed immediately after traumatism.

Standard X-rays must therefore be analyzed with great precision [1]; A–P, lateral and oblique views, and above of all, one should not hesitate in immediately requiring tomograms, should the slightest doubt arise.

Later, after 8 to 10 days, dynamic X-rays will have be done systematically, even if the patient does not complain about important pain anymore. If there is remaining pain, one has to try to localize the acute site where the pain is at its maximal level and require tomograms and/or CT scanning centered on this area. This diagnostic procedure will prevent delayed diagnosis and avoid inadequate treatment.

3. As far as the treatment is concerned, our choice was, twice, the antero-lateral approach because the intervertebral foramen was occupied by a fragment of uncus, because the disc herniation and at last because the diagnosis was delayed. Our choice was the posterior approach in the third case as the lesion was more recent and as there was not disc herniation.

In conclusion, it appears that it is necessary to approach the cervical spine in "all directions" in order to adapt the best treatment.

References

1. Dosch JC (1985) Trauma—conventional radiological study in spine injury. Springer, Berlin Heidelberg New York Tokyo
2. Gehweiler JA, Osborne RL, Becker RF (1980) The radiology of the vertebral trauma. WB Saunders Company, Philadelphia London Toronto

2.14. Relationship Between Osteophyts and Symptoms in the Cervical Spondylosis

N. Nakano and T. Nakano, Sapporo, Japan

It has been said that narrowing of the disc space and the intervertebral foramen in cervical spondylosis may produce neurological deficits. Therefore, it has been stated that the disc height should be regained and the spurs should also be excised in the surgical treatment.

On the other hands, there are many patients with these changes who respond conservative treatment, or who moreover, do not demonstrate any clinical symptoms.

All cervical spine X-ray films belonging to the 781 patients who visited this hospital with symptoms were examined in order to know the extent to which these changes were related to the symptoms they displayed.

Age and changes of the cervical spine: Changes in the cervical spine in the male cases were found to be 43% in the fourth decade, 48% in the fifth, 54% in the sixth and 77% in the seventh decade. In the female cases the same tendency was found.

Narrowing of the disc space and intervertebral foramen: Narrowing of the disc space was found in 5.4% at C3/C4, 16.8% at C4/C5, 51.6% at C5/C6 and 23.1% at C6/C7.

Narrowing of the intervertebral foramen was found in 8.5% at C3/C4, 16.4% at C4/C5, 33.1% at C5/C6, and 25% at C6/C7.

Sex and narrowing of the disc space: Narrowing of the disc in males was found in 3.5% at C3/C4 and 42.7% at C5/C6 in the fourth decade, but 9.7% at C3/C4 and 77.4% at C5/C6 in seventh decade.

In females 2.4% at C3/C4 and 31.6% at C5/C6 in fourth decade and 30% at C3/C4; 65% at C5/C6 in the seventh decade.

There was no significant difference between the male and female results.

Sex and narrowing of the intervertebral foramen: Narrowing of the intervertebral foramen was almost the same as in narrowing of the disc space in both males and females.

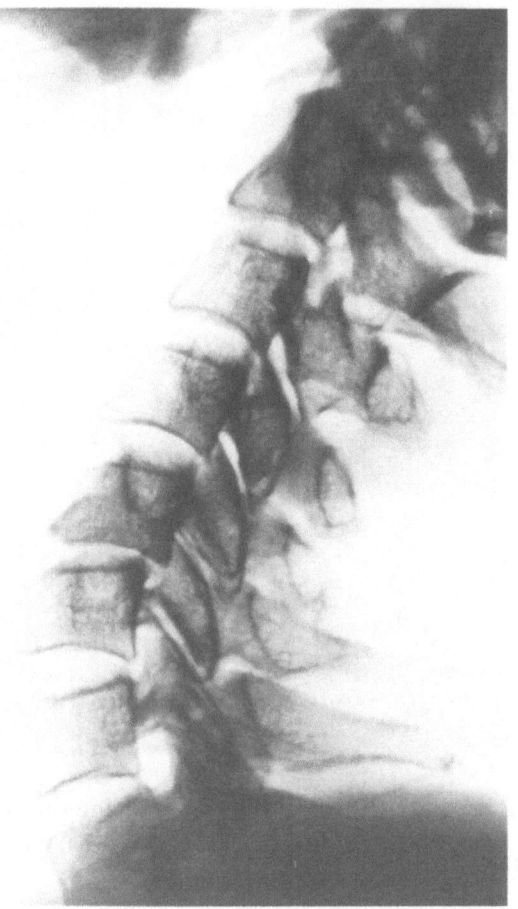

Fig. 1. Case 1, X-ray showed instability and disc narrowing at C 5/C 6 but symptoms were only occasional neck pain. He has a wide spinal canal

Illustrative Cases

Case 1: T. N., 56-year-old male. He was sent to this hospital for the surgical treatment. X-ray films showed instability and disc narrowing at C 5/C 6 but his only symptom was occasional neck pain. Therefore, he has been treated conservatively. His symptoms are not so severe because he has a wide spinal canal (Fig. 1).

Case 2: E. M., 54-year-old male. Anterior interbody fusion was done without removing the spurs 10 years ago. The posterior spurs were seen in the X-ray film but he has settled into daily life without any difficulty (Fig. 2).

Case 3: T. H., 54-year-old male. He had severe pain in the right upper extremity for three months, and after failure of conservative treatment was

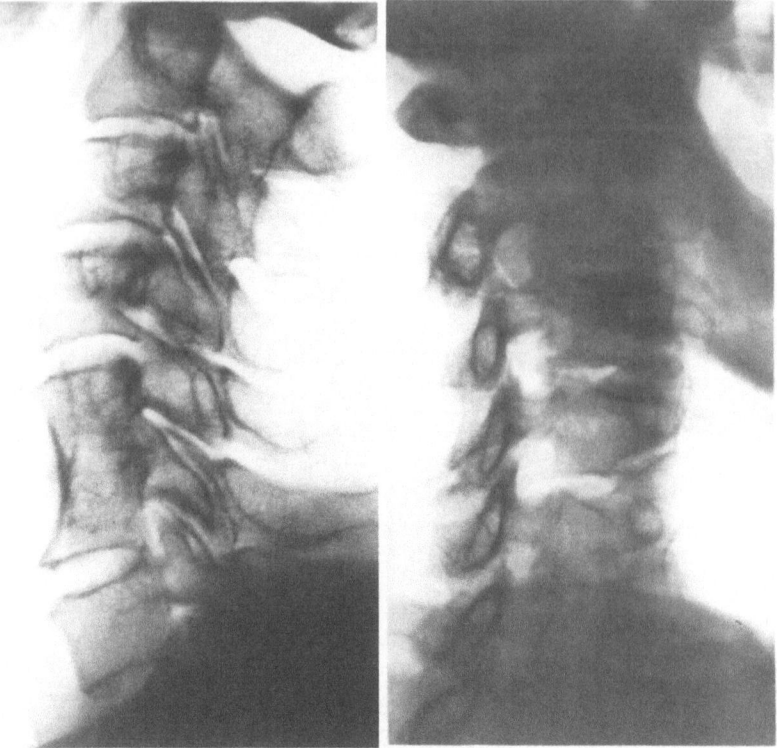

Fig. 2. Case 2, in a X-ray ten years after anterior interbody fusion, the posterior spurs were still seen but he has no symptoms

sent to this hospital. Anterior interbody fusion was done without excising the spurs but all his symptoms were improved after surgery. Narrowing of the disc space and spurs were still seen in the five year postoperative X-ray film, but he has no symptoms at all (Fig. 3).

Case 4: S. Y., 68-year-old female. Interbody fusion was done at C 5/C 6 without regaining the disc space fifteen years ago but she has no difficulty in daily life except occasional discomfort of her shoulders even with narrowing of the disc below the fused disc (Fig. 4).

Discussion

In general, narrowing of the disc space and spurs may cause clinical symptoms and many surgeons have tried to regain the disc space and also excise the spurs. However, such surgical intervention may aggravate symptoms in some cases. On the other hand, patients with these changes

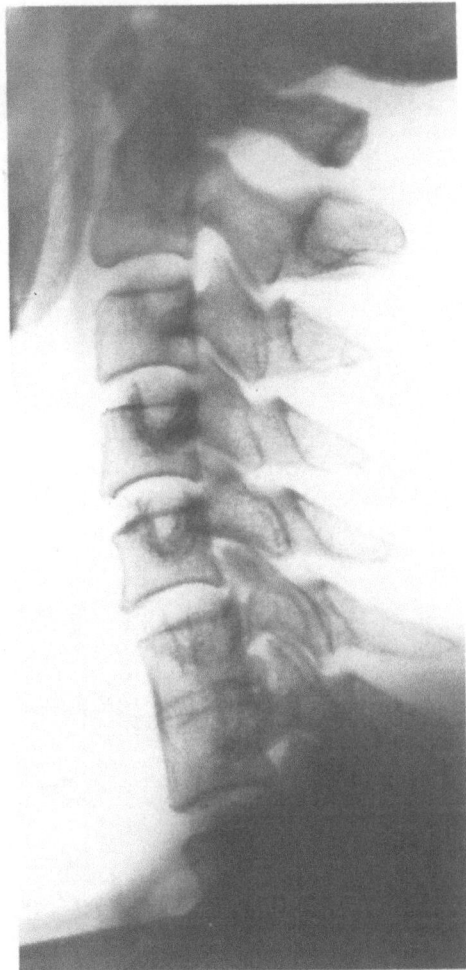

Fig. 3. Case 3, anterior interbody fusion was done without excising the spurs but all
his symptoms improved

respond to the conservative treatment. In this study, only 51 cases out of 791 patients (6.7%), underwent surgical treatment, the rest of them responded to the conservative treatment.

As the surgical procedure, modified Cloward's technique was used, but the disc space was not regained and spurs was not excised.

Results, however, of this operation were as follows; excellent 77%, good 14.8%, fair 6.6% and poor 1.6%.

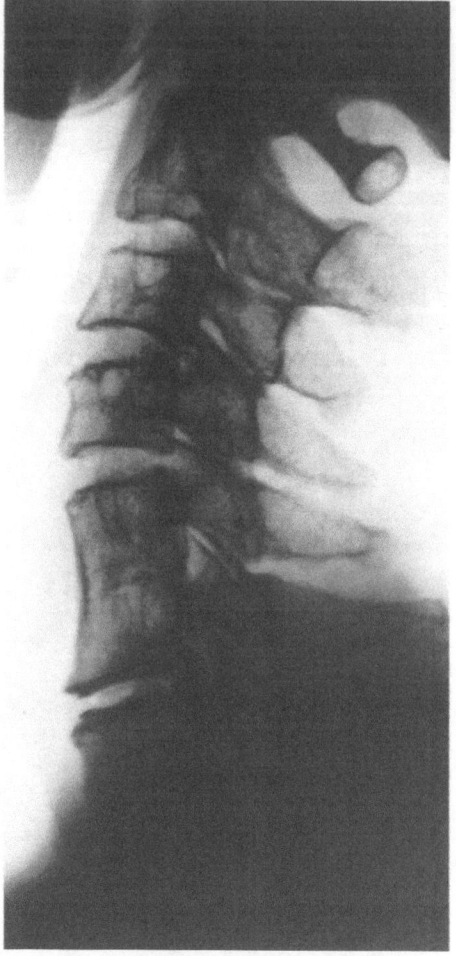

Fig. 4. Case 4, interbody fusion was done at C 5/C 6 without regaining the disc 15 years ago, but she has no difficulty in daily life

Conclusion

It has been concluded by this study that spurs may produce neurologic deficits as well instability and disc protrusion, however, even if spurs are not removed, satisfactory results are obtained by removing other factors.

2.15. Relationship Between Clinical Results and CT After Cervical Spinal Canal Laminoplasty

N. Nakano and T. Nakano, Sapporo, Japan

Since 1978, cervical spinal canal laminoplasties have been performed on fifty-five patients with cervical radiculomyelopathy. Of these patients, thirty-one [two developmental, eleven multiple spondylotic lesions, eighteen ossification of posterior longitudinal ligament (OPLL)] had follow-up studies lasting more than two years, average four years and six months.

Surgical Technique

Under general anesthesia, the patient was placed in a prone position with skull traction. Partial laminectomies were done just medial to the facets by an air drill and this was also used to thin the opposite laminae, near the facets, which were then fractured. This maneuver was performed from C 3 to C 6 in most cases. The laminae were then elevated to the right side, like an opened book. The spinal processes were sutured to the right side of the fascia in order to keep the spinal canal open; then fatty tissue was placed over the dura.

Illustrative Cases

Case 1: K. M. A fifty-eight year-old male had numbness in both hands, including all fingers. The condition worsened until he had difficulty using chopsticks, and he was unable to walk. He was brought by ambulance and admitted to this hospital. An axial tomography revealed OPLL and myosil myelography showed a filling defect from C 3 to C 6. Postoperative axial tomography showed that ossification still occupied a large portion of the spinal canal, but clinical results improved from five points to seventeen points (using the Japanese Orthopaedic Association criteria) over a six year period. In a CT six years after surgery, the dura seemed to be pressed but unlike most, it was not round. Movement of the neck is slightly limited but he has no difficulty in daily life (Fig. 1).

Case 2: T. Y. A sixty-six year-old male had numbness of all extremities until he became unable to walk or use chopsticks. Both of his hands were atrophied and he could not open his fingers. There was atrophy in both shoulders. An axial tomography revealed OPLL. A laminoplasty was done

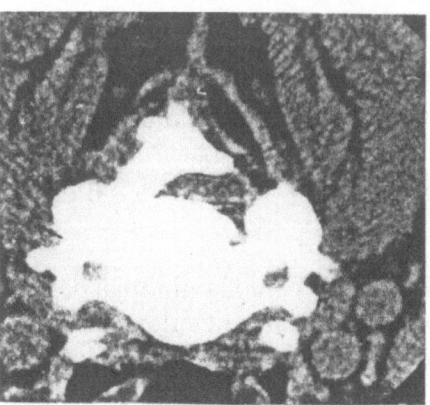

Fig. 1. Case 1, in this CT six years after surgery, the dura seemed to be pressed but clinical results improved from five points to seventeen points

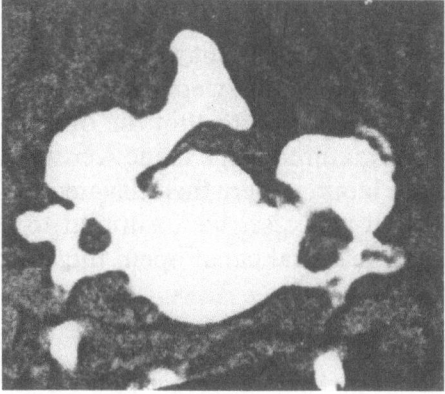

Fig. 2. Case 2, in a four year postoperative CT, ossification still occupies a large portion of the spinal canal but the clinical score improved from three to sixteen points

from C3 to C7. The clinical score improved from three to sixteen points within four years after surgery. Movement of the fingers became normal and the atrophy of the hands diminished. In a four year postoperative CT, ossification still occupied a large portion of the spinal canal. A part of the dura goes into the gap made by the partial laminectomy, but he has no difficulty in his daily life except a slight numbness in his hands (Fig. 2).

Results

Results were evaluated using the Japanese Orthopaedic Association criteria, and a percentage improvement was obtained. Follow-up studies were done on thirty-one patients, observed for more than two years, on average four years and six months.

The overall results of laminoplasty were as follows: Preoperative score was 6.4 and postoperative score was 14.4 and percentage improvement was 77.4%. No case worsened following surgery.

Discussion

Since 1978, we have done laminoplasty by a simple method: a partial laminectomy on the left side and an induced fracture on the right side of the laminae. Then the spinal canal was opened to the right like a book, and a free fatty tissue graft was done to prevent scar tissue going into the spinal canal. Partial laminectomy was always done on the left side. Even when the right side was symptomatic, satisfactory results were obtained.

A fifty-nine year-old patient with OPLL could not close his right hand. Preoperative CT scan showed OPLL on the right side but a partial laminectomy was done on the left side. However, as soon as he awakened from anesthesia, he found he could close his right hand. The spinal cord in a postoperative CT myelography was not round, but he did not have any trouble at all.

A three year postoperative CT of a sixty-five year-old male showed that a large portion of the spinal canal was occupied by OPLL. His symptoms were improved from 0 to thirteen points.

The right lamina fracture sites healed well in all cases and instability was not observed. There was no invasion of scar tissue into the gap which was covered with soft tissue. Therefore, bone grafting was not necessary to obtain stability of the spine.

The recovery from symptoms was quicker than expected, especially when the preoperative period was short. On the other hand, after laminoplasty, even this small enlargement of the spinal canal brought relief. Therefore, improvement may be not due to the degree of enlargement of the spinal canal, but seems to be due to improvement in blood circulation in the spinal canal.

Summary

Since 1978, Cervical Spinal Canal Laminoplasty have been performed on 55 patients with cervical radiculomyelopathy and followed up with studies from two years to six years and two months, which average four years six months in thirty-one cases.

Overall results were as follows: Preoperative score was 6.4, postoperative score 14.4 and the percentage improvement was 77.4%.

Cervical Spine I
© by Springer-Verlag 1987

2.16. Spondylolysis of the Cervical Spine

D. Grob and F. Magerl, St. Gallen, Switzerland

I. Introduction

The occurrence of cervical spondylolysis is extremely rare especially in comparison to its frequency in the lumbar spine. We found only 44 previously reported cases. In our clinic, we have seen 4 cases between 1970 and 1984.

The most common places for defects of the vertebral arch are shown in Fig. 1. The explanation for these deformities is a disturbance in chondrification and ossification in such a way, that the development starts from two isolated nuclei that never fuse [5]. In addition to this teratogenic theory, the localization of the lysis in the lumbar and the cervical spine suggests that a mechanical factor may be involved as well [6]. Both the lower cervical spine and the lower lumbar spine are situated at the base of a mobile, weightbearing lordosis and are thus most susceptible to damage in the posterior parts of the vertebrae [3].

II. Cases

Cases 1 and 2 show a bony defect in the interarticular portion of the sixth cervical vertebra, case 3 had the unilateral lysis on the left portion of the arch of C 4 and patient no. 4 proved to have both lysis in the interarticular portion of C 3 and a complex malformation between the occiput and C 3. This particular case was seen in our emergency room after an accident involving the cervical spine; the actual symptom was acute neck pain after the accident. Case 2 and 3 were referred to us because of chronic cervicobrachialgias. Both patients had a history of bilateral muscular neck pain that had existed for several years and proved to be resistent to every kind of conservative treatment; ; just one (case 1) was involved in a motor vehicle accident with a so-called whiplash injury of the cervical spine, one year before. Since that time he had experienced severe neck pain without neurologic symptoms.

In the two cases with the lysis in C 6 (case 1 and 2) the complaints were severe enough to justify an anterior fusion, one between C 6 and C 7, one including the C 5/C 6- and the C 6/C 7-level because of excessive instability in both segments. The patient with the unilateral lysis of C 4 has continued complain of neck pain but did not feel that the symptoms warranted surgical intervention. Shortly after the accident case 4 was completely asymptomatic, as he had been before the accident in spite of the deformation of the upper cervical spine.

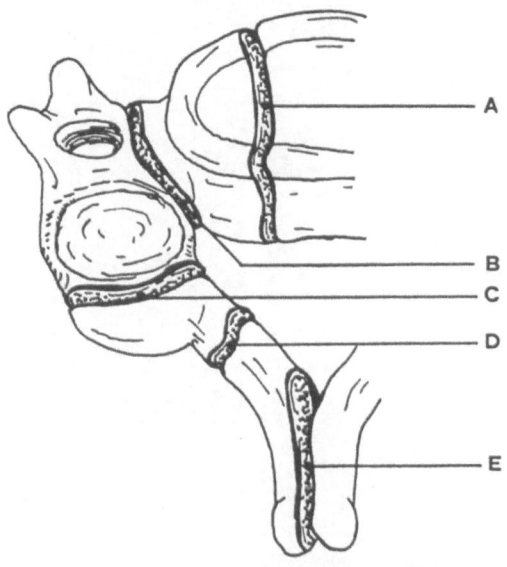

Fig. 1. Localization of possible cleavages of the vertebral arch: *A* Retrosomatic lysis, *B* defect of the pedicle, *C* lysis of interarticular portion, *D* retroisthmic lysis, *E* spina bifida

III. Discussion

The etiology of the isthmic defect is still subject to controversy. The frequent concommitant malformations such as spina bifida or hypoplastic adjacent articular processes favors the teratogenic theory. However, the localization in the most heavily loaded parts of the vertebral column [3] and the nonexistent spondylolysis in very young children [2, 6] tends to support the mechanical theory. Wiltse [6] postulates a fatigue fracture as a possible etiology for the lysis in the lumbar spine. In our opinion, a congenital predisposition may lead to this lysis in the cervical spine. The mechanical factor in the cervical spine is probably less causative then in the lumbar spine, the load of the two different areas being unequal.

The clinical picture of cervical spondylolysis varies from an incidental finding to severe pain. The symptoms described in the literature and in our

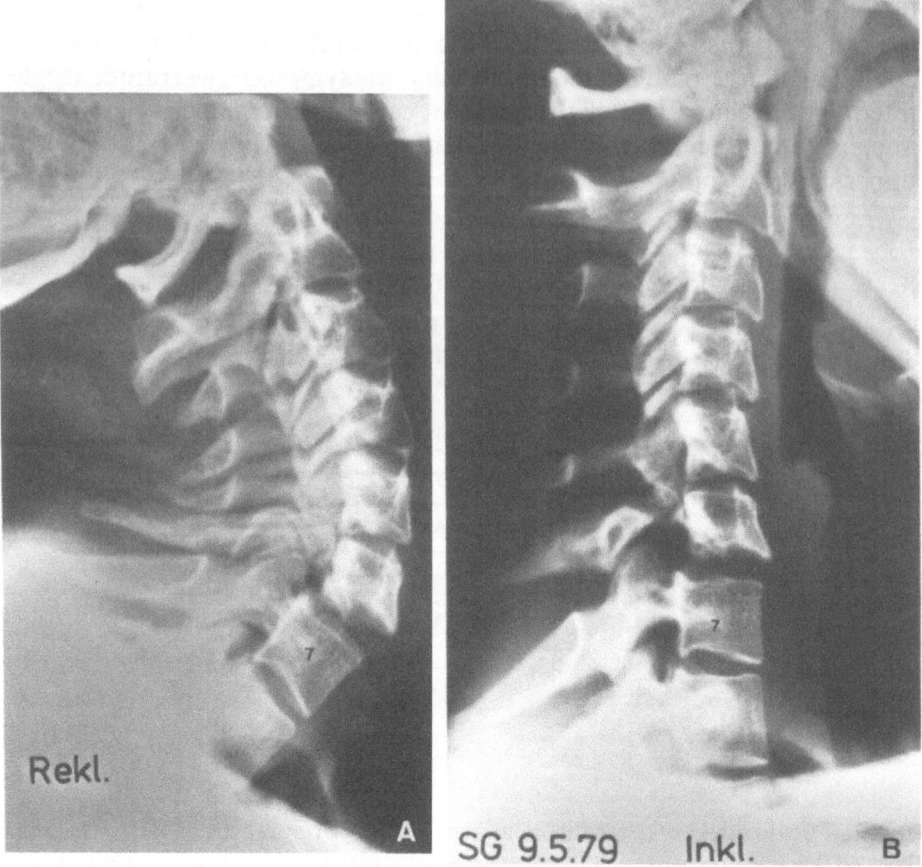

Fig. 2. Instability shown in the functional X-rays of the level of cervical spondylolysis. The defect of C6 causes a slight slipping forward of the body C6 over C7, in addition, the widening of the intervertebral space anteriorly proves the hypermobility

own 4 cases are nonspecific and obviously related to the concomittant instability of the corresponding segments (Fig. 2). The therapies reported vary from simple bedrest to the operative stabilization.

The lysis in the cervical spine is a rare finding. Care must be taken not to misinterprete the lysis as a fracture [1].

References

1. Böhler J (1968) Die Fehldeutung einer cervikalen Spondylolisthesis als Luxationsfraktur. Z Orthop 104: 609–612
2. Charlton OP, Gehweiler JA, Morgan CL, Martinez S, Daffner RH (1978) Spondylolysis and spondylolisthesis of the cervical spine. Skeletal Radiol 3: 79–84

3. Louis R (1982) Chirurgie du rachis, anatomie chirurgicale et voies dabord. Springer, Berlin Heidelberg New York
4. Niemeyer TH, Penning L (1963) Functional roentgenographic examination in a case of cervical spondylolisthesis. J Bone Joint Surg 45 A: 1671–1678
5. Töndury G (1958) Entwicklungsgeschichte und Fehlbildungen der Wirbelsäule. In: Die Wirbelsäule in Forschung und Praxis, Bd 7. Hippokrates-Verlag, Stuttgart
6. Wiltse LL, Widell EH, Jackson DW (1975) Fatigue fracture: the basic lesion in isthmic spondylolisthesis. J Bone Joint Surg 57 A: 17

3. Traumatic Instability and Management

Cervical Spine I
© by Springer-Verlag 1987

3.1. Treatment of Cervical Spine Injuries by a Posterior Osteosynthesis with Plates and Screws

R. Roy-Camille, Ch. Mazel, and G. Saillant, Paris, France

The anatomy of the lower cervical spine is not commonly wellknown. When a posterior fixation is desired we can only see the posterior aspect of the posterior arches. Their shape thus provides knowledge of the anterior elements.

I. Anatomy

The vertebral posterior arch includes the spinous process in the middle with the laminae on both sides and the articular masses more lateral. A groove just like a valley is located at the border between the lamina and the articular mass bulging as a hill. The cord is in front of the spinous process and the laminae. The vertebral artery is in front of the valley and the roots at each level come out the canal through the foraminae. They lie at the level of the articular joint as seen from behind. The fixation plates are placed over the articular masses and the screws are implanted into these masses (Fig. 1).

II. Surgical Procedure

It is easy to implant screws into the articular masses when the exact place of the cord, the vertebral artery and the roots is known. By their lateral position, the screws avoid the cord, and by their implantation into the articular masses and their length they avoid the roots in the foraminae. They also avoid the vertebral artery being lateral to the valley in which it flows.

Surgery is performed through a posterior approach. The patient is in prone position the head firmly fixed in a head holder that enables a flexion-extension range motion. A traction device, if necessary, can be fixed to the operating table. After local xylocaine and adrenaline infiltration, the posterior approach is usually achieved with an electrocuter going down to the lateral side of the articular masses in order to facilitate the finding of the reference marks for implantation of the screws.

The biggest problem in performing this fixation is knowing the exact place to drill and where to implant the screws. This point is located at the top

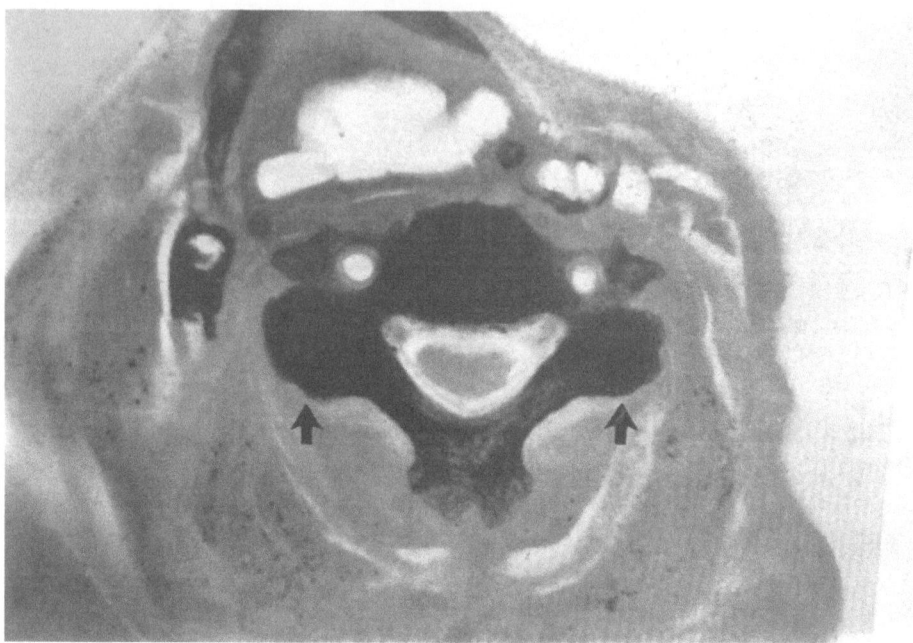

Fig. 1. The cord is in front of the spinous process and the laminae. The vertebral artery in front of the valley. The place to implant a screw is in the middle of the articular mass (arrow)

of the articular mass hill exactly in its middle (Fig. 2). The drilling is done with a 2.8 mm drill when using a 3.6 mm screw. A special drill with a depth gauge prevents it from going too far frontward. A slow motor drill is necessary. The drilling direction is perpendicular to the vertebral plan or 10° oblique laterally but never medially. The lateral obliquity is to increase safety and to avoid the vertebral artery. Performed with such care, we have not noted any complications. It is thus much easier and simplier to implant a screw instead of the wiring technique that is used in some cases and which goes through a hole drilled at the same place into the articular mass. The screws diameter is 3.6 mm and they are 16 or 19 mm long. The plates shape is premoulded to fit the cervical spinal lordosis. They are 2 mm thick, 1 cm wide and the holes are positioned every 13 mm. Usually two plates are symmetrically implanted with 2, 3, 4, or 5 holes depending on the number of vertebrae that have to be fixed.

III. Experimental Study

This study was performed with the help of Rollin Johnson in New Haven at the Veterans Administration Hospital. We have investigated the osteosynthesis mechanical properties in flexion and extension stress.

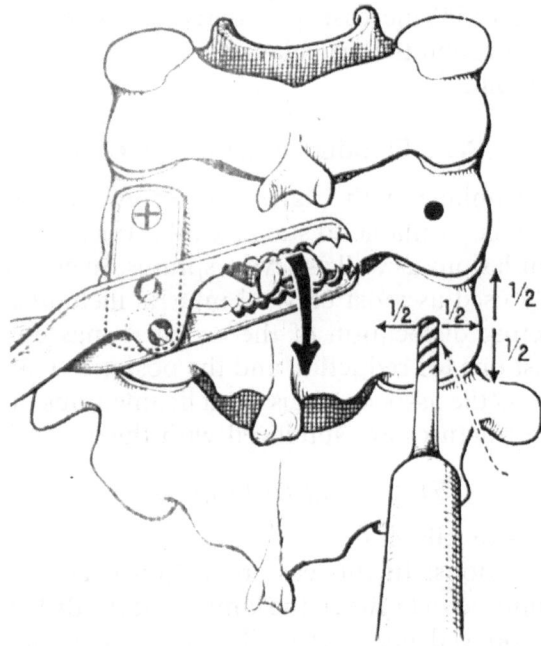

Fig. 2. The place to implant the screw into the articular mass is the middle of it. At the top of the hill. The drilling direction is perpendicular to the vertebral plan or 10° oblique laterally, never medially

Two cervical vertebrae from a fresh cadaver were fixed posteriorly together with a symmetrical pair of two hole plates. The lower vertebra was firmly fixed and stress was applied to the upper vertebra. Displacements were analysed during stress with displacement gauges. The whole experiment was performed in a large glass box in order to keep a constant hygrometric level and to stay as close as possible to *in vivo* characteristics.

Displacements were measured as well as radiographed. All the results have been computerized.

The average breaking load in extension stress is 52.5 kg (515 N). This represents 60% of the load necessary to dislocate two normal cervical vertebrae. These results have been compared with the other methods of cervical posterior fixation. For an extension stress, a posterior wiring of the spinous processes or in the articular masses is inefficient in stabilization the spine. The posterior plates fixation gives an increase of 60% to the normal stability. A methylmetacrylate fixation on the spinous processes gives a 99% increase in stability.

For a flexion stress the posterior wiring between the spinous processes gives a 33% increase in stability, the same wiring but around a complementary bone graft gives a 55% increase in stability, the increase is of 88% when the wiring is going through the articular masses. The plate fixation gives a 92% increase in stability.

IV. Posterior Spinal Plate Fixation in the Lower Cervical Spine Injuries

This surgical technique with plates and screws implanted into the articular masses will be available to stabilize all cervical spine injuries with prevailing posterior lesions as well as severe sprains. In current practice this technique is widely used as most cervical injuries include a dislocation, a fracture, or a fracture dislocation of the articular masses. The posterior approach is the best one for reduction and the posterior plates stabilize the bony lesion as well as the associated disc and ligamentous injuries. We also saw that tear-drop fractures are stabilized with this posterior fixation.

a) Cervical Dislocations

They can be uni- or bilateral.

Unilateral dislocations: In this case reduction is achieved operatively with spatulae introduced in between the laminae at the dislocated level. The first spatula is introduced near the midline against the spinous process. While the first spatula is kept in place a second one is introduced laterally then the first one is placed further on in between the dislocated articular masses. At that moment a tire level manoeuvre enables the reduction, pulling backwards the upper articular mass onto the lower one. The reduction is maintained by the table head holder pushing in extension. A first posterior plate is placed on the dislocated side, then the fixation is completed by a second plate on the other side.

Bilateral dislocations: The same manoeuvre is performed on both sides symmetrically. Once more the stabilization is given by two posterior plates. The dislocations being a one level injury it only needs a fixation of the upper vertebra on the lower vertebra with 2 hole posterior plates.

We always perform this type of treatment on an emergency basis without previous traction. We also prefer open reduction because it allows a much better control and it is performed with extreme smoothness.

b) Facet Joint Fracture and Dislocation

When a facet joint fracture is combined with a dislocation it is usually a fracture of the upper articular facet. Its displacement follows an upper vertebra one. It allows a rotation of the cervical spine and a characteristic subluxation. Two problems have thus to be solved:

— The fixation which is difficult because the stabilization given by the articular facet is missing.

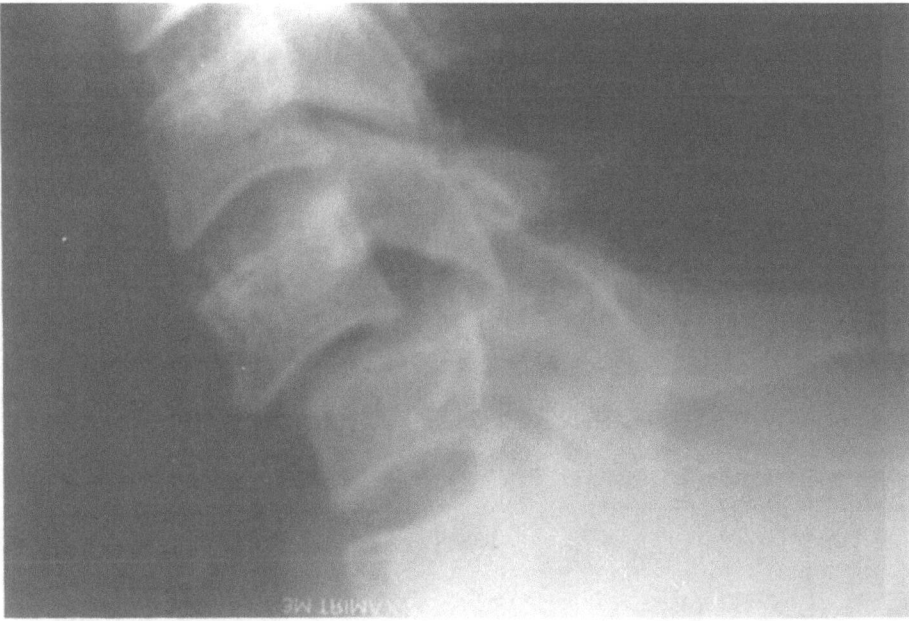

Fig. 3. A) The lateral view easily enables the diagnosis of an C 5–C 6 dislocation. B) The AP view shows that the left C 6 articular mass is horizontal (arrow). This is very specific to the separation fracture of the articular masses. C) and D) The ¾ oblique views demonstrate that the C 6 articular mass separation fracture is associated with a unilateral dislocation. E) and F) The stabilization is given by a "coat-hanger" with a tile plate and a posterior fixation of C 5–C 6–C 7. G) The oblique view shows the quality of the reduction, reconstruction and stabilization. It is interesting to see that the screws are never going into the foraminae

— The cure of a cervico-brachial neuralgia induced by the displacement of the broken fragment into the foramina compressing the root.

Fixation is achieved with a reconstruction of the broken articular facet. Special plates having a tile shape make such a reconstruction possible. It is a real joint arthroplasty. The upper part of the plate is oblique and is slipped between the facet joints, the lower part is fixed in the articular mass. At the beginning of our experience the plate was first used alone, we now prefer to combine a tile plate with a standard one. The plates are placed one on another like a "coat hanger". These combined posterior plates enable us to stabilize the joint being implanted into the upper and the lower vertebrae.

If a fragment is displayed into the foramina producing root compression it is necessary to remove it before performing the "coat hanger" fixation.

c) Separation-fracture of the Articular Mass

This fracture is difficult to stabilize (Fig. 3). There are in fact two fracture lines. The first one is on the pedicle, the second one is on the laminae on the

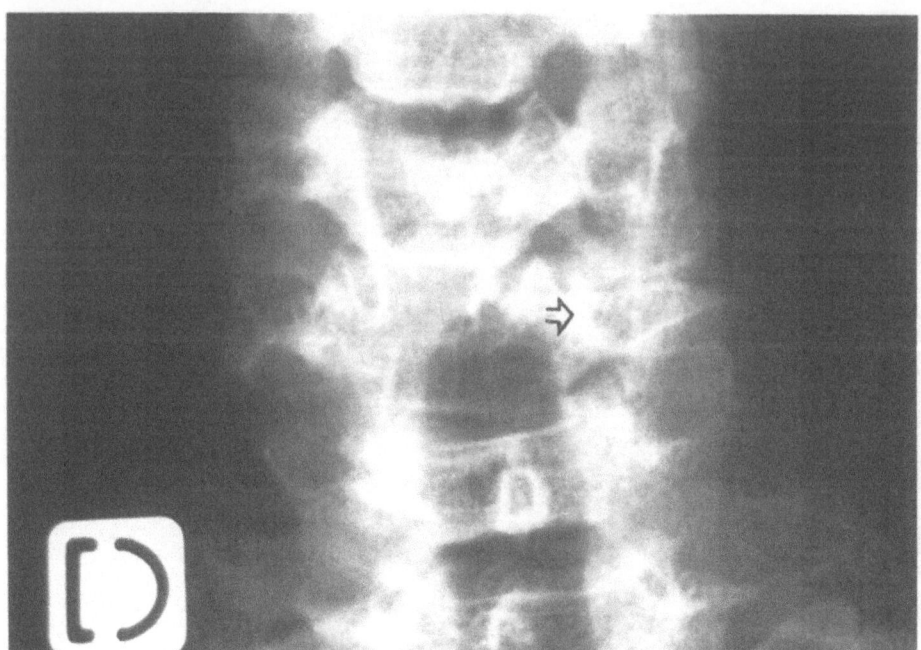

Fig. 3 B

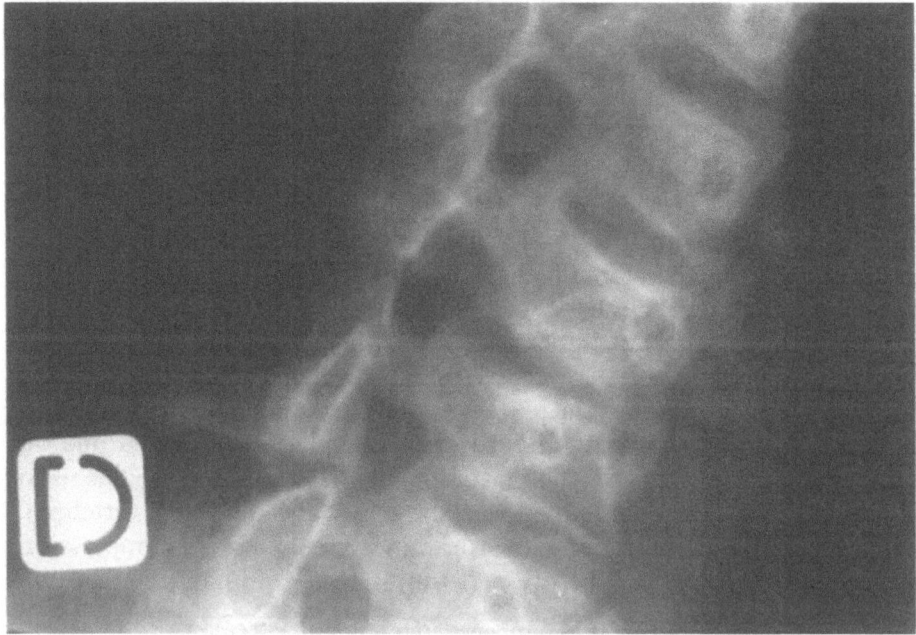

Fig. 3 C

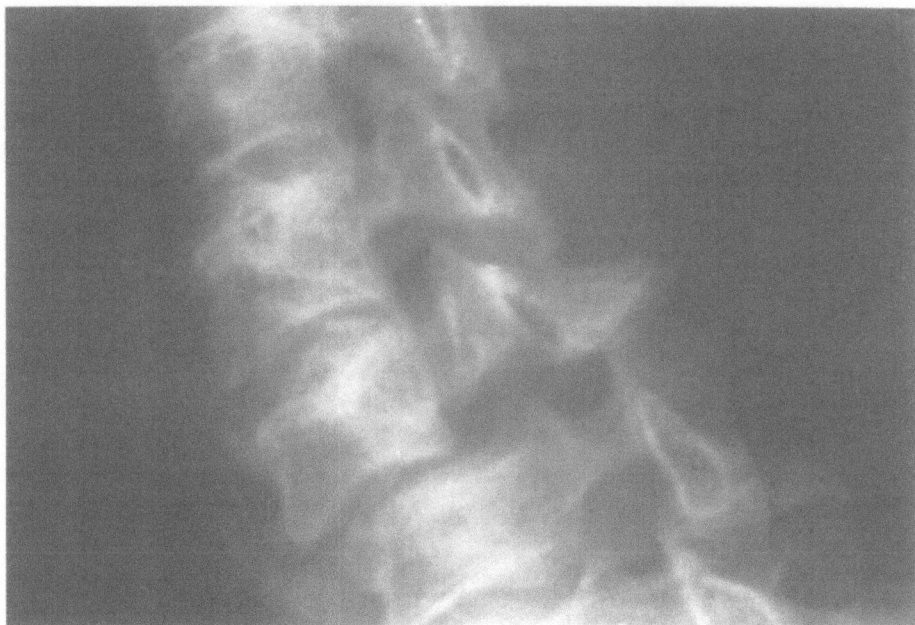

Fig. 3 D

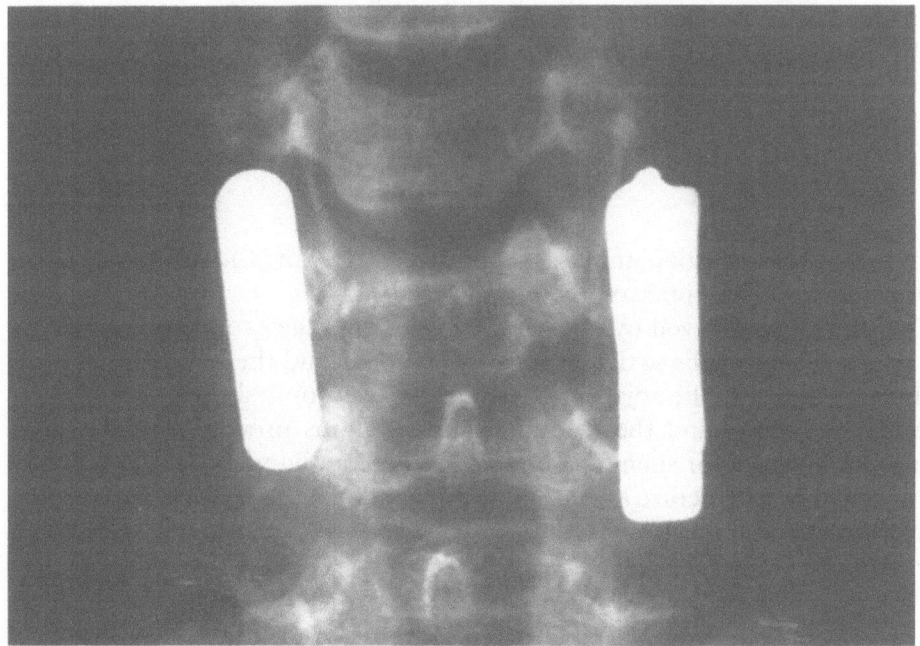

Fig. 3 E

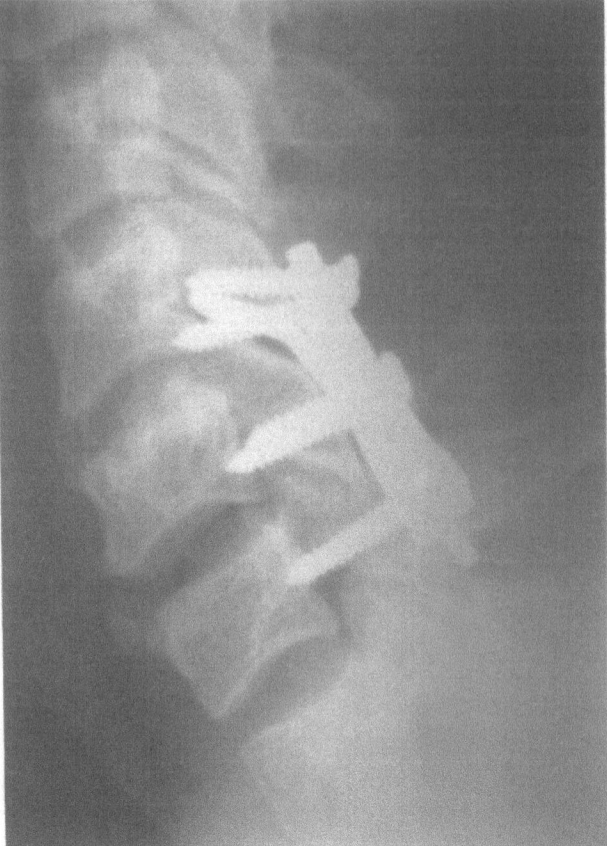

Fig. 3 F

same side. Thus the articular mass is completely free from the vertebra and it will rotate with the upper or the lower vertebra.

The diagnosis is given by oblique views showing the broken pedicle and the displacement of the articular mass. The upper and the lower facets are no longer parallel to the adjacent ones. The AP-view only shows the fracture line on the lamina and the rotation of the spinous process. The correct fixation procedure for such fractures is also a "coat hanger" on the side of the articular mass fracture and a simple plate on the other side. It gives both reduction and stabilization.

d) Tear Drop Fracture

It is more a severe sprain than a fracture. The lesions are more on the disc and the ligaments than on the body with its low anterior corner fracture. Instability comes from a severe sprain. When the injury is mostly posterior

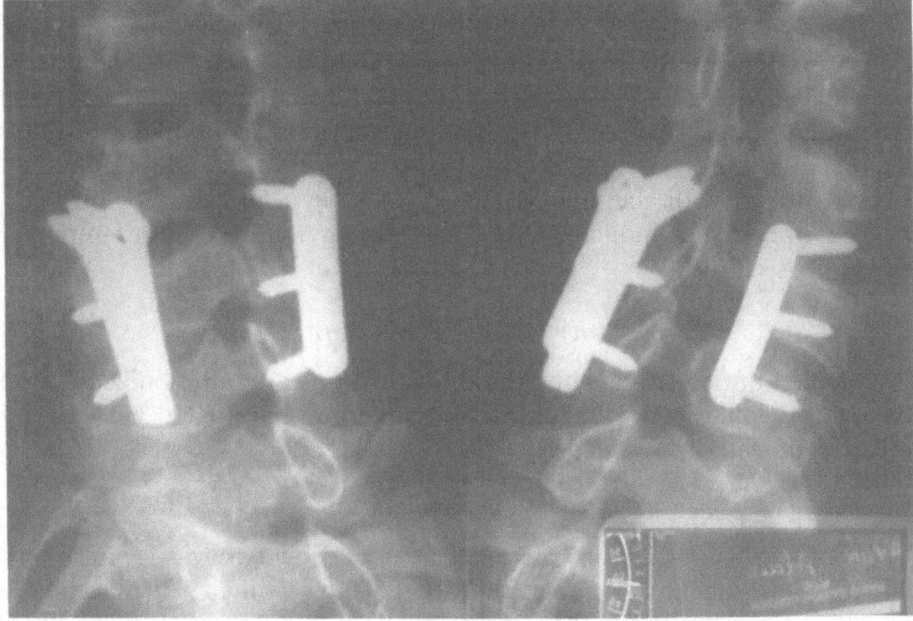

Fig. 3 G

with an interspinous widening and a facet joint posterior opening, the surgical treatment can be performed posteriorly with posterior plates as in the following cases.

e) Severe Sprains

These need to be well investigated. The injury is only a soft tissue one. From the back to the front there is an injury without complete tear of the interspinous ligament, the articular facet joint ligaments, ligamentum flavum, the posterior vertebral ligament, the disc and the anterior vertebral ligament. Induced by the continuous mobilization of the neck the displacement only occurs a few weeks or months later: interspinous widening, facet joint subluxation, disc posterior opening, anterior listhesis of the upper vertebra. The posterior plates and screws fixation is a perfect technique for stabilization of these lesions.

f) Cervical Spine Mal Unions

When there is a local kyphosis with posterior fusion between the articular masses, without any anterior bony bridge, the posterior approach for reduction and fixation with plates and screws is once more well indicated. Preoperative traction shows if there is still any local mobility and surgery will thus be performed. The first step is to remove the callus between the posterior elements then to reduce and to fix the injured level with two plates.

g) Complementary Procedures

The posterior approach and the use of posterior plates enable different associated procedures to be undertaken. A laminectomy is easily performed because the plates are lateral to the laminae on the articular masses. Most of the time fusion occurs simply by the posterior approach and fixation, but a Hibb's fusion on the laminae is always possible if necessary or desired.

The only contraindication to this plating method is an important osteoporosis.

h) Postoperative Care

Simple injuries such as unilateral dislocations are immobilized 6 weeks by a simple collar. More unstable lesions are immobilized 2 to 3 months by a minerva corset.

i) Results

A study of a continuous series of 221 cases of lower cervical spine injuries treated by this technique shows that there is no secondary displacement in 85.2% of the cases. When there is a displacement it is 5° and less in 8.8%, 5° to 10° in 3%, over 10° in 3%.

V. Posterior Spinal Plate Fixation in Upper Cervical Spine Injuries

Plates and screws can also be used for the treatment of upper cervical spine injuries.

a) Occipito-Cervical Dislocations

To stabilize them it is necessary to perform an occipito-cervical fixation and fusion. For this purpose we use special premoulded plates. Their shape is designed to fit the normal curve of the occipito-cervical junction. They are reinforced in their middle at the top of the curve. Two plates are placed, lateral and symmetrical. The fixation to the occiput is done using 13 mm long screws. At cervical level the fixation is achieved with screws into the articular masses as usual. Some plates are short, going down to C 4, others are longer, going to C 5. In most cases an occipito-cervical dislocation is a fatal injury. If the patient does not died, diagnosis is difficult. Thus we have seen a case one year after the trauma with minimum neurological involvement. The computerized tomography was the best complementary examination showing the displacement between the occipital condyles and the atlas. The myelography showed the cord compression against the dens. In such cases with little neurological involvement a simple occipito-cervical fixation and fusion is enough. The bone graft is laid against the occiput and the posterior arches between the 2 plates. In other old cases with neurological involvement, after posterior occipito-cervical stabilization it is necessary to make a dens resection using an anterio-lateral or a transoral approach.

b) Tear Drop Fracture of C 2

If there is important instability, such fractures have to be fixed by an occipito-cervical fusion. In case of a lesser instability a simple C 2–C 3 stabilization is enough. This fixation is then performed with two posterior plates, the screws going into C 2 pedicles and C 3 articular masses.

c) Hangman's Fracture

When the displacement is minimum and the fracture stable, healing will occur with a minerva corset. On the contrary when there is an important disc or ligament injury between C 2 and C 3, or a complete C 2–C 3 posterior dislocation, surgical fixation is necessary. The reduction is best achieved through a posterior approach, the fixation is performed with pedicular screws going into C 2 pedicles and 2 posterior plates to stabilize C 2 and C 3.

The most difficult step of this surgical technique is the positioning of the screws into C 2 pedicles. When C 2 articular mass is seen from behind it can be divided into four quarters. The vertebral artery is in front of the two lateral ones and the lower medial one. The only free quarter is the upper medial. This is the place where the screw should go in. The entry point must be high and medial on the articular mass. The screw will go along the pedicle. Its direction is controlled with a spatula introduced medially into the spinal canal. It enables visualization of the pedicle's medial aspect. The drilling into the pedicle is thus performed under visual control.

d) Jefferson Fractures

The fracture line goes anteriorly through C 1 anterior arch and posteriorly through the posterior arch. Such a fracture line gives an opening of the C 1 ring. Most of the time fusion occurs with orthopedic treatment and a minerva corset. When the displacement is important with a bilateral C 1–C 2 facet joint dislocation, reduction and surgical fixation are necessary. One of the best ways to reach the C 1–C 2 facet joint is an anterolateral approach through the sternocleidomastoid muscle. This approach is done bilaterally, in the supine position, by two surgeons. They will make a dissection going in front of C 1 transverse process and thus easily reach the C 1–C 2 joints. The reduction is obtained by a bilateral push on both sides of C 1 ring. The fixation may be performed with an anterior plate slipped in front of the C 1 anterior arch, after dissection of the retropharyngeal space, or by a bilateral screws going through the C 1–C 2 joints.

VI. Conclusion

Most cervical spine injuries have prevailing posterior lesions. This is why we frequently advocate for a posterior approach and reduction. The quality of the posterior plate and screw fixation is another element in this choice. But we are absolutely aware that anterior lesions exist. In such cases we shall perform a standard anterior approach and interbody fusion.

3.2. Double Hole Plate Fixation of the Lower Cervical Spine

R. STRELI, Linz, Austria

In a former series different types of plates were used for fixation of the cervical spine.

To improve stability in osteosynthesis double perforated plates were used with even and odd number of holes and different lengths.

They are attached to the vertebral bodies with TKFS 6.5 mm diameter screws.

This provides the following advantages:

1. Firm hold due to the spongious screws, which in contrast to small fragment screws, give a firm grip even in osteoporotic bone. A third of a thread perforating the posterior wall of the vertebral body increases stability.

2. With one type of plate it was nearly always possible to insert two screws in one vertebral body.

3. Lateral stability is good.

4. Short segment stabilization is facilitated.

So far 48 cases have been operated upon. The average age was 40 years, the youngest 16 and the oldest 84 years. The first case dated from June 12, 1981. We used 40 steel plates and 8 titanium plates.

So far 23 plates have been removed.

The Surgical Approach

Using a transverse incision in a cervical skin fold from the midline to the right; the skin was dissected 4 cm upwards and downwards. The platysma was cut longitudinally 1 cm medial to the lateral border of the sternohyoid muscle, for cosmetic reasons.

The dissection downwards to the vertebrae is followed by excision of the anterior longitudinal ligament, annulus fibrosus and removal of the disc. Reduction, uncusectomy and the removal of median spurs can now be carried out. Transversectomy can also now be performed using the same approach. Afterwards a 1 mm layer of the adjacent chondral plates is removed to a breadth of 16 mm. The homologous Robinson cube is cut to

R. Streli:

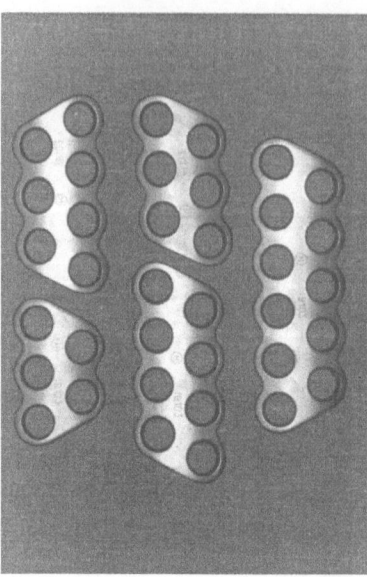

Fig. 1. Titan double perforated plates of different lengths with even and odd number of holes

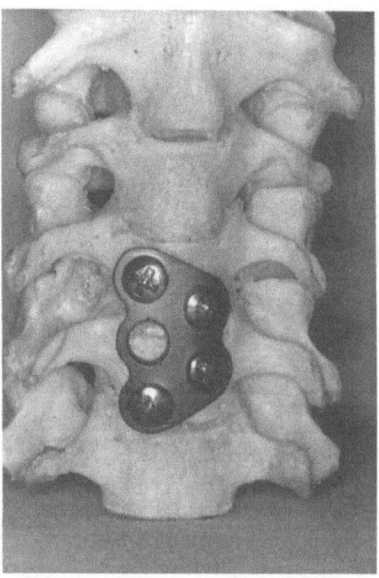

Fig. 2. ⅔ double hole plate mounted on a specimen from a cadaver. One segment spondylodesis. Two TKFS screws in each of the adjacent cervical vertebral bodies

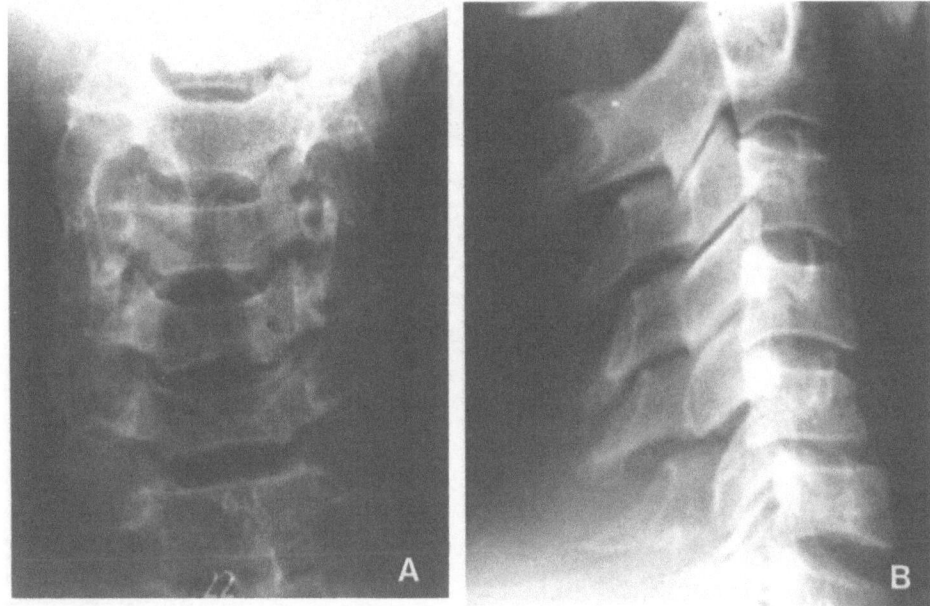

Fig. 3 A, B. Sch. U., 42 years, case 26, UL 24433/83, was thrown to the ground by an enraged horse. This resulted in a fracture subluxation C V/C VI with subtotal quadruplegia. It was not the object to demonstrate the original amount of dislocation. Careful examination with the X-ray intensifier revealed, that the dislocation following the injury was grater than documented in the above X-ray

size and shape and inserted and now the double perforated plate is applied.

Due to its transverse curvature the plate usually fits well to cervical vertebral bodies in different horizontal planes. As a rule lordotic bending is necessary to adapt in the sagittal plane.

The following cases demonstrate the application.

T. H. This 49 years old farmer, who fell into a silo and as a result suffered a dislocation C IV–V. After 7 weeks conservative treatment with a Minerva-cast in a well reduced position there was a recurrence of dislocation and paraparesis superior. After open reduction, removal of the ruptured disc including the extruded parts of it a Robinson spondylodesis followed. A 5/5 double perforated plate was used for osteosynthesis because of the multifragment fracture of C V.

A bony union of C V–VI was obtained without external fixation.

A complete recovery from neurologic deficit and the resumption of normal work as a "mountain farmer" resulted. The plate was removed 14 month after implantation.

A. M. A 45 years old Gynaecologist with a three weeks old rotation subluxation C V–VI. Computerized tomography revealed stenosis of the

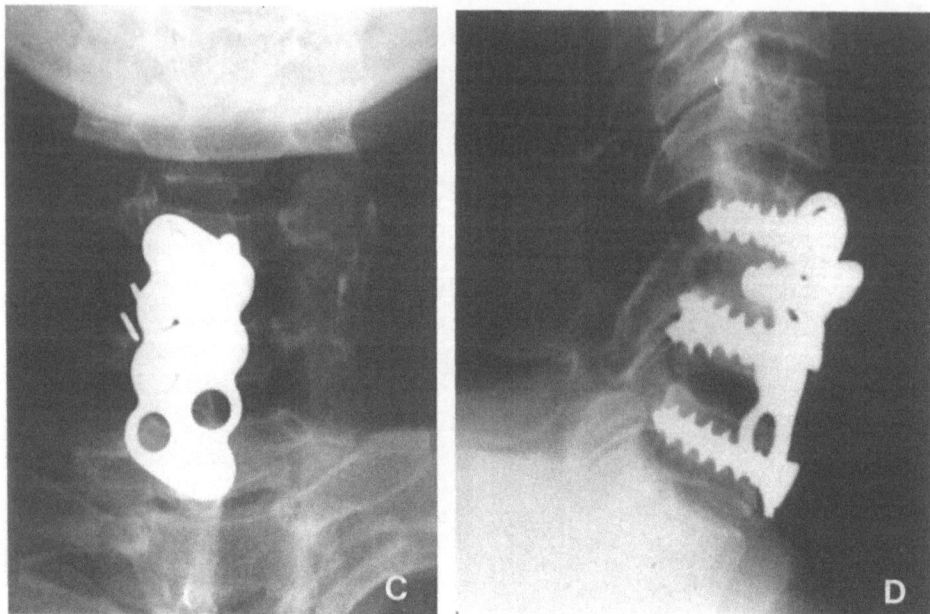

Fig. 3 C, D. AP and lateral view after reduction, Robinson spondylodesis with a
homologous bone block followed by double perforated plate stabilization.
Fragments displaced in the vertebral canal were removed anteriorly. Note further
the overcorrection C V/C VI, *i.e.* increase of distance C V/C VI

vertebral canal, favorized by preexisting spurs. After open reduction,
Robinson spondylodesis and double perforated plate stabilization was
carried out. There was no external fixation.

After six month the plate was removed. A solid bony block C V–VI was
observed. A residue of sensory disturbance in the first interdigital fold right
side remained.

K. E. This 46 years old man suffered from increasing quadruparesis due
to secondary myelopathy caused by posterior median spurs in the course of
cervical spondylosis.

Discs and osteophytes C III–IV and C IV–V were removed and
Robinson spondylodesis performed.

Double perforated plate stabilization C III–V was completed and one
year later both spondylodeses were firmly united and the plate removed.

Both the lower paraparesis and the limp disappeared and the superior
paraparesis improved.

Sch. U. 42 years old champion lady rider (Fig. 3) was repeatedly thrown
to the ground by an enraged horse and suffered a fracture subluxation C V–
C VI with subtotal quadruplegia. Primary reduction and osteosynthesis

were performed. The Robinson spondylodesis united firmly and the plate was removed 17 months later. We think that the early reduction and immobilization of the cord lesion was primarily responsible for the extensive level of recovery. A peronaeus type of neurological deficit remains.

3.3. Unstable Injuries of the Lower Cervical Spine

J. KIWERSKI, Konstancin K/Warszawy, Poland

In the years 1965–1983, 856 patients with spinal injuries in the C 5–Th 1 segment were treated in the early posttraumatic period at the Rehabilitation Clinic at Konstancin. 454 of these patients (53%) had unstable injuries. Table 1 presents the level of injury and mechanism of spinal injury. In the analyzed material the isolated fractures of the vertebrae were mainly of a compression form (84%), while the injury to the intervertebral space was mainly through a flexion mechanism (78%). Unstable injuries most frequently involved the C 6–C 7 intervertebral space.

Table 1. *Level and Trauma Mechanism of Spinal Injuries*

Level of spinal injury	Trauma mechanism			Total
	flexion	compressive	extension	
C 5	33	101	—	134
C 5–C 6	172	2	55	229
C 6	21	129	—	150
C 6–C 7	204	—	52	256
C 7	3	60	—	63
C 7–D 1	21	—	3	24
Total	454	292	110	856

Table 2 presents the degree of spinal cord injury and the type of injury. Unstable (flexion) and stable injuries comprising injuries through extension and compression mechanisms have been distinguished. Partial injuries of the spinal cord have traditionally been classified into three groups [2, 4], similar to Frankel's division [1]:

1. motor paralysis with at least traceable deep sensitivity in feet preserved,

Table 2. *Classification Spinal Cord Injury*

Spinal cord injuries on admission		Type of injury		Total
		stable	unstable	
Complete		144	228	372
	1	68	52	120
Incomplete	2	71	50	121
	3	84	97	181
Without neurological involvement		35	27	62
Total		402	454	856

2. massive pareses (the strength of paretic muscles below 3° acc. to Lovett's scale),

3. pareses of lesser intensity.

It follows from the Table that the difference in the degree of spinal cord injuries in stable and unstable injuries is slight. Complete lesions of the spinal cord in unstable injuries make up to 50% of cases and are slightly less frequent in stable injuries—36% of cases. The quantitative differences in the group of patients without neurological disorders are also small. The great numbers of complete and severe lesions in stable injuries were due to the compression fractures denoted as "explosion" fractures which (as a rule) are accompanied by severe damage to the spinal cord. There was a high frequency of these fractures in our study.

Table 3 presents the incidence of stable and instable injuries in particular age groups. It follows from the Table that stable injuries are more frequent

Table 3. *Incidence of Stable/Unstable Injuries in Different Age Groups*

Age	Type of injury		Total
	stable	unstable	
To 20	97	39	136
21–35	161	94	255
36–50	59	140	199
51–65	49	119	168
Over 65	36	62	98
Total	402	454	856

J. Kiwerski:

found in younger patients as opposed to unstable injuries which are found in older people. The average age of patients with stable injuries was 35 years, whereas in instable injuries it was 46 years. 64% of patients with stable injuries were under 35 years of age, whereas 71% of patients with unstable injuries were over 35 years of age.

Methods of Treatment

The basic methods of treatment together with the types of spinal injuries are presented in Table 4. In total, conservative treatment was applied in 53% of the cases. In stable and unstable injuries conservative treatment was applied in 60 and 46% of the cases, respectively. In the stable injury group the overwhelming majority of the surgical patients were patients with explosion fractures of the vertebral body and surgery aimed at an early decompression of the spinal cord and blood vessels [6].

Table 4. *Treatment of Spinal Injuries*

Type of injury	Treatment				
	conservative			surgical	
	skull traction	collar	func-tional	anterior approach	posterior approach
Stable	146	91	5	155	5
Unstable	187	22	—	224	21
Total	333	113	5	379	26

Skull traction is a method frequently used in the treatment of the discussed injuries, and was applied as the main method of treatment in 39% of cases, and in numerous cases served as a preliminary form of treatment with subsequent surgical decompression of the spinal cord and spinal fusion.

Results of Treatment

Results of treatment are presented in Table 5 and are based on the comparison of the neurological status on admission and on completion of the treatment. The results are presented to compare and to contrast stable and unstable spinal injuries. In total, neurological improvement was achieved in 58% of patients with neurological disorders. Neurological

Table 5. *Neurological Status Before and After Treatment*

Neurological status before-after treatment	Type of injury		Total
	stable	unstable	
C to 3	5	3	8
C to 2	8	6	14
C to 1	6	8	14
1 to norm	1	2	3
1 to 3	36	29	65
1 to 2	18	16	34
2 to norm	12	16	28
2 to 3	48	28	76
3 to norm	62	83	145
3 to 3	21	13	34
2 to 2	6	5	11
1 to 1	8	4	12
C to C	84	139	223
Norm to norm	35	27	62
Mortality in complete	41	72	113
Mortality in partial	11	3	14

(C=complete; 1, 2, 3=Frankel classification [1]; norm=normal neurological status)

improvement was obtained in 62% and 54% of the stable and unstable spinal injuries, respectively. Considerable neurological recovery, of at least two degrees on our scale, was slightly more frequently observed in stable than as opposed to unstable injuries (20 and 16%, respectively). The mortality rate in unstable injuries was about 17% a little higher than in stable injuries (13%). This is probably due to a greater number of patients admitted with symptoms of complete spinal cord injury in the group of unstable injuries [5].

Discussion

In our observations the differences between the stable and unstable spinal injuries with respect to the spinal cord injury and achieved neurological improvement are not great. The differences seem to be much more significant if dislocations are compared with "pure" forms of compression spinal injuries. Both explosion fractures [3] and injuries through extension mechanism [7] are frequently complicated by complete or massive lesions of the spinal cord. The stability of such injuries may also be questioned. Injuries through extension mechanism remain stable provided that the spine is maintained in an "in-between" position. Another hyperextensive movement poses a threat of body displacement since the anterior longitudinal ligament is ruptured. Stability of the spine in an explosion injury is not full, either although the continuity of the ligamentous elements is preserved. The question arises, however, as to whether those ligamentous elements are able to fulfil their tasks since the joint is crushed and often comprises displaced elements.

It seems therefore advisable that, while considering the stability of an injured spine, the above discussed injuries should be considered separately, and not together with typical compression injuries which are definitely stable.

References

1. Frankel HL, Hancock DO, Melzak J, Michaelis LS, Ungar GH, Vernon JDS, Walsh JJ (1969) The value of postural reduction in the initial management of closed injuries of the spine with paraplegia and tetraplegia. Paraplegia 7: 179–192
2. Haftek J, Rudnicki SZ, Kiwerski J (1968) Acute trauma of the cervical segment of the spinal cord. In: Compensation of the spinal cord function. PZWL Warszawa, pp 75–86
3. Kiwerski J (1980) Cervical spine injuries caused by diving into water. Paraplegia 18: 101–105
4. Kiwerski J, Weiss M (1981) Neurological improvement in traumatic injuries of the cervical spine. Paraplegia 19: 31–37
5. Kiwerski J, Weiss M, Chrostowska T (1981) Analysis of mortality of patients after cervical spine trauma. Paraplegia 19: 347–351
6. Kiwerski J (1982) Anterior interbody fusion in treatment of cervical spine traumas. Int Orthop 6: 255–258
7. Kiwerski J (1984) Lesions to the spine resulting from the falling down from the horse cart. Pol Tyg Lek 39: 1063–1065

3.4. Treatment of Unstable Cervical Spine Injuries with Halo Vest

A. NORDWALL, B. LIND, and H. SIHLBOM, Göteborg, Sweden

Traditional conservative treatment of unstable cervical spine fractures has, for ages, been bedrest and skull traction. Primary healing by such conservative treatment has, by different authors, been reported to be between 90–95% [1, 2, 4, 12].

The alternative has been stabilizing surgery by an anterior or posterior approach. This is performed with the aim of obtaining open exact reduction of the dislocation and safe maintenance of the reduced position as well as fast ambulation of the patient. However, in the operative series, there is also a certain incidence of nonunions, and the rate of serious complications has, in some instances, been reported to be quite high, in particular with the anterior approach [6, 7, 11]. On the other hand, Halo vest treatment of traumatic unstable cervical spine injuries combines the advantages of nonoperative treatment with those of active surgical stabilization for maintenance of reduction and early ambulation without complications [3, 5, 8, 9, 10].

This technique has been routinely used at our orthopedic department since 1976. In a prospective, consecutive series, 71 patients with unstable traumatic cervical spine injuries were treated with Halo vest stabilization during the period June 1976 to May 1984. A follow-up was performed one year after the end of the treatment. The age of the patients ranged from 13 to 81 years with a mean age of 37 years. 54 patients had fracture dislocations and 17 had ligament injuries without fractures. The injuries were distributed along the entire cervical spine from C 1 to C 7, including 13 fractures of the odontoid process. 24 patients (34%) had spinal cord injury, 6 of these (8%) were complete tetraplegias and 15 patients (21%) had nerve root symptoms.

Treatment was initiated immediately on admission of the patient to hospital: A Halo ring was fitted after the injury was diagnosed to be unstable. Initial reduction of the dislocation was performed by Halo traction. A vest was fitted and attached to the Halo during traction, usually within 24 hours after the admission. Those patients who were neurologically intact and who did not have any other serious injury were immediately ambulated after the Halo vest application. They were discharged from the hospital on average 10 days after the injury.

Halo vest treatment was continued for 12 weeks. At the end of this time healing was checked by lateral radiograms in functional testing in flexion and extension on three occasions: 12 weeks, 16 weeks and 1 year after the injury. The injury was considered to be healed when there was no or normal motion in the injured segment. In five patients (7%), the Halo vest apparatus could not maintain the fracture reduction and redislocation occurred during the treatment. One of these injuries was surgically stabilized by a posterior fusion, the others were again reduced and stabilized in the Halo vest and healed after full length of treatment. The total healing rate in this series was 92%, *i.e.* 65 patients healed by Halo vest treatment. In 3 patients (4%), there was still instability after 12 weeks of Halo vest treatment and another 3 patients (4%) developed late instability. These injuries were surgically fused. One of these was a type II odontoid fracture. However, 12 of the 13 odontoid fractures did heal, a healing rate of 92% in this fracture which is known to be difficult to heal with conservative methods. All root symptoms in 15 patients resolved completely. 75% of those patients with complete spinal cord injury improved neurologically regaining at least one nerve root level. 63% of the patients with incomplete spinal cord injury regained major motor function, *e.g.* walking ability. There were no neurological deterioration and no other serious complications.

In our hands, the Halo vest proved to be a very effective stabilizing tool for the injured unstable cervical spine. The ease of application, few complications and the fast ambulation that was possible for these patients made the Halo vest very suitable for our demands. It proved to be at least as effective in providing stability as conventional traction methods and superior to these regarding healing rate in particular for odontoid process fractures. These results are in accordance with the experience by others [3, 5, 9, 10]. We found the Halo vest to be an effective and safe alternative to surgical fusion in most cases of unstable cervical spine injuries. The Halo vest will continue to be our method of choice for treatment of these injuries in our department.

References

1. Bedbrook GM (1969) Are cervical spine fractures ever unstable? J West Pac Orthop Assoc 6: 7–29
2. Burke DC, Tiong TS (1975) Stability of the cervical spine after conservative treatment. Paraplegia 13: 191–202
3. Chan RC, Schweigel JF, Thompson GB (1983) Halothoracic brace immobilization in 188 patients with acute cervical spine injuries. J Neurosurg 58: 508–515

4. Cheshire DJE (1969) The stability of the cervical spine following the conservative treatment of fractures and fracture dislocations. Paraplegia 7: 193–203
5. Cooper PR, Maravilla KR, Sklar FH, Moody SF, Clark WK (1979) Halo immobilization of cervical spine fractures. J Neurosurg 50: 603–610
6. Guttman L (1969) Spinal deformities in traumatic paraplegics and tetraplegics following surgical procedures. Paraplegia 7: 38–49
7. Kraus DR, Stauffer ES (1975) Spinal cord injury as a complication of elective anterior cervical fusion. Clin Orthop 112: 130–141
8. Lyddon DW, Jr (1974) Experience with the Halo and body cast in the ambulatory treatment of cervical spine fractures. Ill Med J 146: 458–461
9. Schweigel JF (1979) Halo-thoracic brace management of odontoid fractures. Spine 4: 192–194
10. Seljeskog EL (1978) Nonoperative management of acute upper cervical injuries. Acta Neurochir (Wien) 41: 87–100
11. Stauffer ES, Ketty EG (1977) Fracture—dislocations of the cervical spine. Instability and recurrent deformity following treatment by anterior interbody fusion. J Bone Joint Surg 59-A: 45–48
12. White AA, Southwick WO, Panjabi MM (1976) Clinical instability in the lower cervical spine. A review of past and current concepts. Spine 1: 15–27

Cervical Spine I
© by Springer-Verlag 1987

3.5. Anatomo-pathological Study of Cervical Spine Trauma Treatment and Results

J. P. Lemaire, J. F. Couaillier, G. Braud, and E. Laloux, Dijon, France

On account of the numerous cervical spine injuries and varying treatment concepts, we propose an anatomo-pathological classification in order to try and to improve accurate therapeutic indications.

I. Anatomo-Pathology

The skull acting as a "pendulum" is a peculiar feature of cervical spine trauma, so that the "Major injuring vector (MIV) produces, according to the load component applied, a translation along and rotation around the three axes of the three dimensional coordinate system described by White and Panjabi.

A study of 143 cases allows to describe 5 "families" of trauma according to the direction of injury on the skull.

1. Horizontal Postero-anterior Injury (Fig. 1)

MIV produces flexion (x, flexion axis) and translation, (z translation axis) and leads to:
— anterior displaced dens fracture
— C 1–C 2 dislocation
— bilateral facet dislocation
— unilateral facet dislocation: asymmetrical application of MIV associate axial rotation and lateral bending
— facet subluxation
— herniated disc

Within a facet dislocation, the flexion bending moment acts as a "cap off" of a bottle and successively injures posterior ligaments and discs. The decisive lesion is anterior: posterior ligamentous injury "bolt off" the motion segment and anterior lesions produce dislocation and cord compression. We suggest to treat the decisive lesion: an anterior approach following a closed reduction allows decompression of the cord, and stabilization by a one-level graft and plate fixation.

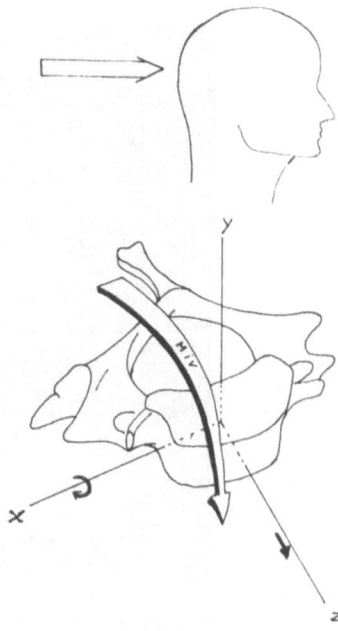

Fig. 1. Major injury rector (MIV) in horizontal postero-anterior injury

2. Oblique Postero-anterior Injury Leads to Tear-drop Fractures

MIV is a flexion bending moment around the X axis, produced by the posteriorly directed force (z axis), and the compression force (y axis). The same mechanism of "cap off" occurs around an anterior hinge located in the anterior part of the disc whereas it is far in front of the spine in dislocation.

This explains the successive body compression fracture, posterior disc and ligamentous tensile failure with posterior subluxation.

Instability, cord compression are present anteriorly; the approach is anterior too.

3. Horizontal Antero-posterior Injury

Produces well described, posteriorly displaced dens fractures, Hangman's fractures and Schneider-syndrom.

4. Oblique Antero-posterior Injury: Fracture—Dislocation (Fig. 2)

The "cap off" mechanism is inversed and occurs in extension. Postero-anterior MIV (z axis) results from an extension bending moment (x axis) produced by injury on the anterior part of the skull combined with a compression force (y axis). The components explain the anterior disc and

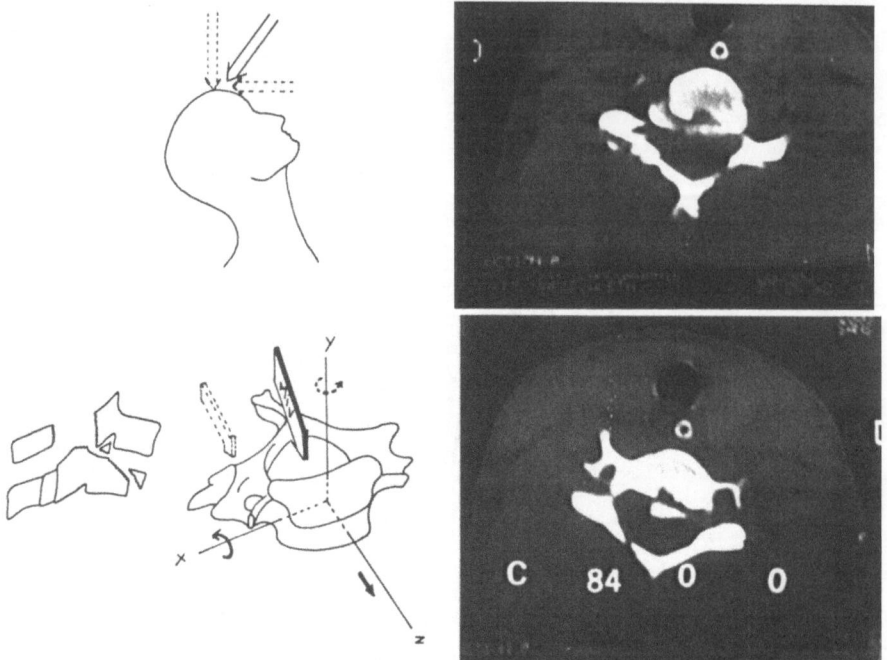

Fig. 2. Oblique antero-posterior injury with fracture dislocation (CT scan)

ligamentous tensile failure, facets fractures, anterior translation and secondary kyphotic evolution.

These lesions need a combined approach: *posteriorly* to remove broken facets and reduce translation; *anteriorly* to decompress the cord and stabilize the reduction by a one-level fusion.

Lateral application of a MIV produces an added rotation about y axis which supports a unilateral fracture-dislocation. In the case of Fig. 3 compression of the cord is not explained by the unilateral facet fracture. Rotation around the y axis and anterior translation tears away the posterior longitudinal ligament with a bony compressing fragment (CT scan). A combined approach is therefore required.

5. Compression Injury Along Y Axis is the Mechanism of Infrequent Lesions such as

— traumatic spondylolysis
— fracture with separation of the articular process

Stability depends on the magnitude of the disc torsion injury. Discography can indicate anterior fusion either isolated for spondylolysis or combined with posterior osteosynthesis for fracture with separation of the articular process.

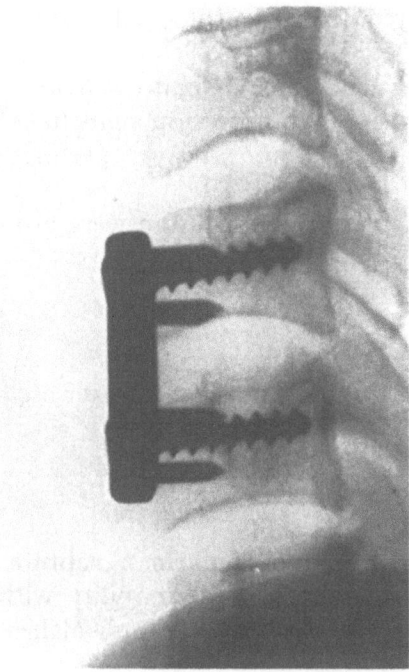

Fig. 3. Anterior fusion by our special designed metal plate

II. Treatment

63 cases with 66 cervical spine injuries treated between 1980 and 1985, were analyzed.

75% needed a surgical treatment and usually by an anterior approach:
— 27 cases of isolated anterior approach (56.2%)
— 7 cases of combined approach (14.6%) and
— 14 cases of isolated posterior approach (29.2%)

71% of the anterior surgery was justified by the biomechanical concept and by the neurological status. Cord compression factors being always anterior.

Anterior fixation of the lower cervical spine required a special designed plate with four pins at each end which was screwed into the vertebral bodies (Fig. 3). The very good stability allowed little immobilization by a simple cervical collar.

III. Results

The results confirmed our opinion without any morbidity:

The anterior graft was always fused after three months. Full activity was recovered after five months when neurological status was normal. We report two vicious consolidations with a slight kyphosis of 10° without functional complication.

26 patients suffered from neurological deficits (54.2% of operated patients):

— 9 cases of cord compression signs (34.6%)

— 17 cases of radicular compression signs (65.4%)

Anterior approaches were always performed producing 92% improvement.

The 9 patients with cord compression were grouped according to the Frankel classification:

A: 3 cases result 2 A*, 1 E

C: 2 cases result 2 E

D: 4 cases result 4 E

(* one tretraplegic patient ranged in A after a combined approach for fracture-dislocation is now a paraplegia A)

IV. Conclusion

All cervical spine trauma results in a rupture of the physiological extension preload, and creates hypermobility with kyphotic evolution. Anterior column injury is the decisive lesion which supports instability and compression cord.

Therefore surgical treatment should be anterior. There is little indication for isolated posterior surgery.

Cervical Spine I
© by Springer-Verlag 1987

3.6. Functional Results of Anterior Interbody Fusion in Injuries to the Lower Cervical Spine

H. Mestdagh, R. Debroucker, J. Letendart, J. P. Delcour,
and H. Reyford, Lille, France

In the last 40 years numerous authors have emphasized upon the importance of early surgical stabilization for unstable traumatic lesions of the subaxial cervical spine, but literature remains scanty as far as the biomechanics of a surgically blocked cervical spine is concerned [1, 6]. In a previous study, one of us developed an X-ray technique to measure the global and segmental mobility of the lower cervical spine in healthy adults [2, 4, 5]. The same method was applied to patients who had a cervical spine arthrodesis. It allowed us to assess the remnant range of motion of the head and neck after operation and to appraise accurately the behavior of the different intervertebral levels above and below the operation site.

Material and Method

Between 1961 and 1980, 106 patients underwent an intersomatic fusion by means of a bone graft applied to the anterior surface of the vertebral bodies. Up to 1969, a dowelled or wedged bone graft between 2 adjacent bodies, according to Cloward was used, thereafter Robinson technique was employed. The patients who had associated blading were discarded from the study. 63 patients were reviewed with a follow-up of 10 years (min 4 years, max 27 years). Each of them was submitted to a careful clinical examination of the head movement, then to a radiological check up:

Movement in the sagittal plane was studied by superimposing the contours of a given vertebral body on lateral films in extreme flexion and extension and measuring the angle between the lines drawn along the inferior margins of the overlying vertebra.

Movement in the coronal plane was studied in the same way with AP radiographs in extreme lateral tilting. The angle between the lines running through the inferior edges of the pedicles of the upper vertebra defined the range of mobility with respect to the lower one.

The rotation angular shift was calculated from the linear displacement of the tip of each spinous process on PA radiographs by means of a trigonometric ratio (Fig. 1).

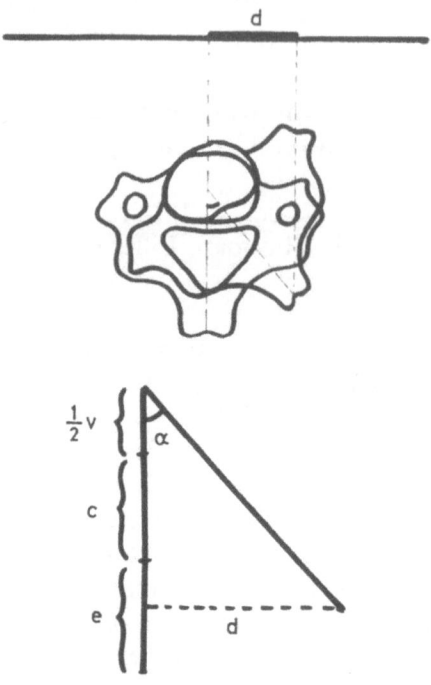

Fig. 1. The trigonometric ratio for calculating the angular rotation of a cervical vertebra. *v* Sagittal diameter of vertebral body, *c* sagittal diameter of bony canal, *e* length of spinous process, *d* linear displacement of the tip of the spinour process.

$$\text{Hence, } \sin \alpha = \frac{d}{\frac{1}{2} v + c + e}$$

Results

Clinically, we have globally observed
— reduction of 25% of the sagittal mobility of the head and neck;
— trivial modification of lateral flexion;
— reduction of 25% of rotation.

Using a strict quotation scale (Table 1), we have classified our results into 3 groups:
— 40 patients retained a good mobility of the head and neck;
— 12 had restricted motion;
— 11 had stiffness.

Dynamic X-rays allowed us to outline the behavior of the fused cervical spine.

At the level immediately above the graft, a "compensatory motion" was often encountered on the lateral X-rays but not so far as to offset the lack of motion assumed by the fused intervertebral disc; this accounts for the slight restriction in flexion-extension.

Rotation was also found restricted despite the poor involvement of the lower cervical spine because no compensatory motion is to be expected except at C 0–C 1 and C 1–C 2.

Below the graft, there was an obvious reduction of mobility in the three spatial planes. At the level immediately underlying the graft, osteophytic spurs developed in 33% of the cases; narrowing of the intervertebral space occurred at times after a long delay.

Table 1. *Quotation of Mobility and Functional Results*

	1 point	2 points	3 points
Flexion	0–2 cm	2–4 cm	> 4 cm
Extension	60°	> 30°	< 30°
Lateral flexion (each side)	40°	> 20°	< 20°
Rotation (each side)	> 80°	> 60°	< 60°

6–10 points: good mobility: 40 cases. 11–13 points: restricted mobility: 12 cases; 14–18 points: stiffness: 11 cases.

Discussion

In view of the long follow-up time in our series, we may now point out certain factors which we feel important in the outcome of the late functional results.

I. Type of Lesion

In 1982, we have stated [3] that in respect to the impact on the mobility of the cervical spine, the traumatic lesion could be rated in increasing order of gravity:

— sprain, disc protrusion,
— bilateral dislocation, tear drop fracture,
— unilateral dislocation with interlocking of the articular facets.

The postoperative stiffness is thus not proportional to the extent of the apparent displacement on the X-rays but more likely depends on the associated soft tissue damage.

II. Quality of Reduction

In order to assess the morphology of the operated cervical spine, a residual displacement index K was attributed to each patient. It was expressed by the angle formed by the intersection of the posterior borders of the injured vertebra and its lower partner. When K was greater than 10° (in our former cases), the range of motion of the head and neck was reduced by half; in contrast when K was less than 10°, reduction of motion reached at most ⅓.

III. Site of Fusion

The remaining mobility is poor after multiple intervertebral fusion or arthrodesis abutting on a congenital vertebral block. More often fusion involved only one intervertebral space. One must then oppose:

Upper fusions (C 2–C 3, C 3–C 4) which, though involving less mobile levels, yield stiffness of the neck especially in rotation, due to the lack of "compensatory motion" by underlying levels. It is important however to point out the eventual occurrence of hypermobility of the cervico-occipital hinge in flexion-extension, especially in young patients.

Lower fusions (C 4–C 5, C 5–C 6, C 6–C 7) which though involving more mobile levels, are well tolerated, due to the overlying hypermobility in flexion-extension.

IV. Age of Patients

If the fusion does not seem to lead to a genuine cervical spondylosis which commonly occurs in the last decades of life, it may however precipitate the evolution of a prior spondylosis in the patient over 50 years old.

Conclusion

Surgical intervertebral fusion does not seem to jeopardize seriously cervical motion and produce long term extensive osteoarthritic changes; however, the overlying compensatory hypermobility is not enough to reconstitute the integrity of motion of the head and neck. So although frequently overlooked, postoperative reeducation of the paravertebral neck muscles is mandatory to improve the final functional outcome.

References

1. Decoulx P, Decoulx J, Leclair HP (1966) La greffe antérieure dans les fractures du rachis cervical. Acta Orth Belg 32: 571–588
2. Gonon GP, Mestdagh H, Deschamps G, Dionnet J, Fischer LP (1981) Etude cinématique de la colonne cervicale dans le mouvement de flexion-extension. Ann Kinésithér 8: 1–9

3. Mestdagh H, Decoulx J, Debroucker R, Letendart J, Delcour JP, Mairesse JL (1982) Traitement chirurgical des traumatismes graves du rachis cervical inférieur. Techniques, indications, résultats. Lille Chir 37: 3–22
4. Mestdagh H (1976) Morphological aspects and biomechanical properties of the vertebroaxial point (C 2–C 3). Acta Morph Neerl Scand 14: 19–30
5. Minne J, Depreux R, Mestdagh H (1970) Les mouvements de rotation du rachis cervical inférieur. Bull Ass Anat 149: 929–935
6. Ramadier JO, Bankart M (1964) Fractures et luxations du rachis cervical sans lésions médullaires. Rev Chir Orthop 50: 3–55

Cervical Spine I
© by Springer-Verlag 1987

3.7. Anterior Stabilization with the Trapezial Osteosynthetic Plate Technique in Cervical Spine Injuries

W. Caspar, Homburg/Saar, Federal Republic of Germany

Trapezial plate osteosynthesis is an advanced technology for anterior internal stabilization in cervical spine injuries and for the treatment of neck instability due to nontraumatic causes.

It has been developed since 1979 and was first applied in November 1980 in a trauma case.

This technique is based on two principles:

— first, reconstruction of the anatomical integrity of the spine by realignment, fusion, and cord and nerve root decompression, and

— second, strong fixation by plate osteosynthesis to keep the spine in an optimal position until the process of bony healing is completed.

This technique relieves pain, prevents further injury, and late sequelae to the cord and roots resulting from repetitive microtraumas due to instability and offers optimal healing conditions to all traumatized structures in a drastically shortened period of time compared to nonoperative treatment.

Anterior metal plate stabilization operations have been carried out for over a decade, but have not found wide spread use, even though this technique is optimally advantageous from many aspects, various reasons for this include:

— an absence of a standard operative technique,

— lack of suitable materials for plating as well as,

— lack of suitable instruments for exposure and plate fixation.

This could then often result in technical problems, thus causing various complications, the most serious being worsening of neurological condition and recurrent instability due to screw loosening, the major problem of plate osteosynthesis.

To improve this situation, we have developed a standardized operation technique and designed a trapezial plate, and an instrumentation that takes into account the particular requirements in this area as well as rectifying the problems previously mentioned (Fig. 1).

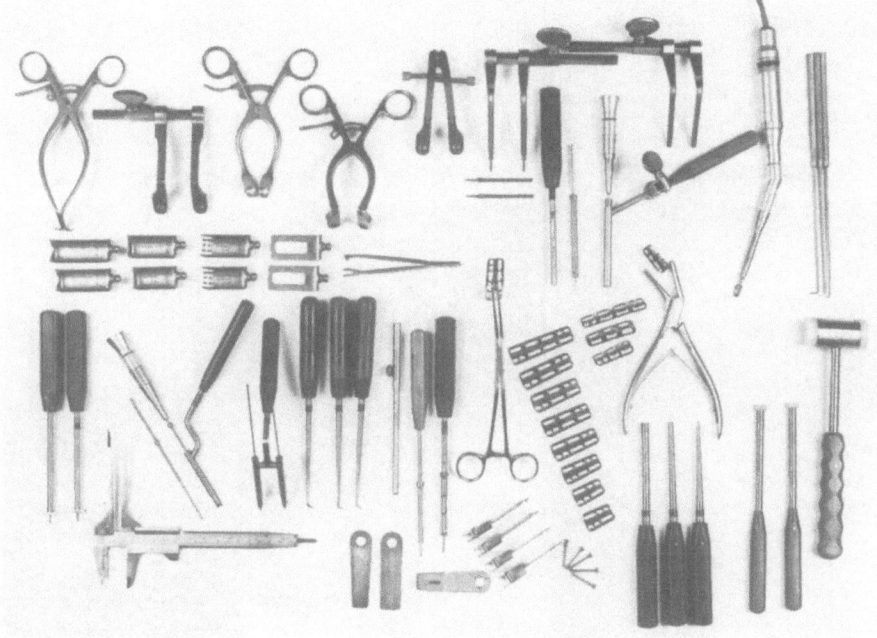

Fig. 1. Surgical instrumentation for anterior cervical interbody fusion and plate stabilization. Consisting of: various soft tissue and muscle retractors with a wide variety of exchangeable blades of a blunt, pronged, toothed, and fenestrated design shown in a selection, vertebral body distraction system, Microtron motor system, graft holders and impactors, tappers, precision caliber, single and dual drilling guides, depth gages, K-wires, threader, special drills and screws, selection of trapezial plates with and without fixation pins, straight and prebent, plate bending pliers, plate holding and insertion instruments, plate fixation tappers, selection of special bi-cortical screws (Swiss pattern) 3.5 mm diameter from 10–28 mm length in 1 mm increments, special screw driver with screw holding mechanism

This technique can be applied from the C 2 to the T 1 level utilizing different fusion and plating techniques such as:
— single and multi-level fusion with 4, 6, and 8 whole plates,
— subtotal body replacement and plating,
— and total body replacement and plating.

To avoid screw complications, intraoperative X-rays guidance, use of the specially designed measuring devices, depth gauges and screw insertion instrumentation are indispensable for proper and safe bi-cortical screw placement.

Only by binding both the anterior and posterior vertebral body cortex is sufficient screw torque obtained, thus preventing screw loosening.

Up to now, we have been using this technique for 4 years in 62 traumas

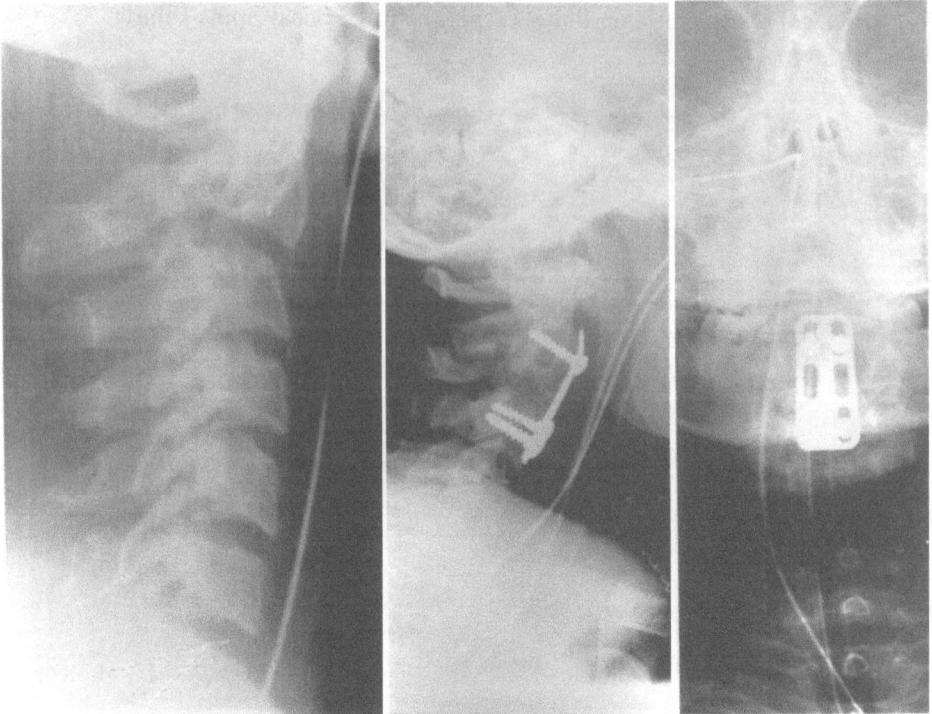

Fig. 2a. C2/C3 fracture subluxation (hangman's fracture). Middle, right: After reduction by traction, autograft interbody fusion and trapezial plate stabilization. Note: To obtain the normal lordotic curve, the plate has been bent over the total length; in addition the upper end has been sharply bent to follow the natural curve of the C2 body

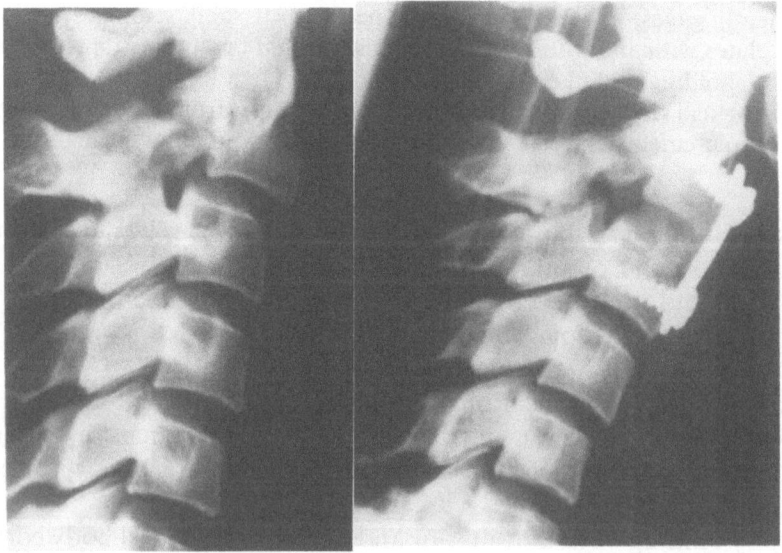

Fig. 2b. C2/C3 bipedicular fracture subluxation treated by anterior interbody autograft fusion and trapezial plate stabilization. Note: The optimal adaption of the pedicle fracture from the anterior approach

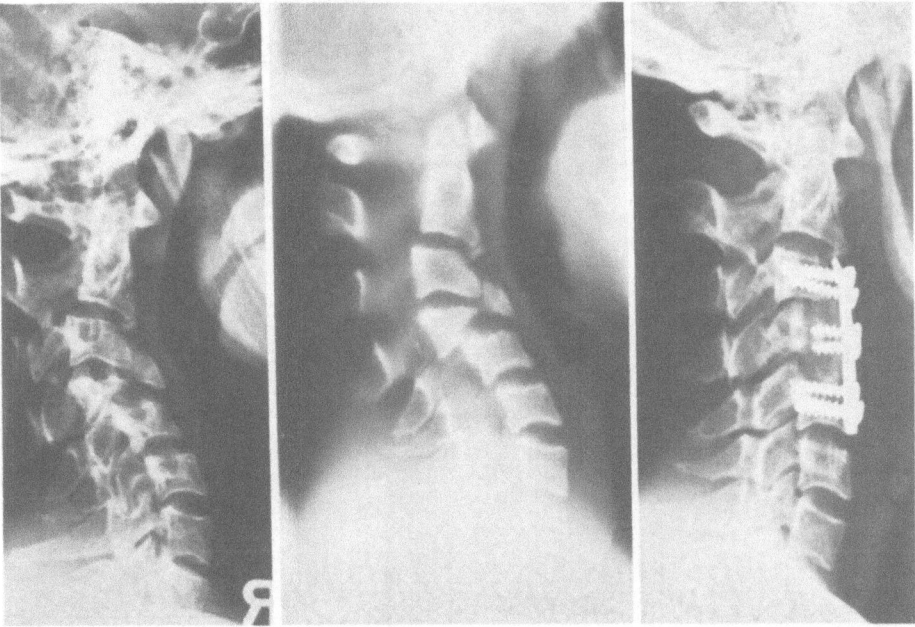

Fig. 3. A severe spine injury with cord symptoms with a compression fracture of C 4 and a posterior displacement compromising the spinal canal, an impressive angulation and a hyperlordotic curve below the level of the lesion. This (untreated) patient came to our attention two months following injury. Reduction by traction was no longer possible. Operative treatment consisted in total removal and bone graft replacement of the C 4 body and C 3–C 5 plate stabilization. Correction of the angulation was only possible by the tremendous strength (step by step) offered by the vertebral body distraction system. Postoperative course was normal and the patient recovered totally from his neurological deficits within 2 months. Discharge from hospital care was 2 weeks postoperative with a soft collar for 2 months. Note: The intermediate pair of screws are merely graft holding screws without a stabilizing effect

and 30 other indications. It has turned out that this technique is capable to solve virtually any problem occurring in cervical spine injuries such as a single level, bi- and multi-level instability with and without subluxation, single and multi-body compression or burst fractures. Furthermore reduction of a severe kyphotic angulation or locked facets unable of being reduced by traction is also possible by an anterior approach in most cases using the vertebral body distraction system.

Up to now, the clinical results were very satisfactory and clearly superior to those of conservative therapy. In our trauma series there was no case of neurological compromise due to the surgical procedure. Solid high quality fusion was obtained in 50 evaluated cases in approximately half the time

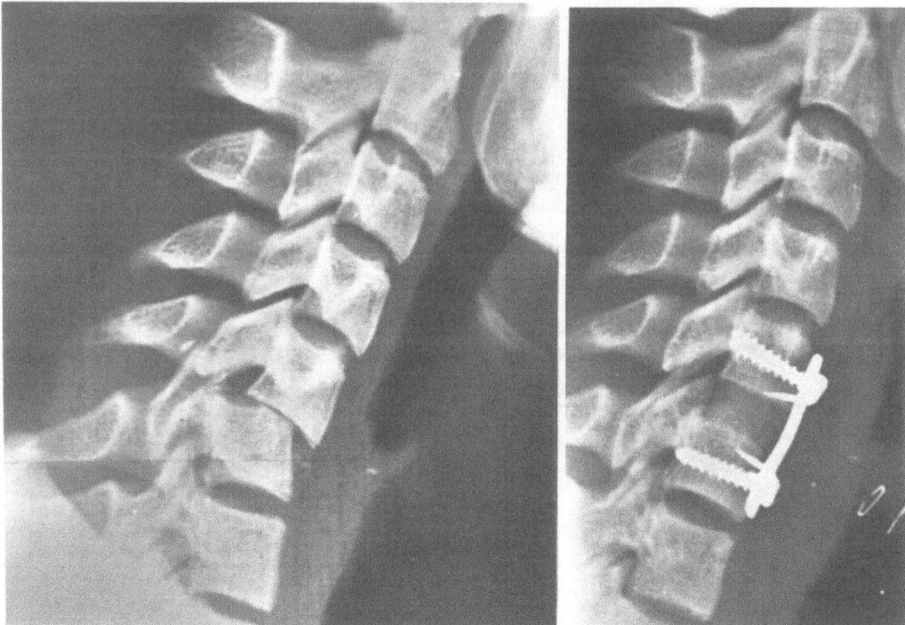

Fig. 4. A single level traumatic posterior ligamentous instability without neurological deficits. Realignment by traction and stabilization with anterior interbody autograft fusion and trapezial plate. Note: Plate adjustment- and fixation-spikes in C 5 and C 6

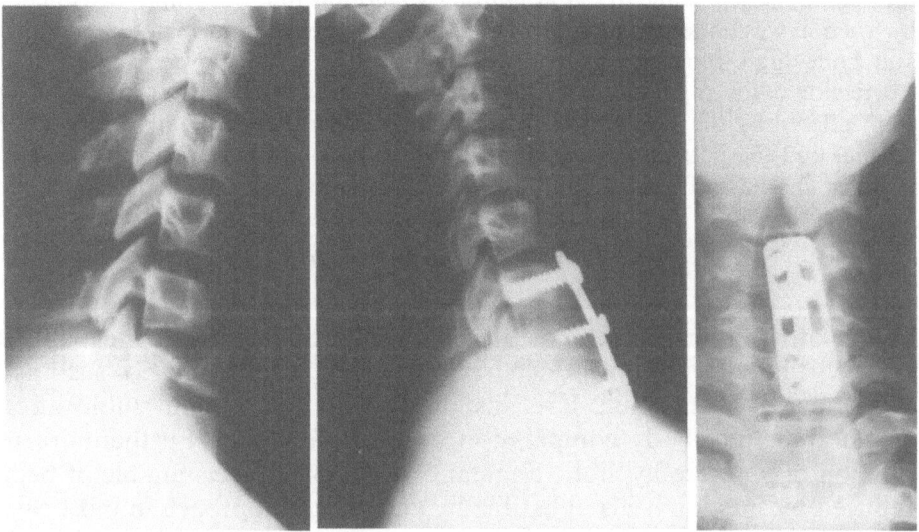

Fig. 5. C 7 burst fracture with posterior body displacement and primary complete sensory-motor transverse lesion. Total C 7 vertebral body replacement (autograft) and plate stabilization C 6–T 1. The vertebral body replacement is held by additional fixation screw thus preventing micro-movements between the graft and the adjacent bodies

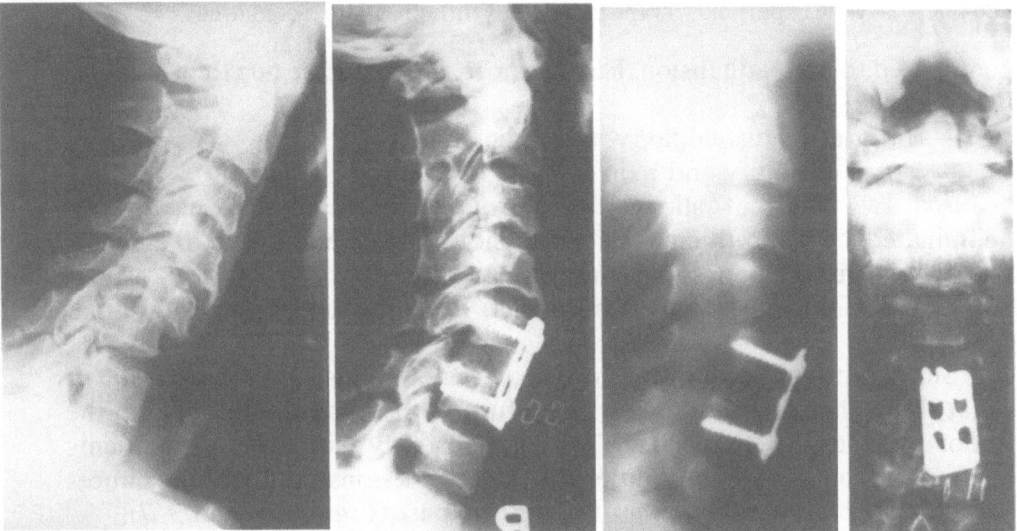

Fig. 6. A C 5/C 6 fracture subluxation with locked facets unable being reduced by traction. Anterior operative realignment by the vertebral body distraction system, autograft fusion and plate stabilization. Note: The special cortical screws (swiss pattern) pass through the whole diameter of the vertebral body, binding the anterior as well as the posterior cortex (bi-cortical screw) as shown in the midline tomogram. Only in this fashion the needed optimal screw torque is obtained thus preventing screw loosening, screw protrusion or screw extrusion

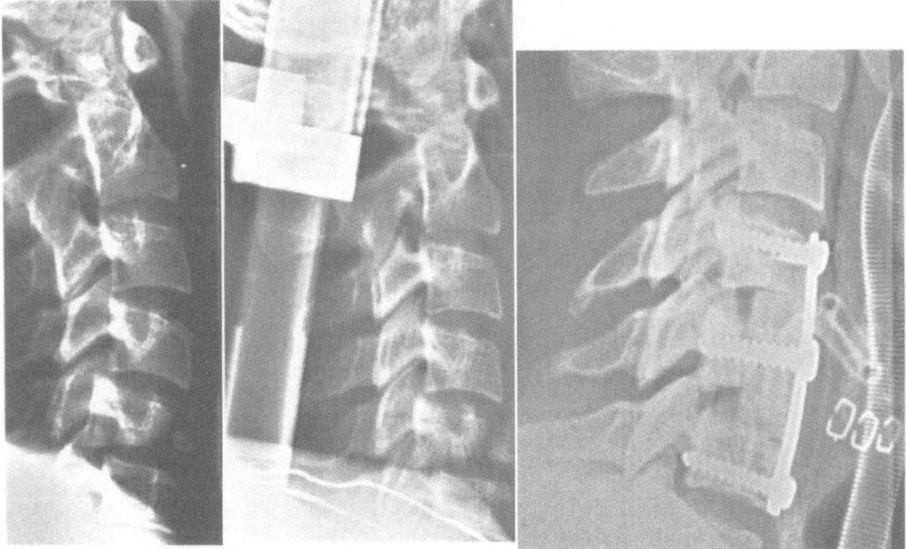

Fig. 7. An example of subtotal vertebral body replacement and plate stabilization in a case of C 5 body tear-drop fracture. Note: The anterior one half of C 5 body has been removed as well as the adjacent discs. The intermediate pair of screws pass through the vertebral body replacement (autograft) into the remaining C 5 body thus binding both tightly together, thereby giving additional stability and at the same time offering best conditions for a rapid fusion process

compared to nonplate fusion. Furthermore, late sequelae due to instability, such as

— progressive myelopathy and radiculopathy,
— spine disability and pain,

caused by recurrent slipage and progressive angulation have been eliminated by the optimal decompression, realignment, and the maintenance of realignment this technique can offer.

Complications were rare, and as yet, have had no effect on the final outcome.

Summarizing almost five years of experience in this field, it can be stated that this technique might have, in the future, the potential to open up the door to much better results. This is particularly true for those patients suffering from severe disabilities due to cord lesions, and whose chances seem to be considerably better than in the past (Figs. 2a, b and 3–7).

3.8. Anterior Cervical Fusion—Indications and Results

M. A. Correia Martins, Oporto, Portugal

Summary

42 acute unstable injuries of the lower cervical spine were treated in our Department with stabilization by anterior fusion and fixation with plates and screws. The radiographic studies showed fusion after 3 months. The final result was good and early ambulation was possible.

Incorrect diagnosis and inadequate immediate treatment following acute cervical trauma often leads to serious disabilities. The prime goal of the treatment is to obtain a stable and functional spine and to enable the patient to lead a normal life.

Posttraumatic instability depends on which structures have been damaged. Thus, lesions of the body of the vertebrae always consolidate although there may be an occasional kyphosis, whereas lesions of the discs or ligaments are more serious because of their long-lasting instability. The following are the more unstable lesions: dislocations, fractures with dislocation, serious sprains, fractures of the body with marked anterior compression, tear-drop lesions. Where there is instability, the cervical spine was stabilized surgically [1–3].

When a fracture can be reduced preoperatively, we greatly prefer the anterior approach as, among other advantages, it gives us better access, makes anesthesia easier, and enables us to quickly fuse only one disc. However, when this is impossible we use the open reduction by posterior approach and then a Rogers wiring procedure.

Anterior cervical fusion sacrifices the common anterior vertebral ligament, often the only intact anatomical structure, but the resulting temporary instability disappears to all intents and purposes when we perform an osteosynthesis with an anterior cervical plate [4–6] (Fig. 1). The advantages of this are (1) it is safe and easy to perform, (2) the fixation is very solid, and (3) the patient is soon ambulatory and released from hospital. We currently use the Robinson [7] or the Bailey [8] techniques. The screws are directed towards the center of the vertebral body and do not invade the posterior cortex (Fig. 2), which guarantees a good fixation.

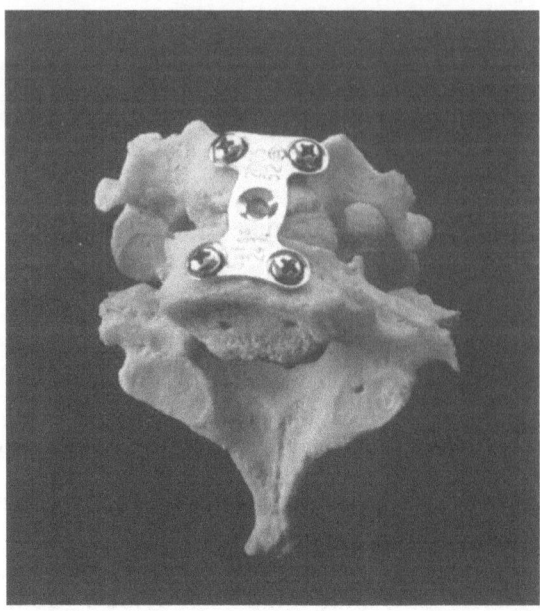

Fig. 1. Specimen showing the osteosynthesis with anterior cervical plate and bone graft

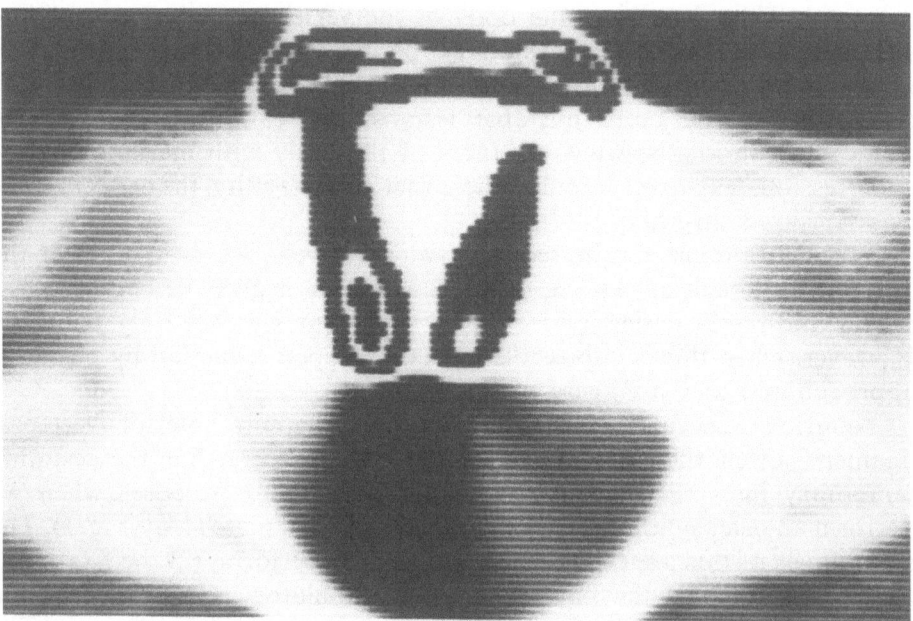

Fig. 2. CT scans of cervical vertebra. The screws ensure stability and need not reach the posterior cortex

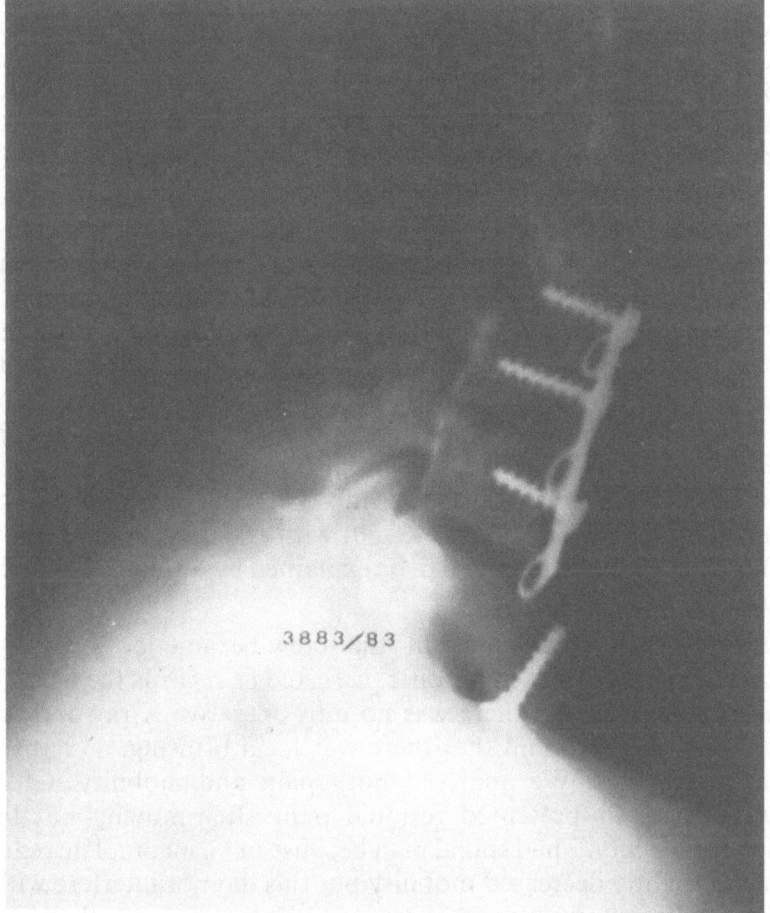

Fig. 3. One month after osteosynthesis; loose screw which resulted from a technical error. No sequelae

From 1979 to 1984, our Department used the anterior approach to treat 42 patients with acute traumatic lesions of the cervical spine. 30 patients (19 men and 11 women) with ages ranging from 12 to 68 years (peak incidence 40–50 years) and with a follow-up of one to six years, were seen again.

Causes of the accidents:

Road accidents .... 14 cases
Falls .... 13 cases
      from trees 5
      from scaffolding 5
      pedestrian 2
      from a circus trapeze 1
Tractor accidents .... 2 cases
From diving boards .... 1 case

67% were dislocations with or without fractures, 17% were tear-drop lesions, 13% were fractures involving the anterior corner of the vertebra, and 3% were serious sprains. The lesions were distributed as follows: 33% (10 cases) C 5–C 6, 17% (5 cases) C 6–C 7; 13% (4 cases) C 4–C 5; 7% (2 cases) C 3–C 4; 20% (6 cases) body of C 5; 10% (3 cases) body of C 4.

The mean delay between admission and placing of the anterior plate was of 16.8 days (0–42). Out of 15 dislocations, the orthopedic reduction was done seven times under an image intensifier and with myorelaxing agents.

Neurological deficit. 6 patients were classified as Frankel Group A. None improved, even though 2 were operated on within six hours. Two patients died during the first month from pulmonary complications. Of the 12 patients in group D, 4 remained in this group and 8 went to group E.

Length of hospitalization. The length of hospitalization of the patients with neurological deficits varied, depending on the number of beds available in the rehabilitation unit. Regarding those with no neurological deficit, hospitalization averaged 32 days (13–60) with osteosynthesis, and 45 days (34–58) without. This difference can be explained by different postoperative procedures.

Local complications. In 1 patient, the screw became loose because of a technical error (Fig. 3) and in another, we erred as regards the level. This is explained by the fact that there was no intraoperative X-ray and that the subjacent disc was torn and that there was local bruising.

Functional results. We analysed both pain and mobility. Of the 30 patients reviewed, 1 presented residual pain after moving but had no alteration in mobility, 2 had spinal pain because of an incomplete reduction, and 2 had a slightly decreased mobility but this did not interfere with their lives. The final results were good and very much the same whether we used a plate and screws or not.

References

1. White AA, Southwick W, Panjabi M (1976) Clinical instability in the lower cervical spine. A review of past and current concepts. Spine I: 15–27
2. Webb JK, Broughton RBK, McSweeney T, Park WM (1976) Hidden flexion injury of the cervical spine. J Bone Joint Surg 58 B: 322–327
3. Louis R, Goutallier D (1977) Fractures instables du rachis. Symposium Rev Chir Orthop 63: 415–181
4. Oliveira JC (1978) Estabilização cervical post-traumática—tendéncias modernas. Rev Ortop Traum I B 9: 89–100
5. Gassman J, Seligson D (1983) The anterior cervical plate. Spine 8: 700–707
6. Senegas J, Gauzere JM (1976) Plaidoyer pour la chirurgie antérieure dans le traitement des traumatismes graves des cinq dernières vertèbres cervicales. Rev Chir Orthop 62: 123–128

7. Bailey RW, Badgley CE (1960) Stabilization of the cervical spine by anterior fusion. J Bone Joint Surg 42A: 565–594
8. Robinson RA, Riley LH (1975) Techniques of exposure and fusion of the cervical spine. Clin Orthop 109: 78–84

Cervical Spine I
© by Springer-Verlag 1987

3.9. Incomplete Dislocations of the Lower Cervical Spine with Unilateral Articular Fracture—the Value of Arthrodesis by Anterior Operative Approach

Ph. Vichard, Besançon, France

This paper describes a lesion of the mobile spinal segment associated with a unilateral articular fracture which undoubtedly facilitates both displacement and reduction but nonetheless also brings about a certain degree of instability which has not been given enough emphasis in the literature.

History

The articular fracture has been described as well as the articular locked facets which it replaces as a result of an incomplete dislocation of the cervical spine.

In France, R. Judet [6] and R. Roy-Camille [8] do not discuss at great length their clinical findings but rather the therapy prescribed by this particular anatomical form. They suggest using a tile plate which is put into place by the posterior operative approach. The posterior approach is absolutely necessary when articular locked facets have not been reduced by orthopedic manipulation or skull traction. In the case of reduction, however, one may use the anterior presternomastoid approach which has been well known and documented for quite some time: Chipault [1], Robinson and Smith [7], Dereymacker and Mulier [4], Cloward [2], Sicard [9] and P. Decoulx [3].

In the light of our own experience, we feel that these incomplete dislocations (associated with a unilateral fracture) which are easily reduced as we have just observed, fully warrant this anterior operative approach with arthrodesis.

In order to demonstrate the merit of this method and the originality of the symptomatology, we will discuss nine clinical studies collected over a period of five years in the Department of Orthopaedics-Traumatology at the University Hospital Center in Besançon.

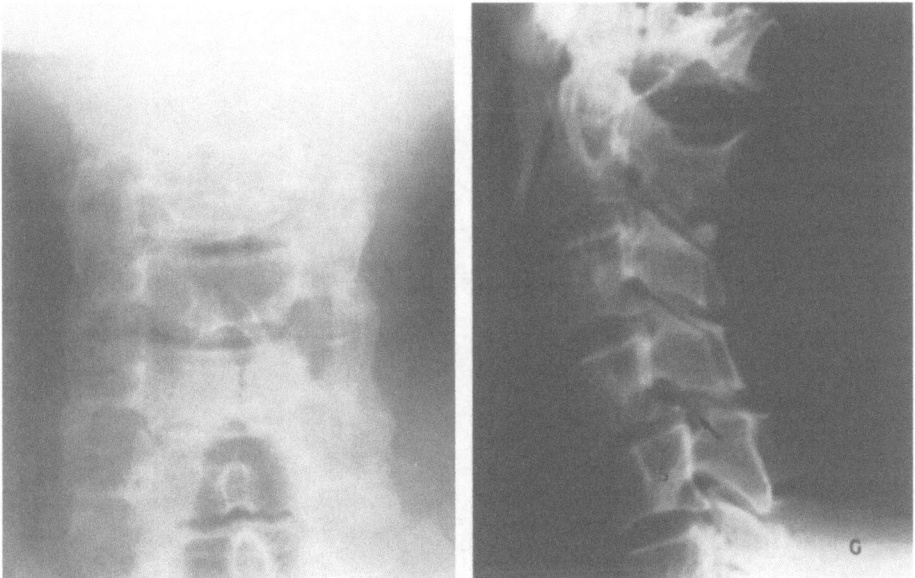

Fig. 1. Lateral radiograph demonstrating an incomplete dislocation of C4–C5 with a fracture of the left upper articular process of C5 and discal compression

Casuistics

Sex	6 men, 3 women
Average age	33 years old
Seat of the lesions	4 incomplete dislocations C6–C7
	2 incomplete dislocations C5–C6
	2 incomplete dislocations C4–C5
	1 incomplete dislocation C3–C4

In seven cases, we were dealing with an upper articular fracture of the subjacent vertebra, and in two cases, a lower articular fracture of the suprajacent vertebra. There were some cases of direct association with other osseous lesions of the suprajacent segments (pedicle, lamina, spinous process).

Circumstances: car accidents in all cases.

Clinical findings:

— cervical pain and restriction of varying amplitudes may be unrecognized in a clinical picture of polytraumatism;

— frequent occurrences of paresthesias whose topography in the fingers is directed towards the injured level. These occurrences may be intermittent.

Plain radiography, tomography, flexion radiographs, and CT scan have provided the radiologic findings. The clinical studies, however, do not discuss medullary complications *which are possible.* In our series, this

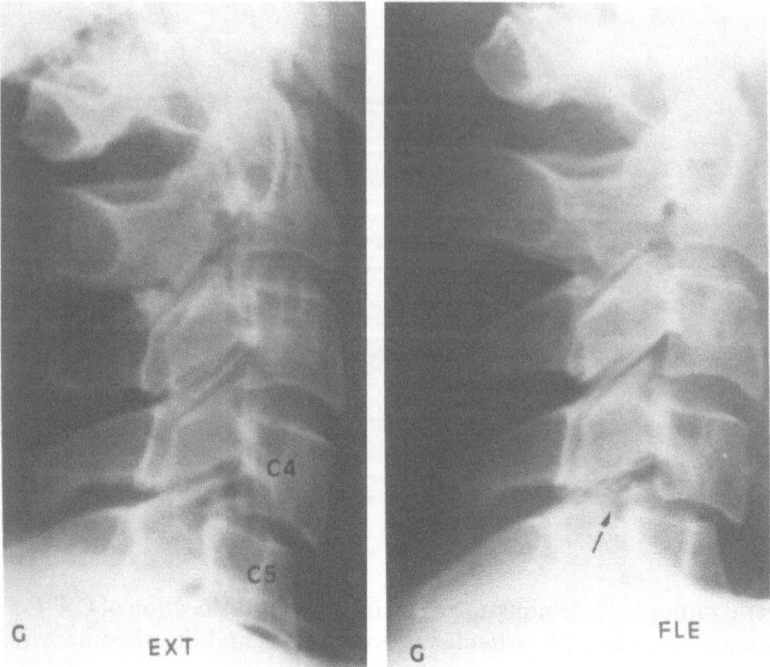

Fig. 2. Dynamic films show, in extension, a partial reduction of the lesion; whereas, in flexion, the dislocation and discal compression are clearly accentuated

complication is ruled out because of the immediate dispatching of the injured patient on their admission to the University Hospital Center.

The various *treatments* carried out are as follows: orthopedic therapy: 0; osteosynthesis by posterior operative approach: 3; arthrodesis and synthesis by anterior operative approach: 6.

Mechanism

There is a clear indication of lesions resulting from hyperflexion, and accompanied by a rotatory component, thereby accounting for the unilateral impairment of the joints.

Clinical Findings

The factor of instability has been reported. It is obvious that both pain and restriction of amplitude, although variable, are nonetheless virtually constant. However, one must observe that paresthesias which indicates the injured level may disappear during the reduction phases, giving thus the impression that the initial examination was inaccurate.

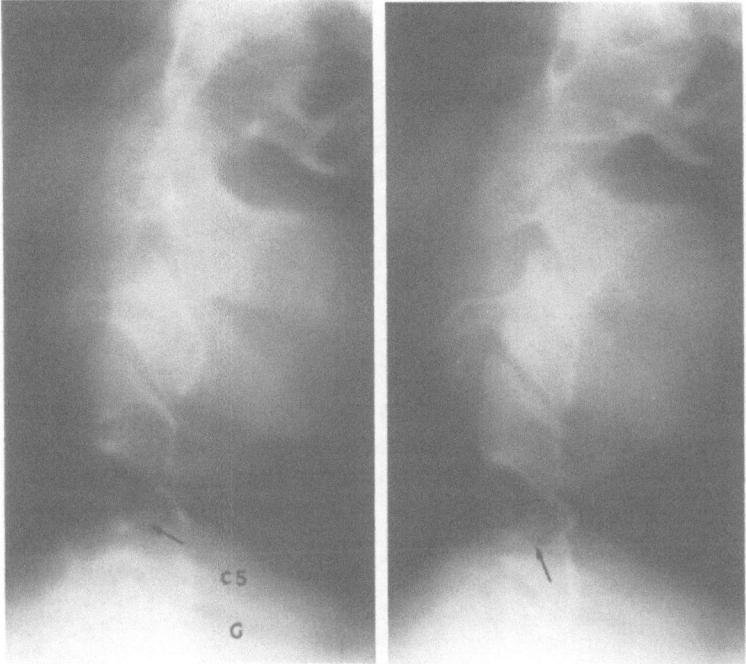

Fig. 3. Fracture of the articular process of C 5 is confirmed by lateral tomography

Radiologic Findings

Careful examination of our clinical studies revealed the following signs:

1. *On plain radiography:* The *frontal view* indicates bayonet deformity of the spinal processes as in the case of articular locked facets.

The *lateral view* shows articular compression affirming discal impairment. This indication remains constant, unlike the bayonet and incomplete dislocation, shown laterally on either side of the vertebral bodies and in the joints, the appearance of which is quite different above and below the injured plane. This difference can be attributed to rotation.

2. Inasmuch as most of these symptoms are, in fact, intermittent, the value of *extension and flexion lateral radiographs* to induce or reduce displacement becomes clear. On plain radiography, the articular fragments are not often easily recognizable. It is for this reason that lateral tomography would appear more useful.

3. *The CT scan,* which we have for quite some time considered to be valuable in the case of this type of upward-extending lesion, sometimes enables us to see the articular fragment and to do a differential diagnosis with the fractures-separations of the articular pillar (Roy-Camille), the symptomatology of which is also unstable.

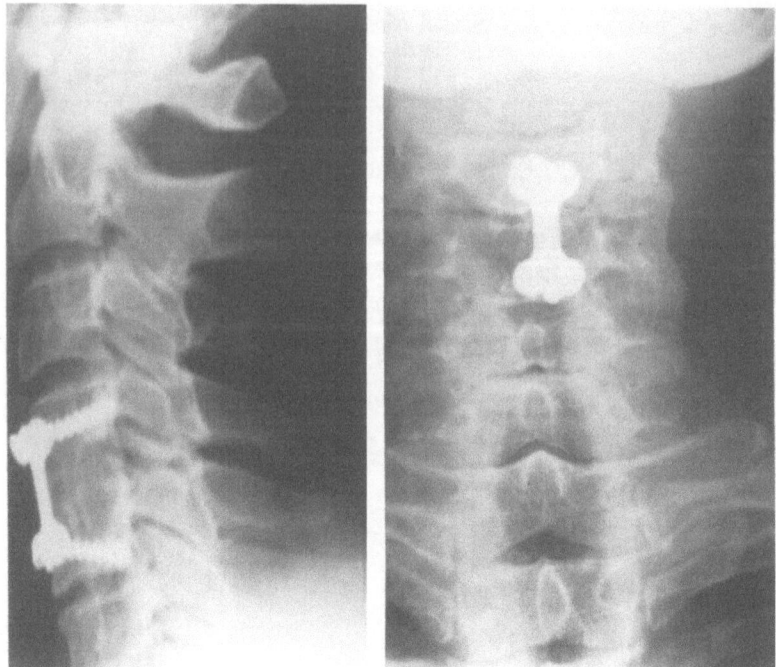

Fig. 4. X-ray views after three months (see Fig. 3)

Treatment

Conservative treatment, regardless of its nature, involves the risk of prolonging displacement and paresthesias, therefore failing to solve the discal problem.

Very soon after traction, the posterior approach may be carried out directly. Restoration of the joint is not possible, and its replacement by a tile splint often illusory. Immobilization of several levels using plates appears illogical. It implies secondary removal of the material and does not solve the discal problem.

In our own experience, we systematically choose the presternomastoid approach, provided that the diagnosis was certain. If displacement does not easily yield to hyperextension induced by a wooden block placed under the patient's shoulders for a few hours, we apply skull traction using Gardner's tongs.

The presternomastoid approach with the patient placed in supine position enables the surgeon to remove the disc while preserving the joint posterior vertebral ligament. The vertebral borders are refreshed by use of a drill. A cube, taken from the homolateral iliac crest and measuring $0.8 \times 10 \times 10$ mm on an average, is impacted in the interspace. Skull traction or hyperextension is discontinued. A Senegas plate is screwed onto the two vertebrae. The patient is placed in a Minerva jacket for 2 months. This jacket may be removed once a week for the purpose of washing and dressing.

Results

6 anterior approaches with osteosynthesis and arthrodesis = 6 successes (Figs. 1–4).

3 posterior osteosyntheses with:

— in the first case, persistence of pain and paresthesias;

— in the second case, persistence of paresthesias and pain accompanied by an incomplete reduction;

— in the third case, persistence of an incomplete dislocation with stiff and painful kyphosis which resulted in a secondary anterior arthrodesis.

Conclusion

We are presently on the look for this type of lesion which is not always obvious and whose symptomatology lacks stability. As we see it, the best treatment seems to be the presternomastoid approach with arthrodesis and osteosynthesis of the injured level. This technique provides a solution to the discal problem, obstructs the only injured level, and does not require removal of the material.

References

1. Chipault A (1894) Etudes de la chirurgie médullaire. Alcan, Paris
2. Cloward RB (1962) Treatment of acute fractures and fractures of the cervical spine by vertebral body fusion. J Neurosurg 18: 201–209
3. Decoulx P, Decoulx J, Duquennoy A, Leclair HP (1968) Fractures luxations du rachis cervical. Indications et techniques de l'arthrodèse antérieure. J Chir 96: 423–438
4. Dereymacker A, Mulier J (1956) Nouvelle cure chirurgicale des discopathies cervicales. La méniscectomie par voie ventrale, suivie d'arthrodèse par greffe intercorporéale. Neurochir 2: 233–234
5. Gardner WJ (1973) The principle of spring loaded points of cervical traction. J Neurosurg 39: 543–544
6. Judet R, Judet J, Roy-Camille R, Lerah JC, Saillant G (1970) Fractures du rachis cervical: fracture-séparation du massif articulaire. Rev Chir Orthop 56: 155–164
7. Robinson RA, Smith GW (1955) Antero-lateral disc removal and body fusion for cervical disc syndrome. Bull John Hopk Hosp 96: 223–224
8. Roy-Camille R, Saillant G (1972) Chirurgie du rachis cervical. Luxations fractures articulaires. La Nouvelle Presse Méd 1: 37

9. Sicard A (1960) L'arthrodèse du rachis cervical par voie antérieure. J Chir 80: 145–154

10. Smith GW, Robinson RA (1958) The treatment of cervical spine disorders by anterior removal of the intervertebral disc and interbody fusion. J Bone Joint Surg 40 A: 607–623

11. Verbiest H (1962) Anterior operative approach in cases of spinal cord compression by old irreductible displacement or fresh fracture of cervical spine. J Neurosurg 19: 389–399

Cervical Spine I
© by Springer-Verlag 1987

3.10. Stable Dorsal Fusion of the Cervical Spine (C 2–Th 1) Using Hook Plates

F. Magerl, D. Grob, and P. Seemann, St. Gallen, Switzerland

A new technique of stable posterior cervical fusion has been developed by the senior author (F. M.) and applied at our clinical since 1979. The purpose of this paper is to describe the principals of this technique and to discuss its indications and applications.

1. Indications for the Hook Plate Fixation

The indications are traumatic disco-ligamentous instabilities of the cervical spine and the various indications of cervical fusion other than trauma. In the treatment of significant vertebral body fractures, the posterior approach may be used as a supplement to anterior surgery. The technique is applicable from the second cervical to the first thoracic vertebra.

2. Operative Technique

The hook plate (Fig. 1) has a thickness of 1 mm and is available in seven lengths from 16 mm to 33 mm. The two shortest plates have one screw hole, the others have two. Normally, to fix the plates, 3.5 mm AO cortical screws are used.

The hook of the plate is placed beneath the lamina, immediately medial to the facet joint into a small notch (Fig. 2). This prevents the hook from slipping into the joint. In the superior adjacent vertebra, the plate is anchored with a screw. The direction of the screw is important to the safety of this procedure. The screws are inserted close to the junction between the articular process and the lamina, parallel to the joint surface and directed laterally at 20–30 degrees (Figs. 2 and 3). Two goals are thus achieved, namely good hold of the screws and minimal danger to the vertebral artery and nerve roots. By tightening the screws the facet joints are pressed together. In order to prevent hyperlordosis a pressure-resistant cortico-cancellous bone graft is applied between the spinous processes before to tightening the screws (Fig. 3). This graft also plays an important bio-

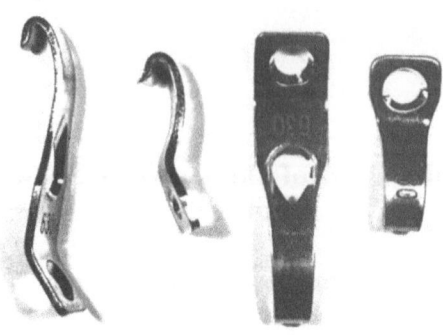

Fig. 1. Design of hook plates

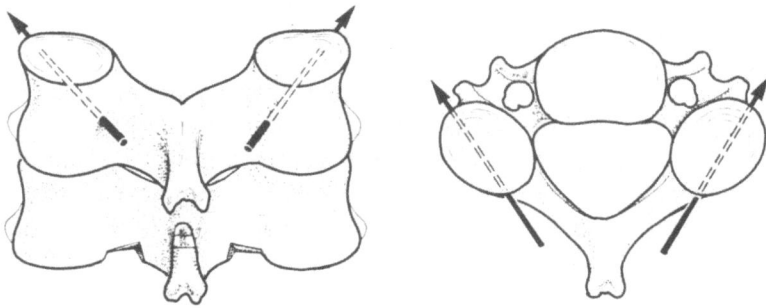

Fig. 2. Direction of the screws. The notches for the hooks in the lower lamina and for the H-graft in the lower spinous process are shown

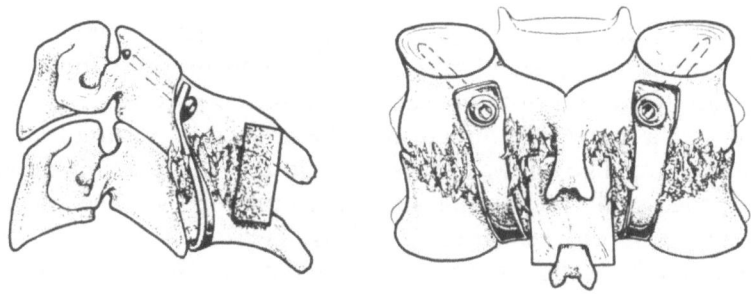

Fig. 3. Hook plate fixation. The screws lie parallel to the joint surfaces. The plates are twisted to adapt to the bone surface. A H-graft is placed between the spinous processes. Cancellous chips are applied

mechanical role by forming the third buttress of the fixation, the two others being provided by the facet joints. Since the hook plates lie within triangle formed by the two facet joints and the graft in the horizontal plane, the system is stable in all directions. By tightening the anchoring screws, the plate is held in tension. Therefore, this fixation corresponds to a prestressed compound system (Fig. 4).

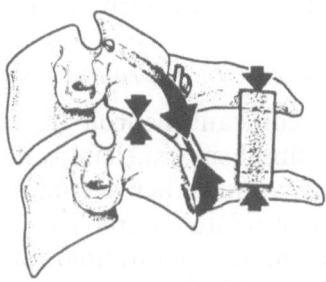

Fig. 4. Biomechanics of the hook plate fixation. The two facet joints together with the pressure resistant interspinous H-graft form a triangular 3-buttress system. Since the resulting force vector created by the plates lies within this triangle, the fusion is stable in all directions

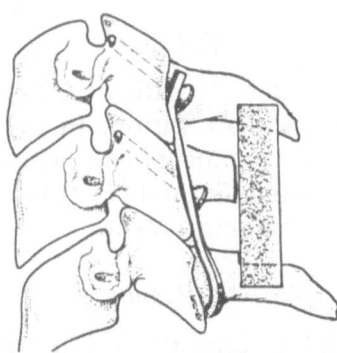

Fig. 5. Hook plate fixation over two motion segments (cancellous chips are not shown)

The second hole may be used as an additional anchorage for the plate to the lower vertebrae. However, it is mainly meant for the fixation of two motion segments. When spanning three vertebrae, the technique is in principle the same, except that the spinous process of the middle vertebra is removed and the plates are additionally anchored by screws to the middle vertebra (Fig. 5).

3. Reduction of Dislocations

3.1. Dislocations without Neurologic Complications

In these cases closed reduction is preferred, using skull traction. Surgery is delayed for several days until reduction is achieved. In order to prevent disc herniation which might occur during the operation, myelography is carried out prior to wound closure. The agent is instilled at a lower lumbar level and the spinal canal is assessed using image intensification.

3.2. Dislocation with Neurologic Complications

In the presence of significant neurologic complications immediate reduction is carried out using heavy skeletal traction or open reduction if necessary. Posterior stabilization is then accomplished as soon as possible. Since extrusion of disc material into the spinal canal necessitates an anterior approach, preoperative computerized tomography is essential. In dislocations in which no disc material is found within the spinal canal, posterior surgery is carried out, including myelography.

4. Postoperative Treatment

Postoperatively the neck is immobilized by a semisoft collar for three months. Ambulation and physiotherapy are started immediately.

5. Cases

From 1979 to 1984 a total of 40 patients (33 males and 7 females) have been treated with the hook plate fusion. In 29 cases the indication for surgery was acute trauma. 15 patients had neurologic deficits of varying degrees. Posttraumatic chronic instability existed in 7 cases. In 4 patients miscellaneous nontraumatic indications for posterior fusion were present.

6. Results

All patients were followed until the fusion was solid. 36 patients were evaluated after an average of 29 months. All fusions healed with no loss of reduction. In 34 patients the neurologic state remained unchanged or improved. In 2 patients the neurologic deficit increased.

7. Complications

Postoperative neurologic deficits occurred in the two cases mentioned above. In the first case, disc material extruded into the spinal canal following posterior open reduction. In spite of immediate anterior decompression the patient remained tetraplegic and died several months later. In the second case an anterior spinal artery syndrome developed gradually four days after closed reduction and posterior fusion. The upper level of the syndrome was below the level of the injury and fusion.

Neither of these complications are related to the hook plate fixation. The first case is a complication caused by the reduction. The second is of unknown etiology, as it developed four days after surgery. This patient had extensive degenerative changes at multiple levels of the cervical spine.

8. Discussion

As Ulrich, Wörsdörfer, Claes and Magerl demonstrated (see chapter 1.10, page 65), the stability of the hook plate fixation in disco-ligamentous injuries of the cervical spine is equal to that which otherwise can only be obtained by a combined anterior and posterior fusion. This is one reason, why we prefer this technique in the treatment of cervical dislocations. However, the technique is not advisable as the sole treatment of vertebral body fractures. In these cases we use anterior fusions supplemented by posterior stabilization as necessary. Placing the screws in a divergent fashion is safer than sagittal positioning as far as injury to the vertebral artery or nerve roots is concerned.

The approach to reduction of dislocations in the cervical spine is still subject to controversy. The advantage of the anterior approach is that extruded disc material may be removed easily. On the other hand, fragments of articular processes compressing nerve roots can only be removed posteriorly. In our opinion the latter is much more frequent than the former. For this reason and for greater stability, we prefer the posterior approach. Partial fractures of articular processes do not reduce the stability significantly.

When reducing cervical dislocations the possibility of spinal cord compression by extruded disc material is an ever present danger. We believe that by using the methods described, the risk can be minimized. This danger does not exist in nontraumatic cases. On the contrary, the possibility of creating a slight lordosis widens the disc space.

Acknowledgment

This study was supported by research grants from the ASIF-foundation.

3.11. Traumatic Quadriplegia in Cervical Spine Stenosis

J. P. Carret, L. Fischer, P. Roussouly, and G. Sun, Lyon, France

Introduction

A traumatic quadriplegia in the cervical spine stenosis is usually shown in cases such as this:

After a traffic accident, a 40–50 years old man, presents a neurological state of complete or incomplete quadriplegia with a simple cervical X-ray as well as normal dynamic X-rays.

The myelography, tomography, and CT scan reveal a cervical spine stenosis usually degenerative with compression of the radicular spinal cord composits.

Cases and Methods

The elements of the study are represented by a twelve case series. This type of lesion does not seem unusual because between 1978 and 1983, 40 cases of quadriplegia have been treated as a result of fracture or cervical dislocation.

These observations concern eleven males and one female. Two patients are 30 years old, 9 are between 40 and 50, and one is 78.

Reasons of the injury: horse fall: 1 case, stairs fall: 2 cases, high place fall: 3 cases, traffic accident: 6 cases.

The neurological lesions were a complete quadriplegia in 4 cases and uncomplete quadriplegia in 8 cases.

Methods

a) The medical treatment: has been used in 3 cases and consists of anti-edemateous agents (Mannitol, Solumedrol, Soludactone). Cardiac and respiratory troubles sometimes need assisted ventilation during a few days.

b) The surgical treatment: used in 9 cases: 2 laminectomy; 6 anterior decompression either limited to the Cloward technique [1] more extended to Senega's method [2, 3]; one case, both have been done.

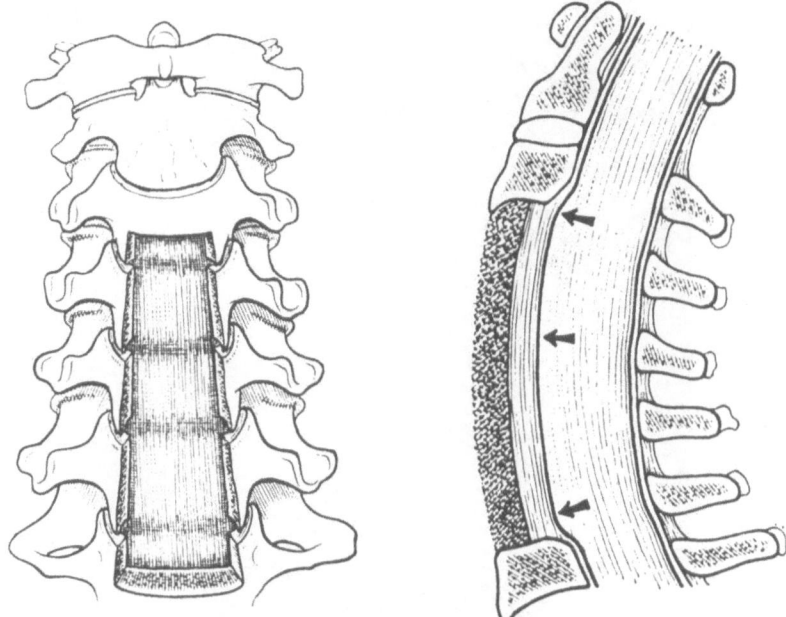

Fig. 1. Diagram of the anterior medullar decompression according to the Senegas method [2, 3]

Results

1. General Results

In this short series, we can notice a total recovery from neurologic problem troubles in 7 cases, a partial recovery in 3 cases, 2 deaths: one from pulmonary embolism, the other one from a heart-attack.

2. Results in Relation to the Initial Neurological Symptoms

In most of the quadriplegia cases, the incomplete ones are the most successful: *Complete initial quadriplegia*, 4 cases: no complete recovery, 2 incomplete, 2 deaths. *Incomplete initial quadriplegia*, 8 cases: 7 complete recoveries, 1 incomplete, no deaths.

3. Results Depending on the Type of Treatment

a) Medical treatment: used 3 times in this series with 2 complete recoveries (in incomplete quadriplegia) and with one death from pulmonary embolism.

b) The surgical treatment: used 9 times, with 5 complete recoveries, 3 incomplete recoveries, 1 death from a heart-attack.

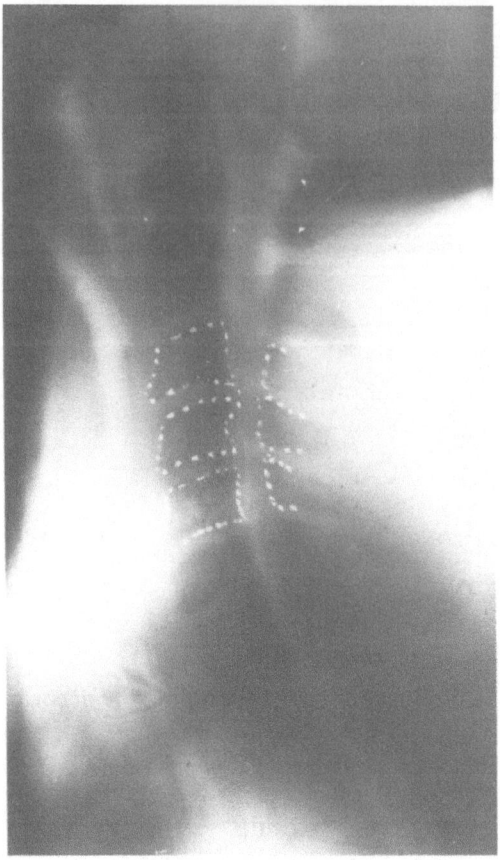

Fig. 2a

Fig. 2. M. S., 60 years old, posttraumatic tetraplegic. No apparent fracture. C 3–C 4, arthrosic cervical spine stenosis shown on the myelography (a). Postoperative X-ray showing the anterior decompression with C 3–C 4 arthrodesis (b)

Discussion

This series is too short to claim to give any final conclusions because it is just based on 12 observations.

But in the case of traumatic quadriplegia on cervical spinal stenosis, this series appears important.

1. Medical Treatment

Its purpose is to fight medullar edemous and avoid problems concerning quadriplegia.

Fight medullar edemous: this appears early after the traumatism. It can sometimes occur, spontaneously. Frequently, it becomes complicated due to secondary histological destructions more or less reversible.

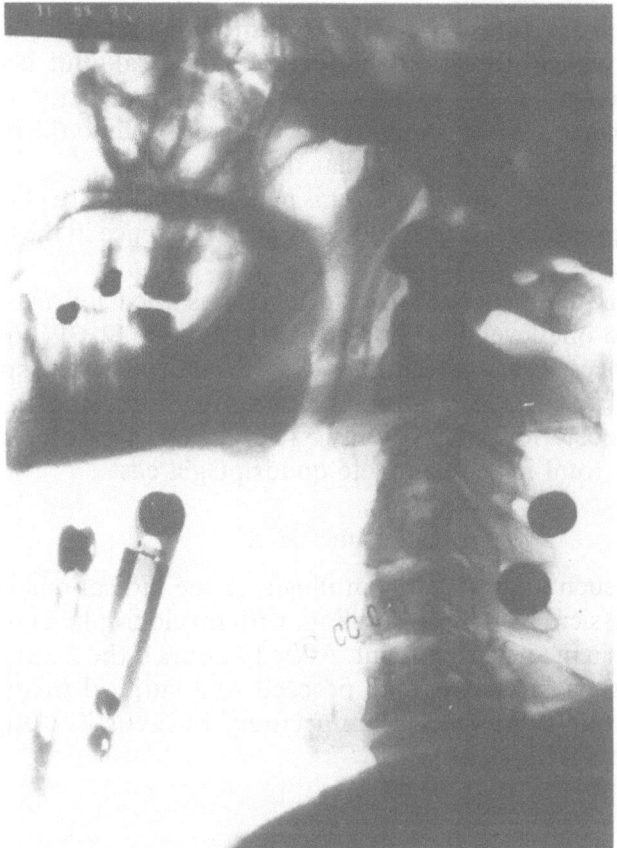

Fig. 2b

The treatment is based on an osmotical therapy (Mannitol 20% to adult: 100 cm³ every 4 or 6 hours; depending to age). The term of this treatment is generally 48 hours.

Corticoides: they have a preventing and curative effect. We use the Solumedrol 40 mg twice a day for 2 days and later given in smaller dosage.

Anti-aldosterone: we use Soludactone twice a day for 5 days.

One must watch for complications relating to any quadriplegia: the prevention of cardiac and respiratory troubles, digestive hemorrhage, stress ulcer, and infection, mostly urinary infection.

2. Surgical Treatment

There are two possible approaches: the posterior decompression and the anterior decompression.

a) The posterior decompression. The laminectomy partially cuts off the stenosis to expand the spinal cord and protect if from anterior osteophytes.

Its technical process has changed with time but remains quite extensive, more in the vertical direction than in a transversal. But it only gives a posterior freeing leaving in place the cause of anterior compression. However, the medullar ischemic troubles increase due to the pulling on the radicular vessels during the medullar decompression.

b) The anterior decompression. This makes it possible to eliminate all the anterior compressive elements and leave an large space in the cervical spine for all the stenosis.

Two techniques have been used in this series: the Cloward technique [1] just limited to one level and the Senegas technique [2, 3] (Fig. 1).

In one of these cases presenting a very extended cervical spine stenosis, we have used to a double approach: anterior (according to the Senegas method) and posterior (laminectomy). The recovery was interesting because it was almost total in the complete quadriplegia case.

Conclusion

Faced by such a lesion, we can illustrate the indications in this way:

After a classical X-ray examination, with myelography and CT scan, we first start with a medical treatment. After 12 hours if the treatment does not give good results in recovery we proceed to a surgical treatment. At the beginning we often performed a laminectomy, but actually we agree with the Senegas method (Fig. 2a, b).

References

1. Cloward R (1958) The anterior approach for removal of ruptured cervical discs. J Neurosurg 6: 602
2. Senegas J, Gauzere JM (1976) Plaidoyer pour la chirurgie antérieure dans le traitement des traumatismes graves des cinq dernières vertèbres cervicales. Rev Chir Orthop 62 [Suppl] 2: 123–128
3. Senegas J, Guerin J (1975) Technique de décompression médullaire antérieure dans les sténoses canalaires étendues. Rev Chir Orthop 61 [Suppl] 2: 219–223

Cervical Spine I
© by Springer-Verlag 1987

3.12. Fracture Separation of the Articular Process of the Inferior Cervical Vertebra: a Comprehensive Review of 13 Cases

J. M. Fuentes, J. Benezech, B. Lusszie, and J. Bloncourt,
Montpellier, France

The fracture separation of the articular process was first described by Judet and Roy Camille [6]. Usually this type of fracture is unilateral and concerns the inferior cervical spine (C 3–C 7). In some cases one can see an anterolisthesis on the lateral view of the X-rays mirroring the unilateral luxation of the flexion rotation fractures. In other cases with no displacement the lesion is difficult to identify while further displacement can occur eventually.

French authors [1, 3, 7–9] refer for this lesion to the Judet and Roy Camille's paper [6] whereas British authors [5] refer to Forsyth's description of the "horizontal facet" related to a compression extension rotation injury. This author stresses the fact that some dislocations by hyperextension mechanism look like luxation by flexion mechanism with defect on the myelogram caused by the articular process fracture. In 1964 this same author identified among 159 cervical spine injuries a 50% rate of hyperextension mechanism. Pure hyperextension does not exist. It is combined most of the time with compression mechanism leading to a fracture line running through lamina and pedicles of the vertebra. The whole anterior lesions (common anterior ligament, disc and small anterior tears of the vertebra) described by Taylor and Blackwood [10] and posterior arch lesions allow the anterior displacement. The radiological diagnosis is based upon the "horizontal facet" given by the displacement of the inferior articular above the subluxation. Harris [5] puts this type of lesion among hyperextension mechanisms associated with asymmetrical compression when the head is rotating or laterally tilting.

The fracture separation of the articular process seems to be a sort of dislocation fracture in hyperextension of the inferior cervical spine and would be limited to lesions without displacement.

Own Cases

We have collected, from 1975 to 1985, 13 cases. The most extensive series published seems to be Marie Anne's 30 cases [7].

Our series includes 8 males and 5 females. The average age was 32 ranging from 18 to 55. These 13 cases represent 9% of cervical spine trauma with neurological deficits. This fracture would be more frequently found according to Judet: 16% of inferior cervical fracture [6]. A single case in a 5-year-old boy has been reported by Badelon and Bensahel [1].

Etiology and Mechanism

Hyperextension associated with compression and rotation is the main mechanism and explains the unilateral aspect of the fracture.

A severe traffic accident was the cause in 10 cases, a fall in 2 cases and a sports accident (rugby) in one case.

From a clinical point of view we note:

— in 5 cases: neck pain was the only symptom;

— in 4 cases: radicular pain was present with sensory and motor involvement in the same (2 cases);

— in 4 cases: neurological deficits were present: brachial diplegia (1 case), Brown-Sequard-syndrome (1 case) and complete tetraplegia (2 cases).

The radicular involvement is due either to the anterolisthesis when a displacement is present or to an tilting of 30 degrees anterior of the articular process. Judet [6] reported a possible vascular syndrome due to vertebral artery compression.

The lesional levels concerned: C 3 in 2 cases, C 4 in 1 case, C 5 in 6 cases and C 6 in 4 cases.

The C 4 level with C 4–C 5 dislocation is stressed by Forsyth [4]. C 6 is reported once by Badelon [1] and in Judet's series [6] one notes: 3 cases involving C 3 (1 C 2–C 3 dislocation and 2 C 3–C 4 dislocation), 1 case involving C 4 (without dislocation), 2 cases C 5 (1 C 4–C 5 dislocation and 1 C 5–C 6 dislocation), and 3 cases C 6 (1 without dislocation and 2 with C 6–C 7 luxation). In Marie Anne's series [7] C 3 is involved 5 times, C 4 twice, C 5 12 times, C 6 10 times, and C 7 once. Therefore the inferior cervical spine (C 5, C 6, C 7) is predominantly involved (73%) followed by C 3 (19%) and C 4 only in 8% of the cases.

Associated Lesions

Anterior displacement is frequently found (6 times in our own series) and generally inferiorly of the fractured vertebra. A similar finding is reported by Marie Anne [8] except in one case where the dislocation was above the fracture. The displacement could appear immediately or later. When the fracture separation is bilateral (2 cases) a highly unstable spondylolisthesis appears (Marie Anne [8]).

Radiological and Pathological Findings

A standard X-rays examination shows 4 direct signs of fracture separation of the articular process:

1. fracture of the lamina on the AP view. 2. fracture of the pedicle on the oblique view. 3. tilting of the articular process on the lateral view. 4. anterolisthesis of the vertebral body (3 mm) on the lateral view.

Indirect signs can be found: desaxation of the spinous process which affects the rotation of the vertebra; oblique and lateral aspect of the vertebra coexisting on the same lateral view; hyperextension indicates tearing of the antero-inferior wedge of the vertebral body.

Diagnosis can be difficult if the rotation is minor and horizontalization of the articular process can be missed. Misdiagnosis is dangerous since the lesion is quite unstable and susceptible to further displacement. (1 case in our series, 6 out of 9 in Judet and Roy Camille's [6]). Therefore tomographic examination and CT scan are necessary when some clinical or radiological features suggest this lesion [2]. The pedicular fracture is difficult to visualize on a conventional X-ray. It runs most of the time through the vertebral artery canal and is represented crossing behind.

Asymmetrical compression is the main factor when the cervical spine is in neutral position but the disco-ligamentary lesions are caused by the hyperextension and correspond to the mentioned lesions [5, 10] including rupture of the anterior ligament and disc.

Personal Classification (Fig. 1)

Type 1: fracture separation without displacement (disc integrity). Cervico brachialgia or neck pain belong to this group.

Type 2: fracture separation associated with rupture of the disc and anterior ligament without displacement. A neurological deficit is possible.

Type 3: same lesion plus anterior displacement of 3 mm.

Type 4: double disc lesion (2 levels) above and below the articular fracture. This type could explain some luxation above the level of the fracture and would cause further kyphosis described by Roy Camille [9] after posterior surgical approach.

Differential diagnosis has to be made with incomplete fracture and crushing fracture of the articular process when no displacement exists.

If there is a displacement one must know other causes of lateral anterolisthesis [3]: unilateral luxation and superior edge fracture of the articular process by flexion rotation. Congenital cervical spondylolysis can be difficult to differentiate but the fracture line is located through the isthmus and spina bifida is frequently found.

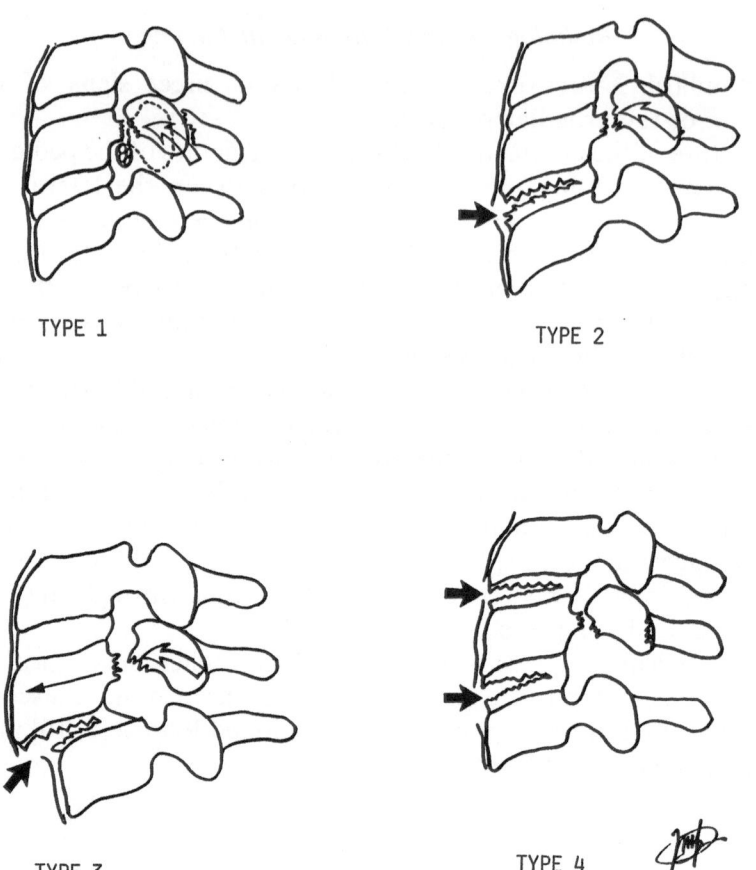

Fig. 1. Personal classification

Treatment

The fracture separation of the articular process is quite unstable and should be identified early.

Posterior fusion with wire fixation has been proposed by Forsyth [4].

Roy Camille [9] stresses the great difficulty in achieving a complete reduction (48% of cases) and proposes a posterior approach with metal plate fixation. An orthopedic immobilization by cervical brace is advised by Badelon [1] for children.

Our personal series includes 12 out of 13 surgical approaches under cervical spine traction.

A posterior approach was performed in 2 cases and anterior approach in 6 cases. In these cases an anterior interbody fusion was carried out and an originally designed metal plate was placed over one (5 cases) or two discs (1 case).

A combined anterior and posterior approach has been performed in 4 cases: in one stage (3 cases) and in two stages (1 case).

Complete reductions were always achieved.

An anterior approach seems to be justified since the potentially unstable lesions are anterior. A complete reduction seems more consistently achieved by this approach but may require a combined approach in some cases.

Summary

The authors report their experiences with 13 "fracture separation" of the articular process of the inferior cervical spine (C 3–C 7). These types of fracture seem to be correlated to a complex mechanism including extension compression rotation and can be considered as a variety of hyperextension fracture dislocation.

This type of fracture is quite unstable and has been subdivided into four groups.

Anterior approach and/or combined anterior and posterior approaches are required to achieve a good reduction and stabilization.

References

1. Badelon O, Bensahel H (1984) Fracture séparation du massif articulaire du rachis cervical chez l'enfant. Rev Chir Orthop 70: 83–85
2. Bloncourt J (1982) Exploration moderne des traumatismes du rachis. Scanner rachidien et épidurographie. Thèse pour le doctorat en Médecine, Montpellier
3. Dosch JC (1984) Le syndrome d'antélisthésis cervical latéralisé: diagnostic. Etiologie. Traumatisme du Rachis, CEPUR, Luxembourg, Octobre 1984
4. Forsyth HF (1964) Extension injuries of the cervical spine. J Bone Joint Surg 46-A: 1792
5. Harris JH (1978) The radiology of acute cervical spine trauma. The Williams and Wilkins Co, Baltimore
6. Judet R, Judet J, Roy Camille R, Zerah JH, Saillant G (1968) Fracture du rachis cervical: fracture séparation du massif articulaire. Rev Chir Orthop 54: 765–780
7. Marie Anne S (1978) Fracture séparation des massifs articulaires du rachis cervical (A propos de 30 cas). Thèse en Médecine, Paris
8. Marie Anne S (1979) Les fractures séparation des massifs articulaires du rachis cervical inférieur. In: Rachis cervical traumatique non neurologique. Premières journées d'Orthopédie de la Pitié. Masson, Paris, pp 116–122
9. Roy Camille R, Saillant G (1970) Ostéosynthèse des fractures du rachis cervical. Actual Chirur Orthop Hop R Poincaré. Masson, Paris 8: 175–194
10. Taylor AR, Blackwood W (1948) Paraplegia in hyperextension cervical injuries with normal radiographic appearances. J Bone Joint Surg 30 B: 245

3.13. Traumatic Spondylolisthesis of the Axis

W. R. Francis, Houston, Texas, U.S.A., J. W. Fielding, New York, N.Y.,
U.S.A.,
R. J. Hawkins, London, Ontario, Canada, J. Pepin, Ann Arbor, Michigan,
U.S.A., and
R. Hensinger, Ann Arbor, Michigan, U.S.A.

Traumatic spondylolisthesis of the axis involves bilateral fractures of the pedicles and may be caused by vehicular and diving accidents, or other deceleration injuries. The lesion, which has been called "hangman's fracture", is characteristically produced by hyperextension and axial loading, but has also been described as resulting from flexion and axial loading.

In 1913 Wood-Jones first described the bony anatomy of the lesion in the dried remains of five individuals hanged with the knot in a submental position. All specimens showed bilateral axis pedicle fractures and Wood-Jones postulated that complete disruption of the ligaments and disc between the second and third cervical vertebrae has resulted in transection of the cord and instantaneous death.

In 1965, Schneider et al. described a similar bony lesion seen in patients after vehicular accidents and other sudden deceleration injuries, and drew attention to the common association with injuries to the face or head. Schneider et al. use the term "hangman's fracture", but the mechanics of the two lesions are different. Hyperextension is common to both lesions, but the distraction produced by judicial hangings is absent in the other injuries and is replaced by axial loading. This probably accounts for the very different incidence of neural damage, and "traumatic spondylolisthesis of the axis" (Garber 1964) is a more appropriate term for the lesion.

This series includes 123 patients, of whom 86 were male. The age of the patients was from 9 to 78 years (mean 32.7 years) and follow-up ranged from 12 to 62 months (mean 31.3 months). Patients were seen from 1962 to 1978 in one of four centers: Baylor College of Medicine, Houston, Texas; St. Luke's Hospital, New York; The University of Michigan Hospital Center, Ann Arbor, Michigan; and the University of Western Ontario, London, Ontario, Canada. All patients were assessed personally by at least one of the authors.

The commonest cause of this injury was a motor vehicle accident (78%). Falls with the face forward and diving accidents accounted for 21%. All conscious patients suffered pain, usually localized to the upper part of the back of the neck, but neuralgia in the distribution of the greater occipital nerve was recorded in only seven patients. 79% of these wounds were frontal or apicofrontal, thus supporting the concept that the mechanism of

Table 1. *Classification of Injury into Five Grades*

Grade	Displacement	Angulation (degrees)
I	< 3.5 millimeters	< 11
II	< 3.5 millimeters	> 11
III	> 3.5 millimeters < 0.5 vertebral width	< 11
IV	> 3.5 millimeters < 0.5 vertebral width	> 11
V	disc disruption	

injury is hyperextension and axial loading. Five patients had wounds of the posterior vertex or occiput suggestive of flexion loading of the neck, and had sustained compression fractures of the third cervical vertebra. Six patients had asymmetrical injuries of the pedicles suggesting rotational or lateral flexion forces at the time of injury. In 26 patients, no point of impact could be established.

Thirty-nine patients had other injuries of the cervical vertebrae (Table 2). Nine patients had additional fractures of the spine below the neck and 46%

Table 2. *Distribution of Other Spinal Injuries Associated with Traumatic Spondylol-isthesis of the Axis*

Multiple levels	3
Odontoid	4
C 1 arch	10
C 1 lateral mass	3
C 1 Jefferson	2
C 2 lateral mass	3
C 3 compression	5
C 3 arch	6
C 3–C 6	6
Thoracic and lumbar compression	6
T 12–L 1 fracture-dislocation (paraplegia)	1
L 5–S 1 fracture	2

of patients had other major injuries. Significant neurological deficits occurred in only eight patients, 6.5% of the series. All but two of these patients gained complete neurological recovery within 22 days. One patient developed paralysis of the left arm five weeks after injury, three weeks after the application of the halo support. Traction neurapraxia was diagnosed and the brace removed. The fracture healed and there was complete neurological recovery. One patient suffered paraplegia as a result of fracture dislocation at T 12 and was not included in this analysis.

The radiographs of all but fifteen patients revealed typical bilateral fractures of the pedicles of the axis with fracture lines traversing either the pars interartucularis of the foramina transversaria. All patients with displacement of the fractures also had anterior displacement of the body of the axis. Only twelve patients had undisplaced fractures. Nine patients had fractures involving the body of the axis. This group of fractures differs mechanically from the typical injury in that the posterior fragment of the body of the axis may compress the cord against the posterior elements of the atlas as in an atlantoaxial dislocation. No patient sustained a single unilateral fracture.

In 117 of the 123 patients the injury could be diagnosed on lateral radiographs, and oblique views were needed in only four patients. Tomography was useful in only two cases in lieu of oblique views. Tomography was used to confirm the diagnosis of 30 consecutive cases early in the study but was discontinued because of the reliability of diagnosis from lateral radiographs.

Thirty-five patients were managed primarily in cervical or cervicothoracic supports and allowed to walk. Eighty-eight patients were treated by traction, and 43 of these were in traction for an average period of six weeks, ranging from 4 to 12 weeks. These patients were treated in traction for an average of 8.1 days, ranging from 3 to 13 days (Table 3). These patients were then allowed up, wearing a halo-pelvic brace from four to seven weeks, with

Table 3. *Incidence of Nonunion Related to Method and Period of Treatment*

	Traction 4 to 12 weeks (mean 6 weeks)	Traction 3 days to 3 weeks (mean 8.1 days)	Other treatment
Union	39	44	33
Nonunion treated surgically	4	1	2
Total	43	45	35

a cervicothoracic brace for a further four weeks. The period of bed rest and the type and rigidity of bracing support could not be correlated with the speed or incidence of union, though accuracy of reduction was not as well maintained in less rigid devices.

Healing occurred in 116 patients (94.5%) in under 16 weeks, regardless of the regime of treatment, and occurred as early as eight weeks after injury in six patients. The average time for healing was 11.5 weeks. Seven patients were operated on; of six patients with nonunion, four had anterior fusion of the bodies of C 2–C 3, and two had posterior fusion of C 1–C 3. One patient had a posterior fusion at C 2–C 4 performed after union of the pedicles because of persistent pain and a flexion injury at C 3–C 4 level which created an unstable kyphosis. Patients were kept in traction during operation and for 7 to 10 days afterwards. They were then allowed up in a Minerva cast or halo-vest for 8 to 12 weeks. Union occurred in all seven patients in 9 to 15 weeks with complete relief of symptoms.

Displacement did not appear to influence healing, being present in only two of the patients who required operation. When flexion was the mechanism, injury was of grade II or grade IV. Five of the patients with disruption of the C 2–C 3 interspace showed this only after traction had been applied. They were placed in this group and not in that indicated by the initial lateral radiograph.

It is possible that more patients would have been classified as having grade V injury if they had been subjected to distraction. Because of the risk involved, it is not recommended that traction should be used to establish the degree of ligamentous injury. The distribution of patients in the various grades (Table 1) in relation to those failing to unite, is given in Table 4. Six of the seven patients requiring operation showed angulation on initial radiographs.

Table 4. *Incidence of Nonunion Related to the Grade of Injury*

Grade	Number of patients	Number with nonunion
I	19	0
II	9	3
III	46	0
IV	42	1
V	7	2

3.14. Dens Fractures: a Multi-center Study

Ch. R. Clark, Iowa City, Iowa, U.S.A., and
A. A. White, III, Boston, Massachusetts, U.S.A.

The treatment of dens fractures is controversial. No single method of management has yet become universally accepted. The major controversy centers around fractures occurring at the base of the dens.

No large, long-term study is available which truly answers the question of appropriate initial management of these fractures. *The Cervical Spine Research Society* addressed this issue with a multi-center study [1].

Because of its clinical applicability as well as its anatomical significance, the Anderson and D'Alonzo classification was selected as the basis for this study [2]. *Type I* is an oblique fracture of the tip of the dens and is very unusual. *Type II*, a common injury, is a fracture of the junction of the dens with the body of the axis. The *Type III* fracture is one in which the fracture goes deep into the body of the axis. Additional factors such as direction, angle, and degree of displacement of the fragments were also considered.

Patients with pathological fractures and fractures occurring in children less than ten years of age were excluded. Diagnosis was established by appropriate radiographic studies.

Treatment modalities were documented including type, duration, and result.

Stability and union were determined radiographically. Criteria for union included trabeculation across the fracture site and no movement on lateral flexion/extension radiographs. A fracture was considered stable if there was no evidence of displacement on lateral flexion/extension radiographs regardless of bony union. Date forms and radiographic reports were compiled by each participating member of the society and forwarded to the senior author for compilation and analysis.

One hundred and fifty-six cases met the above criteria and were evaluated. There were 106 Type II fractures and, fifty Type III fractures. Patients sustaining Type II injuries averaged 42.7 years, and patients with Type III injuries averaged 43.9.

72% of the Type II injuries occurred in males and 28% in females. The majority of Type III injuries also occurred in males. Virtually all injuries were the result of either a motor vehicle accident or a fall.

Displacement and angulation were analyzed. Thirty-six displaced Type II fractures had a mean AP translation of 5.8 mm and eleven Type III fractures had a mean translation of 4.5 mm. Twenty-eight Type II fractures averaged an angular deformity of 13.3 degrees and twelve Type III fractures averaged 15.3 degrees. The majority of both types were displaced anteriorly.

Neurological involvement in Type III injuries included two patients with Brown-Sequard syndrome, three patients with hemiparesis and seven patients with quadriparesis. Neurological involvement in Type III injuries included hemiparesis in one patient and quadriparesis in three patients.

Following the initial treatment of *all* Type II injuries 64% were united however 36% were nonunited. In Type III injuries 72% went to union, 15% were nonunited and 13% were malunited.

Management of the fractures varied considerably. Results according to specific treatment modality will be discussed according to fracture type.

Treatment modalities for Type II injuries ranged from no treatment to surgery. Anterior fusions included transoral and anterolateral approaches and generally were fixed internally with a screw. All cases not treated originally or treated with an orthosis went on to nonunion. 68% of patients treated with a halo device were united following the initial treatment. However, 26% were nonunited and 6% were malunited. One patient with an anterior cervical fusion went on to nonunion. 96% of patients treated with a posterior cervical fusion went on to solid union and one developed a nonunion.

Looking at Type III fractures: All of the patients who were not treated initially went on to nonunion. 18% of the patients treated with an orthosis were nonunited, and 36% were malunited. All patients treated by bedrest, anterior or posterior cervical fusion went on to solid union. One patient treated with skeletal traction had a malunion. Of the patients treated with a halo device 86% united, one developed a nonunion and one patient displaced the fracture whilst in the device and required surgical fusion.

Significant displacement was defined as 5 mm or more of translation in the AP plane and/or 10 degrees or more of angulation. A chi-square analysis of Type II fractures evaluating the dependence of significant displacement and union demonstrated a statistically significant rate of nonunion/malunion in Type II fractures with displacement ($p < 0.05$). A chi-square bivariant analysis failed to reveal a statistically significant relation between union and displacement for Type III fractures.

Thirty-one patients with Type II injuries required further treatment including anterior or posterior cervical fusion. All of these united solidly except one patient who had an increased neurological deficit following an attempted open reduction and posterior fusion for an old fracture. Ten patients with Type III injuries required further treatment and all of these patients went on to solid union.

Four patients with Type II injuries died suddenly following their injuries. Two additional patients died during follow-up, one secondary to metastatic carcinoma and a second patient died of respiratory failure following an anterior cervical fusion. Two patients with anterior screw fixation of the dens had migration of their internal fixation device with one patient developing an eye palsy. One additional patient treated with an anterior fusion had increased neurological deficit. Complications in patients sustaining Type III injuries including one patient treated in a halo who died twenty-four hours following injury due to a cardiopulmonary arrest.

Based on our multi-center study of dens fractures the following conclusions were reached:

1. Classification of dens fractures according to anatomic level appears to be very useful. In addition displacement is a significant factor.

2. There was a significant rate of nonunion/malunion following initial treatment of dens fractures. 36% of Type II fractures did not unite following initial management. In Type III fractures, 15% were not united and 13% were malunited.

3. The halo device was successful in managing Type II injuries in 68% of cases, whereas a posterior cervical fusion was successful in 96%. However, the complications may be more significant with the surgical mode of treatment.

4. Patients with Type II injuries having significant displacement should be considered for surgical stabilization. Patients managed with posterior cervical fusion had a significantly higher success rate and lower complication rate compared to those patients managed with an anterior stabilization procedure.

5. Type III injuries are not benign. There is a significant rate of malunion and nonunion in patients treated with an orthosis alone. It appears that the halo device is the safest and most reliable form of therapy for the Type III injury. An exception to those mode of treatment may be the impacted Type III fracture in an elderly patient.

References

1. Clark CR, White AA III (1985) Fractures of the Dens: a multicenter study. J Bone Joint Surg, 67-A: 1340–1348
2. Anderson LD, D'Alonzo RT (1974) Fractures of the odontoid process of the axis. J Bone Joint Surg 56-A: 1663–1674

3.15. Dens Transfixation Plate

R. Streli, Linz, Austria

Performing osteosynthesis in dens fractures using an anterior approach has proved to be an interesting challenge. Following studies on cadaver specimens, we first performed medullary nailing in a dens fracture, using a curved nail with U-shaped profile.

Technically it was not difficult to complete this procedure in the case of this 34-year-old theatre nurse (UL 2830/75), although roentgenologically the fracture did not heal satisfactorily. The operation was carried out in February 1975 and was regularly examined for a period of ten years.

In June 1975 we started to use dens plates. These plates were delta-shaped and had a central hole for the dens compression screw. This screw inserted upwards and backwards into the dens and therefore pressed the dens to the plate and simultaneously compressed the fracture according to the parallelogram of forces.

The specimen shown is case no. 1, who died as a result of Ondine's Curse. The osteosynthesis was stable (UL 12759/75). Eighteen cases were operated upon. The average age was 47 years, the youngest being 17, the oldest 72.

12 were males and 5 females. The results obtained were promising. No complications occurred with the exception of case 1. This demonstrates the case of a 24-year-old nurse. The pseudarthrosis was $^4/_5$ resected. The defect has been filled with spongious bone. Full reduction could not be obtained. The stabilization with a dens plate functioned excellently and the pseudarthrosis healed well, the patient was free of symptoms and complaints (UL 11.382/78 and UL 5530/79) and did not show severe limitations of movement 6 years after removal of the plate (the dens plate was 421 days in the recipient). Further observations made clear, that the level of effectiveness could be improved if the anatomical shape of the anterior aspect of the axis was considered. In particular the plate should fit the prominentia mediana Firbas of the axis. The steep position of the facies subarticularis could be used for the temporary transfixation of the lateral atlanto-axial joints.

Therefore a casting mould in metal was made of the anterior surface, using a material with low melting temperature. A positive was then made.

Howmedica produced the dens-transfixation plate according to this shape. The shaft of the plate could be attached to the body of the second and third or in some cases fourth cervical vertebra. The plate is manufactured in vitallium (Fig. 1).

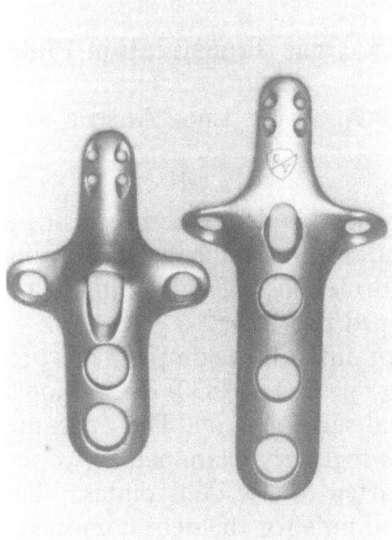

Fig. 1. Dens transfixation plate. Left: short size, lateral extension tilted 30°. Right: normal size lateral extensions tilted 45°, to fit the facies subarticulares axis on both sides

When attached to a cervical spine specimen it can be demonstrated, that the upper extension of the plate lies on the anterior surface of the dens and fracture, and behind the anterior tubercle of the atlas. The screw in the center of the delta, introduced obliquely backward and upwards to the apex of the dens, compresses the fracture and presses the dens against the plate. Screws are inserted for the transfixation of the lateral atlanto-axial joints through the lateral extensions fitting the facies subarticulares. The upper extension of the plate has two small holes for the application of wire sutures left and right of the anterior atlantic tubercle.

The shaft of the plate is attached to the body of the second, third and fourth cervical vertebral using 6.5 mm TKFS screws. This screw has a flat head to avoid bulging out against the pharynx and oesophagus and deep cross slits to provide grip for the screw drivers. The posterior cortex of the vertebral bodies should be perforated with a half thread of the screws (Fig. 2).

The procedure is undertaken in a dorsal recumbent position. It starts with a 6 cm transverse incision from the midline to the right over the fourth cervical vertebra.

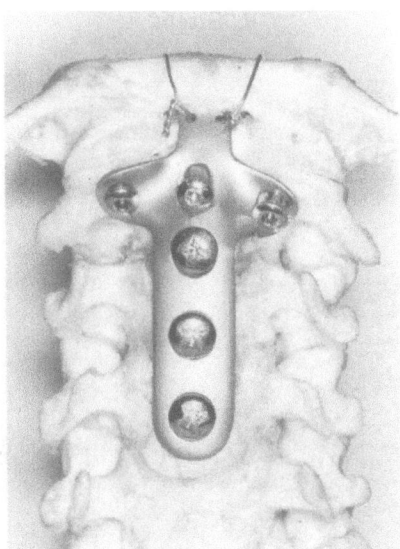

Fig. 2. Dens transfixation plate mounted on a specimen from a cadaver. The left screw is not completely driven in to show its direction 10° lateraly and 10° backwards. Full details in the text

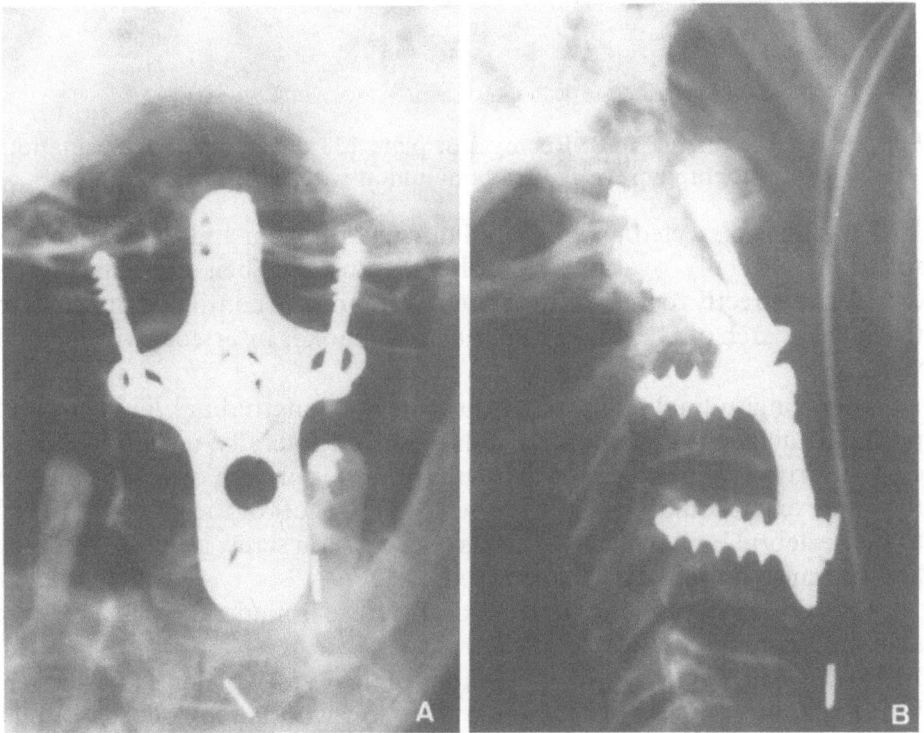

Figs. 3 A and B. G. A., 49 years, DT-Case 23, UL 29528/84. X-ray: short dens transfixation plate AP and lateral view. Operation was carried out nine days after the accident. Full reduction and compression of the dens fracture is demonstrated

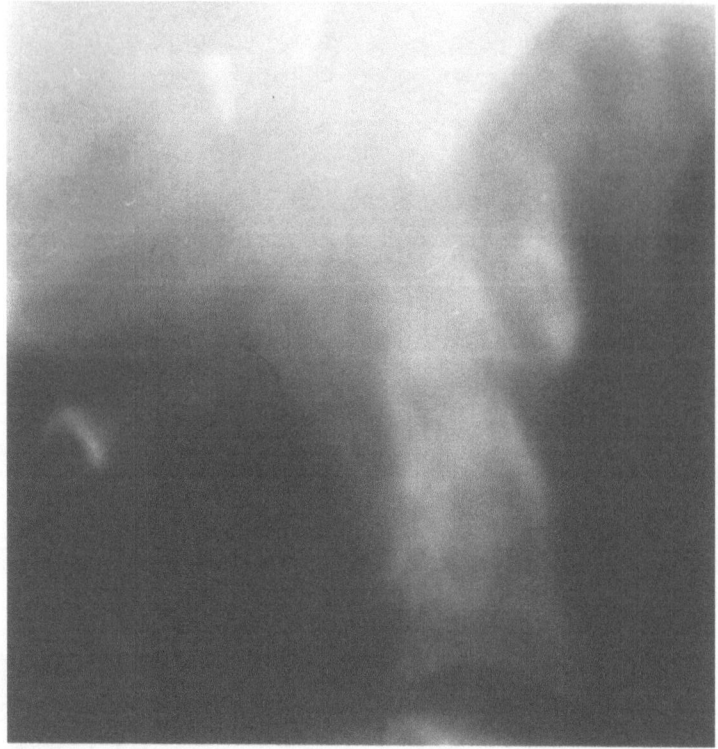

Fig. 4. Same case as in Fig. 3. Removal of plate 133 days after instrumentation. Tomography reveals firm bony union without dislocation

The skin is dissected upwards and downwards 4 cm and the platysma is split longitudinally over the sternohyoid muscle. Then the exposure is carried out directly to the fourth cervical vertebra and continued upwards to the anterior arch of C 1, where a special atlas hook is inserted, giving a good view.

After longitudinal splitting of the anterior longitudinal ligament and partial detachment of the longus colli muscles bilaterally, a slightly curved chisel is driven up between the dens and the anterior arch of C 1. In this slit the upper extension of the plate is inserted. The shaft of the plate is screwed to the vertebral bodies. Then the dens compression screw is applied and the lateral transfixation screws positioned.

A suction drain is implanted. No deep suture is made, the platysma and skin are sutured.

In this case (Figs. 3 and 4) a short plate was applied (DT-Case 23, UL 29528/84). Despite of low grade infection with staphylococcus albus, which was sensitiv to all antibiotics, the fracture healed well. It is also of note, that the patient was diabetic. Usually dens fractures heal in a relatively short time, when stable osteosynthesis in the reported manner is achieved.

As a result of the experience gained from 24 cases we feel encouraged to continue with this simple and safe procedure, which is stable without external fixation and without permanent spondylodesis C 1–C 2.

We have the following ideas for the future:

1. A shortening of the duration of implantation times for people up to 70 years of age.

2. A possible shortening of the implant down to the lower anterior margin of the second cervical vertebra.

3. The use of two or three prefabricated plates fitting the individually varying shapes, lengths and breadth simultaneously.

This would make secondary bending of the plate during operation, which is sometimes necessary, superfluous.

References

1. Ryan MD, Taylor TKF (1982) Odontoid fractures. J Bone Joint Surg 64 B: 416–421
2. Streli R (1981) Kompressionsosteosynthese bei Frakturen und Pseudarthroscn des Dens epistrophei. Z Orthop 119: 675
3. Streli R (1981) Teflon C I/C II Platte. Zbl Chir 106: 244–247
4. Streli R: Unstable fractures of the Dens axis and pseudarthrosis. (Vorgetragen: International College of Surgeons, Wien, October 6, 1982). In: Traumatology of the spinal column (Vècsei V) Proceedings of the I. Viennese Workshop, International College of Surgeons, Austrian Section. Informatica Ges.m.b.H. Vienna, p 203
5. Streli R (1983) Neue Denstransfixationsplatte. Hefte zur Unfallheilkunde 165: 280

Cervical Spine I
© by Springer-Verlag 1987

3.16. Traumatic Lesions of the Upper Cervical Spine

D. S. Korres, K. Stamos, and Chr. Kosmidis, Athens, Greece

I. Introduction

The upper cervical spine due to its anatomical and functional peculiarities always provokes great interest. Its contribution to the support of the head, the performance of various movements and the protection of the spinal cord, has been studied in depth. However, these studies have not prevented the appearance of serious disputes particularly with regards to the biomechanical characteristics of the upper cervical spine.

The position of the upper cervical spine as well as the complexity in the functioning of the existing joints between the occipital, the atlas and the axis renders it prone to injuries. Some, injuries are fatal and therefore do not reach hospital. Alternatively however, it is possible, for people who have survived a serious injury, not to have or to present mild neurological signs.

The clinical picture and the history, will lead us to better investigation and projection of the underlying lesion. However, knowledge of the injuries which can occur in this part of the spine is indispensable in order to proceed to the correct treatment. In certain cases we are facing the particular, but also interesting phenomenon of the coexistence of more than one injury, phylogenically different to each other, a fact which renders their treatment difficult.

II. Material

The present study deals with 91 patients with fractures of the upper cervical spine, among 289 patients with fractures of the cervical spine treated from January 1970 to December 1983 in the Orthopaedic Department of Athens University, K.A.T. Hospital. The percentage of these injuries was found to be 31.5. There were 56 males and 35 females with an average age of 45.8 years. Fifty-three were victims of a road traffic accident, 36 of a fall and two of a different cause.

Their admission to the Clinic varied between some hours to 6 weeks after the accident (63.7% were admitted the first 24 hours).

The average time of treatment in hospital was 22.9 days (1–339). The X-ray study showed 104 fractures, 3 dislocations and 4 fracture-dislocations. Seventeen of these patients had an other fracture at a different level of the spine (18.6%) and 20 out of 91 (21.9%) had another fracture in the peripheral skeleton. Fifteen patients (16.4%) had a neurological lesion. Table 1 shows the type and percentage of those injuries.

Table 1. *Type of Injury of the Upper Cervical Spine*

A. Fractures

1. Atlas: 24 (26.3%)   Anterior arch 1 (1.01%)
                             Posterior arch 19 (20.8%)
                             Jefferson 3 (3.3%)
                             Transverse proc. 1 (1.01%)

2. Axis: 80 (87.9%)   Dens 37 (40.6%)
                             Ring 37 (40.6%)
                             Body 6 (6.6%)

B. Dislocations

   1. Atlanto-axial 3 (3.2%)
   2. Atlanto-occipital 0 (0.0%)

C. Fracture-Dislocations

   1. Atlanto-occipital 1 (1.01%)
   2. Atlanto-axial 3 (3.2%)

III. Results

Eight patients died, and 8 more could not be followed up. So 75 patients were reexamined in an average time of 55.2 months (7 to 164). The combination of the clinical (pain, restriction of movements, neurological status etc) and X-ray presentation gave us an excellent result for 45 cases, a good one for 25 and a moderate result for 5 patients.

IV. Discussion

Studying these 75 medical records, we gave special attention not only to the whole totality of the lesions of each patient but also to the different types of lesions separately:

a) The frequency of 31.5% is rather high, because of the spacial anatomical morphology of the area and its great mobility.

b) The cause of the accident was found to be in relation to the age of the patients. Approximately 58% (58.2%) of the patients, victims of a road traffic accident, were 20 years younger than the victims of a fall.

c) The coexistence at the same time of a lesion in the skeleton (22%) and in the spine (18.6%). The rate of 18.6% of double level fractures of the spine (as it was defined in a previous article) is the highest ever recorded [4]. Sixteen of these patients had a second fracture or dislocation at a lower cervical spine.

d) The low frequency of a neurological lesion. Not a single lesion of the vertebral artery was recorded.

e) The high frequency of the fractures of the dens associated with fractures of the posterior arch of the axis (5 cases or 5.5%) and

f) Total absence amongst our cases of a pure atlanto-occipital disloca- tion, due of course to the severity of this lesion.

Fracture of the Atlas

Examining each type of lesion separately we noticed that the fractures of the atlas (8.6%) were not so frequent, and some of them quite rare (2.7%). These did not present big problems: Anyway we must point out 4 points of particular interest:

1. The failure of diagnosis concerning fractures of the transverse processes or unilateral fractures of the posterior arch of the atlas (a percentage of 22%).

2. The low frequency of the neurological lesions or the absence of injury of the vertebral artery.

3. The high frequency of associated lesions of the atlas, a percentage of 72% (17 cases of fracture of the dens, 3 cases of fracture of the posterior arch of the axis, 2 cases of fracture of the body of the axis and 7 cases of a fracture at a distal vertebra).

4. Complications caused by the traction or by long periods of rest in bed, especially among aged people.

Fractures of the Axis

They were of particular interest especially those of the dens or those of the posterior arch, knowing that those of the body do not present specific problems.

Fractures of the dens represent 13% of cervical fractures in our series. Their main problem is related to the stability and pseudarthrosis (1.6%). Studying 37 records, 28 of them with a follow-up of 55 months we noticed that:

a) the delay in starting treatment, b) a displacement of more than 3 mm not reduced and c) bad immobilization were the main causes of delayed union or fusion in an unacceptable position or, finally of pseudarthrosis. Horizontal fracture—following the Roy-Camille classification [5]—seemed to be the most unstable, presenting the highest rate of pseudarthrosis (3 out of 4 in our series).

Fractures of the posterior arch of the axis (13%) do not present particular problems especially when the displacement was not more than 12 mm and when dislocation did not exist [3].

Stability of the fracture depended on how severe the lesion of the soft tissues was, especially the C 2–C 3 disc, which should be checked with great care. No occurrence of a single pseudarthrosis.

That fact gave us the idea that the outcome of this type of fracture is not related to the time treatment was started or to the initial displacement. No spontaneous bony fusion between C 2–C 3 bodies was found.

Undisplaced fractures of the posterior arch as well as fractures of the body, comprise the type, which produce best results with treatment. On the contrary, fractures involving the facets do not respond so well to treatment. Fracture dislocations or pure dislocations as well as multiple level fractures present some difficult and serious problems. Here the treatment is rather difficult, but the results are rather encouraging.

The combination of fractures of the atlas and axis together in the same case, or the coexistence of an odontoid fracture with a fracture of the posterior arch of the axis, are of a special interest and must not be overlooked [4]. The reason is that the treatment concerning one of them could interfere with the other. For example the presence of a simple lesion could be a stable one but combined to a second lesion could form a very unstable model. The frequency for those cases was found to be rather high (36.2%).

Our results are based on cases treated conservatively, and if we ignore the exception of fractures of the dens, where we had the least satisfying results, we can consider the conservative treatment, when properly applied, as satisfactory.

References

1. Amyes E, Anderson FM (1956) Fractures of the odontoid process. Arch Surg 72: 377–399
2. Boni R (1957) Sombra mi raro caso du frattura del tuberculo anteriore dell'atlande. Rad Med 43: 455–462
3. Effendi *et al* (1981) Fractures of the ring of the axis. JBJS 63-B: 319–329
4. Korres D, Katsaros A, Pantazopoulos Th, Hartofilakidis-Garofalidis G (1981) Double or multiple level fractures of the spine. Injury 13: 147–152
5. Roy-Camille R, Bleanie JF, Saillant G, Judet Th (1979) Fracture de l'odontoïde associée a une fracture des pédicules de l'axis. Rev Chir Orthop 65: 387–391
6. Shatzker J, Robareck Ch, Waddel JP (1975) Non union of the odontoid process: an experimental investigation. Clin Orthop 108: 127–137
7. Sherk HH, Nickolson JT (1970) Fractures of the atlas. JBJS 52-A: 1017

Cervical Spine I
© by Springer-Verlag 1987

3.17. A Combined Fracture of the Anterior and Posterior Arch of the Atlas due to Extreme Lateral Bending: Case Report

B. JEANNERET, Bern, Switzerland

Since Jefferson's description of fractures of the atlas in 1920 [6], combined fractures of the anterior and posterior arch have been attributed to axial compressive forces typically following a blow to the vertex of the skull [2, 4, 6, 7, 9, 10, 12, 14]. These compressive forces are transmitted through the occipital condyles to the lateral masses of the atlas. Due to the obliquity of the atlanto-occipital and atlanto-axial joints, the resultant vertical load produces significant horizontal distraction forces that can disrupt the ring (Fig. 1) at one or more of its weakest points [6]. These are by virtue of the anatomy, the anterior arch near the junction with the lateral masses and the posterior arch at the level of the vertebral artery groove [3, 6, 7, 13, 14]. Separation of the lateral masses may also lead to secondary rupture or bony avulsion of the transverse ligament resulting in an unstable fracture dislocation [7, 8, 11, 14]. In particular, this must be suspected when the frontal radiographs demonstrate bilateral splaying of the lateral masses greater than 6.9 mm [11].

We recently investigated a combined fracture of the anterior and posterior arch of the atlas which, based on the circumstances of the accident, on the autopsy findings and on preliminary experimental results could not be attributed to axial compression but to sudden extreme lateral bending of the neck. To our knowledge, this is the first description of a combined fracture of both arches of the atlas attributed to this type of mechanism.

Case Report

While driving a motor vehicle (30 km/h) and wearing a three-point safety-belt, a twenty-year-old male was struck broadside on the left by a little truck (60 km/h). The car was pushed to a standstill, without turning over. The whole side was caved in at the level of the driver's body and head, the roof was damaged but not pushed in. The driver, still strapped into the seat, died immediately. Due to the obvious death, no resuscitation was performed, no radiographic examinations were done. Postmortem

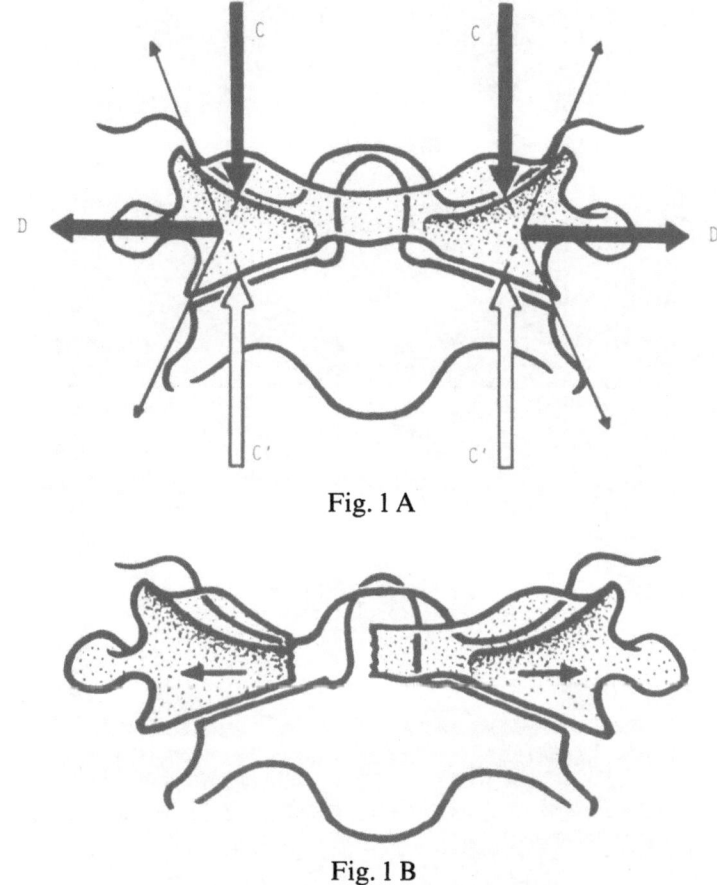

Fig. 1 A

Fig. 1 B

Fig. 1. A) In burst fractures of the C1-ring, axial compressive (C) and reacting forces (C′) produce horizontal distraction forces (D). B) These distraction forces may disrupt the C1-ring and lead to separation of the lateral masses

examination subsequently revealed marked contusions of the left hemi-thorax and multiple glass cuts on the left side of the neck, cheek, temple and ear. The nose, mouth and both auditory canals were filled with blood. The cause of the death was ultimately attributed to contusion of the left side of the body with multiple rib fractures, fracture of the left clavicle and rupture of the aortic arch and spleen with massive hemorrhage into the pleural and peritoneal cavities. Examination of the skull disclosed concentric fractures of the left temporal and parietal bone with radial fissures. Craniotomy subsequently revealed an additional fracture line crossing the base of the skull just in front of both superior petrosal sinus and contusions of the left temporal and parietal lobes. In addition, the atlas had nondisplaced

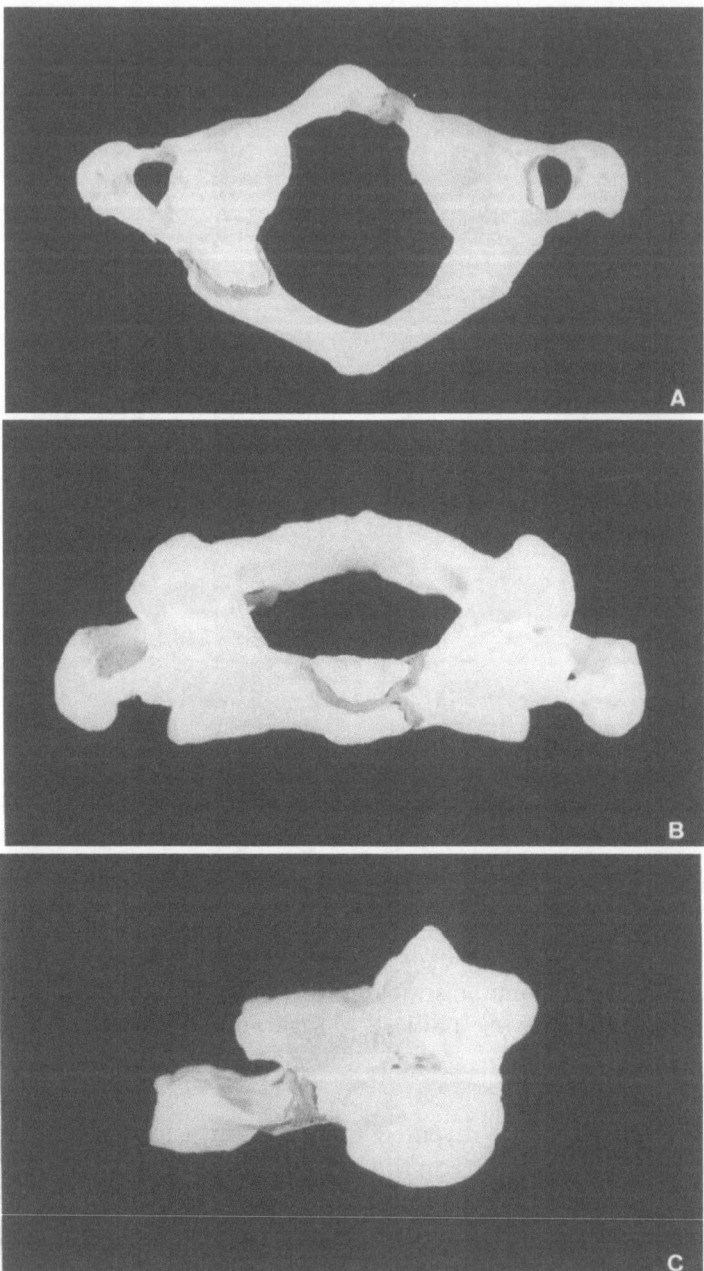

Fig. 2. Autopsy preparation of the atlas; the fracture has been reduced and secured with adhesive. A) Caudal view (the right lateral mass is on the left side of the figure): The anterior arch is fractured on his left paramedian aspect, the posterior arch just behind the right lateral mass. B) Anterioposterior aspect (the right lateral mass is on the left side of the figure): The anterior arch of the atlas presents a fracture of its left paramedian part with a typical cranial butterfly fragment formation. C) From the right side: The posterior arch of the atlas is broken just behind the right lateral mass, at the level of the vertebral artery groove

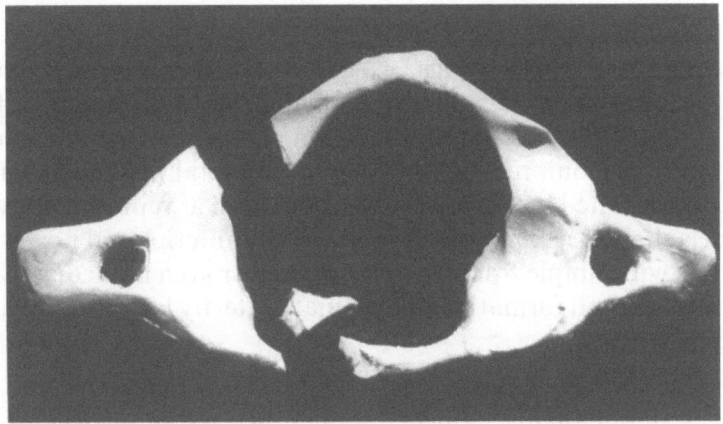

Fig. 3. Compression and bending forces applied simultaneously between both lateral masses resulted in all cases in this fracture pattern

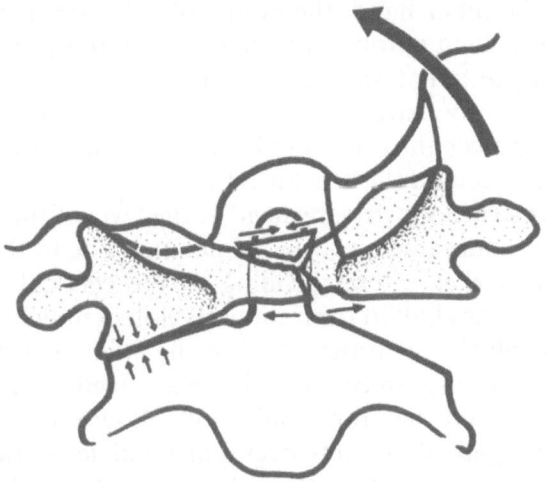

Fig. 4. Fracture mechanism of the combined fracture of the anterior and posterior arch of the atlas in lateral bending injuries (explanation, see text)

fractures of the anterior and posterior arches (Fig. 2 A). Anteriorly, the ring was disrupted through the left paramedian aspect and presented a typical cranial butterfly fragment (Fig. 2 B). The posterior arch contained a simple fracture immediately dorsal to the right lateral mass through the vertebral artery groove (Fig. 2 C). The right vertebral artery, however, was intact. Small hematomas were found in the anterior longitudinal ligament at the level of the atlas, in the atlanto-axial and posterior atlanto-occipital ligaments ipsilateral to the fracture of the posterior arch, in the capsule of the left atlanto-occipital joint, which was intact and around the capsule of the left atlanto-axial joint which was partially disrupted. The alar and transverse ligaments were intact.

Experiment

Prompted by these findings, we attempted to reproduce this fracture pattern on models of the atlas by applying the same forces to them that usually produce butterfly fragments in long bone diaphyseal fractures [1, 5]: *i.e.* bending and compression between both lateral masses. In each of five models, this resulted in the same fracture pattern as reported above (Fig. 3). All models showed a combined fracture of the anterior and posterior arches of the atlas with simple fracture of the posterior arch immediately dorsal to the lateral mass and formation of a cranial butterfly fragment in the anterior arch.

Discussion

Since a "Jefferson mechanism" implies distraction forces in the anterior and posterior arches of the atlas and these forces never produce butterfly fragments [1, 5], our patient's fracture can not be explained by such a mechanism. On the other hand, the events of this motor vehicle accident together with subsequent autopsy information and our preliminary experimental results suggest that this fracture of the atlas was produced by bending forces due to extreme lateral bending of the cervical spine. Although the exact mechanism can not be proven, the following mechanism of injury most likely caused this fracture (Fig. 4): The violent collapse of the left side of the car struck the driver's head at the level of the skull. Since the body of the driver maintained its original position due to the seat belt, this force resulted in marked lateral bending of the cervical spine and in a bending moment to the skull to the right with violent upward pull of the left occipital condyle which was transmitted to the atlas by way of the strong atlanto-occipital capsule. Since the atlas was fixed to the axis by the transverse ligament and therefore could not follow the movement of the skull, the upward pull of the left occipital condyle to the lateral mass produced a bending moment in the atlas ring which ultimately failed: anteriorly by producing a typical butterfly fragment in the compressed superior part, and posteriorly as a simple fracture through the flat vertebral artery groove.

Based on our observations, we believe that combined fractures of the anterior and posterior arches of the atlas are not always the result of compressive forces as stated by Jefferson [6], but may, in some cases, be caused by bending forces due to extreme lateral bending of the cervical spine.

References

1. Alms M (1961) Fracture mechanics. J Bone Joint Surg 43-B: 162–166
2. Baker EG, Krumpelman J, Long JM (1976) Isolated fracture of the medial portion of the lateral mass of the atlas: a previously undescribed entity. Am J Roentgenol 126: 1053–1058

3. Gehweiler JA, Duff DE, Martinez S, Miller MD, Clark WM (1976) Fractures of the atlas vertebra. Skeletal Radiol 1: 97–102
4. Gehweiler JA, Osborne RL, Becker RF (1980) The radiology of vertebral trauma. WB Saunders Company, Philadelphia London Toronto
5. Gozna ER (1982) Biomechanics of long bone injuries. In: Biomechanics of musculoskeletal injury: by Gozna ER, Harrington IJ, Evans DC. Williams & Wilkins, Baltimore London
6. Jefferson G (1920) Fracture of the atlas vertebra. Report of four cases, and a review of those previously recorded. Br J Surg 7: 407–422
7. Jefferson G (1927) Remarks on fractures of the first cervical vertebra. Br Med J 2: 153–157
8. O'Brien JJ, Butterfield WL, Gossling HR (1977) Jefferson fracture with disruption of the transverse ligament. A case report. Clin Orthop 126: 135–138
9. Sherk HH, Nicholson JT (1970) Fractures of the atlas. J Bone Joint Surg 52-A: 1017–1024
10. Sicard A, Picard J, Martin H (1958) Les fractures isolées de l'atlas. J Chir (Paris) 75: 521–538
11. Spence KF, Decker S, Sell KW (1970) Bursting atlantal fracture associated with rupture of the transverse ligament. J Bone Joint Surg 52-A: 543–549
12. Stuhl L, Martin H, Picard J (1959) A propos des fractures isolées de l'atlas. Presse Méd 67: 1879–1882
13. von Torklus D, Gehle W (1970) Die obere Halswirbelsäule. Thieme, Stuttgart
14. White AA, Panjabi MM (1978) Clinical biomechanics of the spine. JB Lippincott Company, Philadelphia Toronto

4. Degenerative Lesions and Management

4.1. Hydroxylapatite Graft Materials for Cervical Spine Fusions

St. D. Cook, Th. S. Whitecloud, M. C. Reynolds, A. F. Harding,
A. S. Routman, J. F. Kay, and M. Jarcho, New Orleans, Louisiana, U.S.A.

Introduction

Hydroxylapatite (HA) is a ceramic material which holds promise as either a replacement for or a supplement to autogenous bone graft material [1, 4]. Previous studies utilizing this material in various applications have shown excellent biocompatibility [1]. The purpose of this paper is to report on the use of bioresorbable and nonbioresorbable HA ceramic materials evaluated as fusion materials in the cervical spines of dogs.

Materials and Methods

Two forms of HA ceramic implants were evaluated. They were a porous surfaced, solid core of nonbioresorbable material and a uniformly porous bioresorbable implant material. Both implant systems were in the form of discs measuring approximately 10 mm by 10 mm in diameter and 3.5 mm thick. The animal model used was the adult greyhound dog, 2–5 years of age, approximately 22–25 kg in weight. Implants were inserted at either the C 3–C 4, C 4–C 5 or C 5–C 6 disc interspace utilizing standard aseptic surgical techniques and an anterior approach. Immediate postoperation radiographs were taken to confirm satisfactory implantation. Prophylactic antibiotics (600,000 units of Procaine Penicillin and 0.75 grams of Dihydrostreptomycin) were administered once a day for four days postsurgery. No external orthopedic device or cervical collar was utilized and unrestricted activity was allowed.

A total of 23 implants, (14 nonbioresorbable and 9 bioresorbable) were evaluated in 13 dogs at time intervals ranging from 1 to 24 weeks. Implant interbody position and progression of fusion were evaluated radiographically at intervals of 3 weeks throughout the implantation periods. In addition, gait analysis using force plates was performed on a periodic basis to assess neurologic function.

At sacrifice, the cervical spines were retrieved *en bloc*. Each operated interspace was isolated and cut at the adjacent mid-vertebral body location.

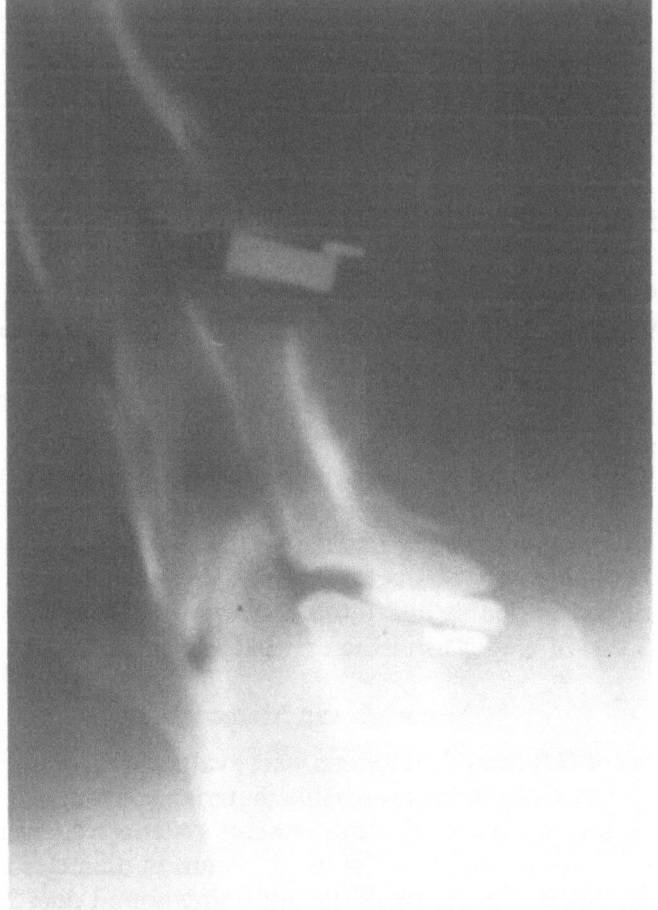

Fig. 1. Immediate postoperative radiograph showing the appearance of the implants within the interspaces (C 4–C 5 nonresorbable, C 5–C 6 bioresorbable)

Preparation of the segments for histologic evaluation was achieved by using standard nondecalcified polymethylmethacrylate embedded ground section techniques [2]. Thin sagittal sections, 50–100 µm thick, were stained with toluidine blue and basic fuchsin for transmitted light microscopy. Non-decalcified microtome sections, 5 µm thick, were also produced using a Jung Model-K Sledge microtome and then stained with toluidine blue, Villanueva bone stain and Krutsay's silver stain [2].

Results

No differences in the fusion rate or the degree of fusion could be detected between the two material systems either radiographically or histologically. In addition, no neurological complications were observed.

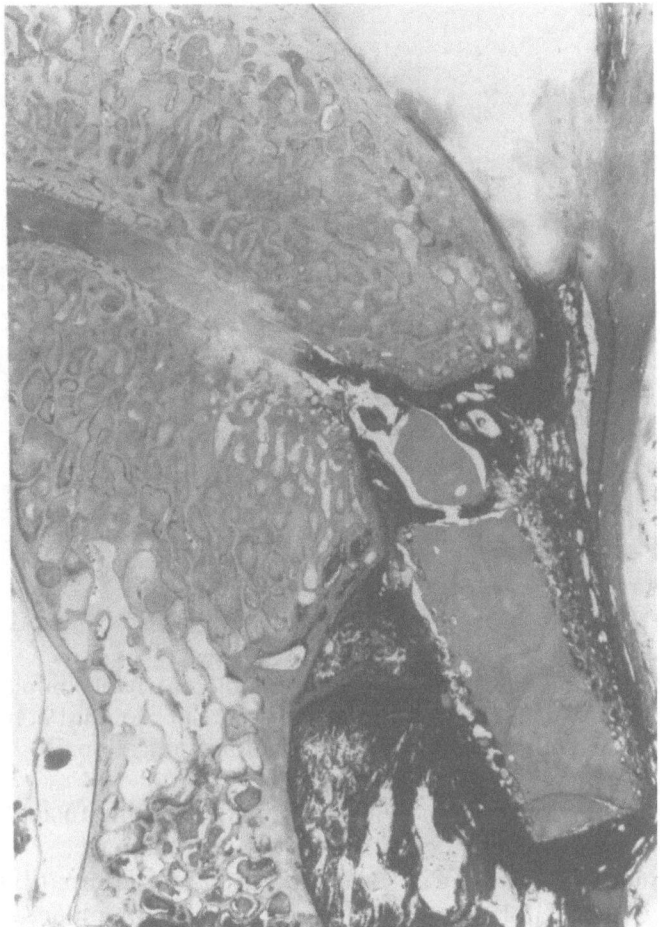

Fig. 2. Photomacrograph of a histologic ground section exhibiting fracture and extrusion of a nonbioresorbable implant into the surrounding soft tissue

Radiographic examination included determination of implant interbody position, progression of spinal fusion and evaluation of implant condition (intact/fractured/extruded). Fig. 1 shows the typical appearance immediately postoperation of implants within the disc spaces. In some cases, fracture of the implant occurred at the time of surgery.

In 9 of 23 cases, fracture with total extrusion of the implant material into the adjacent soft tissue occurred, resulting in a lack of apparent osseous fusion and notable loss of disc space height. In 14 of 23 cases ($\sim 61\%$), the implant materials remained within the interspace, although in most cases implant fracture had occurred. At less than six weeks postoperation increases in apparent bone density, primarily anteriorly, were noted. By 12

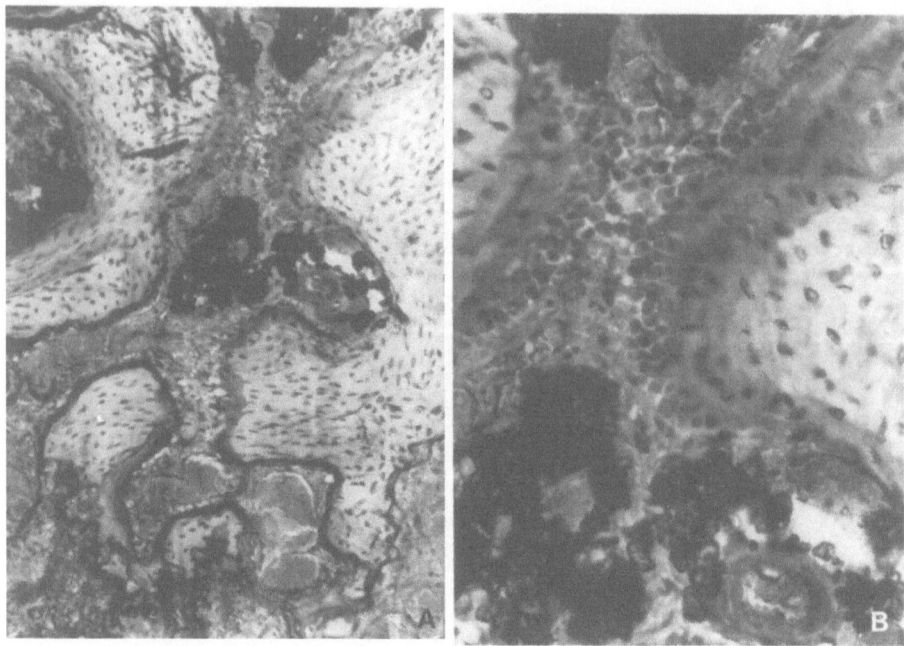

Fig. 3. Photomicrographs of a 3 weeks nonbioresorbable implant exhibiting increased osteoblastic activity within the adjacent subchondral bone. A) Original magnification 20 × ; B) Original magnification 50 ×

and 24 weeks postoperation, evidence of radiographic fusion was marked by increases in radiodensity across the entire interspace.

Histologic evaluation was based upon tissue compatibility and the degree of trabecular bridging and fusion of the interspace. Microscopic examination of the hard tissue specimens revealed no adverse tissue reactions to either implant system. Histologic sections confirmed extensive fracture and extrusion of the implant materials into the adjacent soft tissues (Fig. 2). Examination of these sites often revealed a lack of trabecular bone bridging with the presence of a fibrous union of the interbody space. At 12 and 24 weeks postsurgery, the adjacent vertebral body surfaces appeared biconcave rather than flat most likely the result of resorption of the opposing articulating surfaces.

Evaluation of sections in which parts of the fractured or intact implant remained within the interspace showed considerable osteoblastic activity in the subchondral bone of the adjacent vertebral bodies at early time periods with indications of early signs of fusion (Fig. 3). Extensive fibrous tissue infiltration in and around the implant materials was also noted, with little evidence of resorption of the bioresorbable material at six weeks post-implantation. By 12 and 24 weeks, fibrous tissue was being replaced by new bone and fusions were observed with both implant materials. The HA/bone

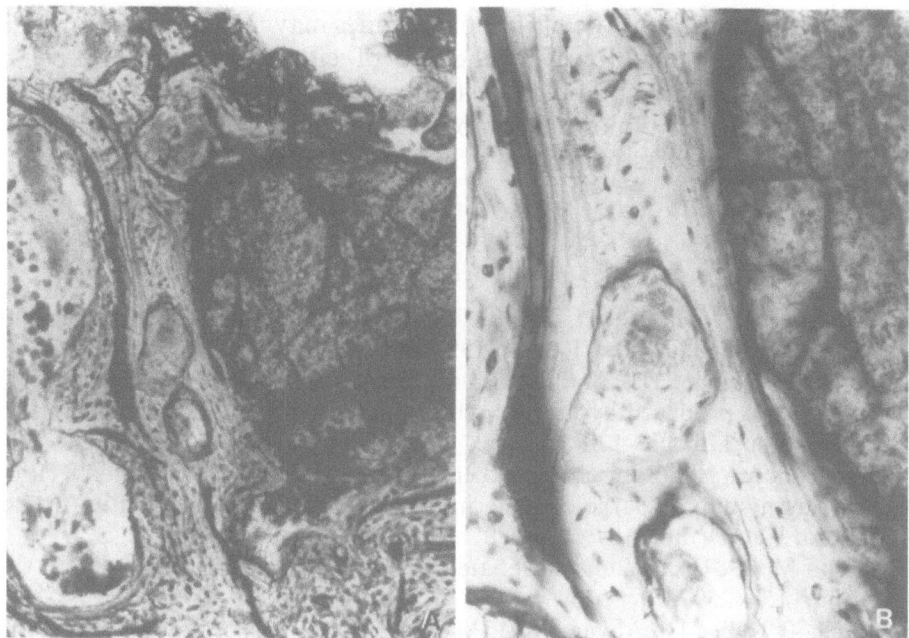

Fig. 4. Photomicrographs exhibiting the HA/bone interface of the nonbioresorbable material at a later time period. A) original magnification 20 ×; B) original magnification 50 ×

interface of the nonbioresorbable materials showed excellent bonding of bone to implant without the presence of any fibrous connective tissue layer (Fig. 4). Also by 12 to 24 weeks, the majority of the bioresorbable HA material was gone and replaced by bone and fibrous tissue.

Discussion

The mechanical loading of the HA implants in canines is most likely severer than that which would be expected in a controlled clinical setting. Unrestricted immediate mobility of the animals may well have been a significant factor in the widespread incidence of implant fracture and subsequent extrusion. The results of the extruded implant materials showing a fibrous rather than an osseous union was probably due to the absence of contact between the HA graft and the subchondral bony plates which has been deemed necessary for acceleration of bone growth and fusion [3]. Conversely, the results of the "successful" implantations, in which whole implants or pieces of the implanted materials remained within the operated interspaces, revealed varying degrees of osseous fusion.

Future studies must optimize the mechanical properties of the ceramic materials if these are to become a viable alternative to autogenous bone grafts. The extremely brittle nature of ceramics may make their use in solid form impractical [5]. However, the use of either nonbioresorbable or bioresorbable HA in a composite system may be an alternative. Mechanical properties as well as biological response time could then be tailored in the manufacturing process to particular needs of the surgical site.

References

1. Cameron HU, MacNab I, Pilliar RM (1977) Evaluation of biodegradable ceramic. J Biomed Mater Res 11: 179–186
2. Cook SD, Skinner HB, Haddad RJ (1983) A quantitative histologic study of osteoporosis produced by nutritional secondary hyperparathyroidism in dogs. Clin Orthop 175: 105–120
3. Hoogendoorn HA, Renooij W, Akkermans LMA, Visser W, Witterbol P (1984) Long-term study of large ceramic implants (porous hydroxylapatite) in dog femora. Clin Orthop 187: 281–288
4. Jarcho M (1981) Calcium phosphate ceramics as hard tissue prosthetics. Clin Orthop 157: 259–278
5. Shima T, Keller JT, Alivara MM, Mayfield FH, Dunsker SB (1979) Anterior cervical discectomy and interbody fusion. J Neurosurg 51: 533–538

Cervical Spine I
© by Springer-Verlag 1987

4.2. A Simultaneous Combined Anterior and Posterior Approach to the Cervical Spine for the Resection of an Osteoblastoma

C. R. WEATHERLEY and J. P. O'BRIEN, Oswestry, U.K.

Introduction

Osteoblastoma of the cervical spine is a tumor well known for its liability to recur following operative resection. This may in part be related to the pathological nature of the tumor, but in part is probably also due to its tendency to involve the lateral elements of a vertebra, thereby making an initial complete resection difficult.

To resect completely such a tumor it is important, therefore, to have a good operative exposure. Such an exposure is provided by a combined anterior and posterior approach. This has been used successfully and will be described.

Case History

A 16-year-old girl presented with a one-year history of pain in the right side of the neck and shoulder. She had a limitation of rotation of the head to the right and localized tenderness over the transverse process of C 6 on this side. Radiography identified an osteoblastoma involving the lateral elements of C 6. A resection of the tumor was carried out from a posterior approach combined with a simultaneous posterior fusion extending from C 5 to C 7.

Three years later, the girl again sought medical advice for a recurrence of the same symptoms. She was again tender over the transverse process of C 6 and had redeveloped a limitation of rotation of the head to the right. Radiographic investigation showed a more extensive involvement of the lateral elements of C 6 (Fig. 1). A technetium bone scan showed increased activity at the site of the lesion, with no abnormality in the rest of the skeleton. Bilateral vertebral angiography was carried out: the right vertebral artery entered the foramen transversarium of C 5, the left vertebral artery was normal. Computerized axial tomography defined the anatomy of the lesion (Fig. 2). Because of the extensive nature of the tumor, it was doubted if a complete resection could be guaranteed using either an anterior

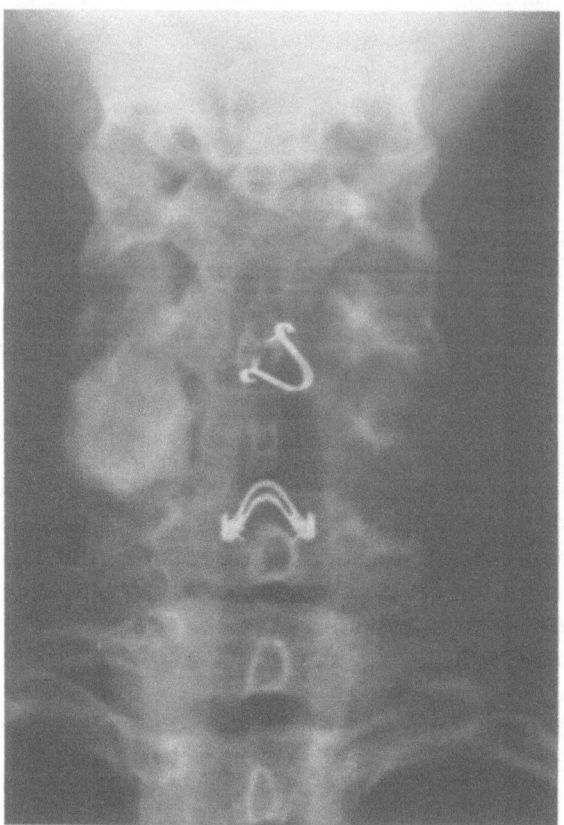

Fig. 1. AP radiograph of the lower cervical spine showing the osteoblastoma involving the lateral mass of C 6 on the right side. (The two clips mark the upper and lower limits, C 5 and C 7, of the posterior fusion associated with the previous operation)

or posterior approach alone. Accordingly, the tumor was resected through a combined approach.

Operative Procedure

Anterior Approach

The operation was carried out under general anesthesia. The patient was placed supine with a sandbag between the shoulders and with the neck extended and the head turned slightly to the left. A transverse skin incision was used on the right side at the C 6 level, beginning lateral to the midline and extending posteriorly to the posterior border of the sternomastoid. The underlying platysma was divided vertically in the line of its fibers. With lateral retraction of the sternomastoid and the carotid sheath, and anterior approach was made to the sixth cervical vertebra (Fig. 3). The level was

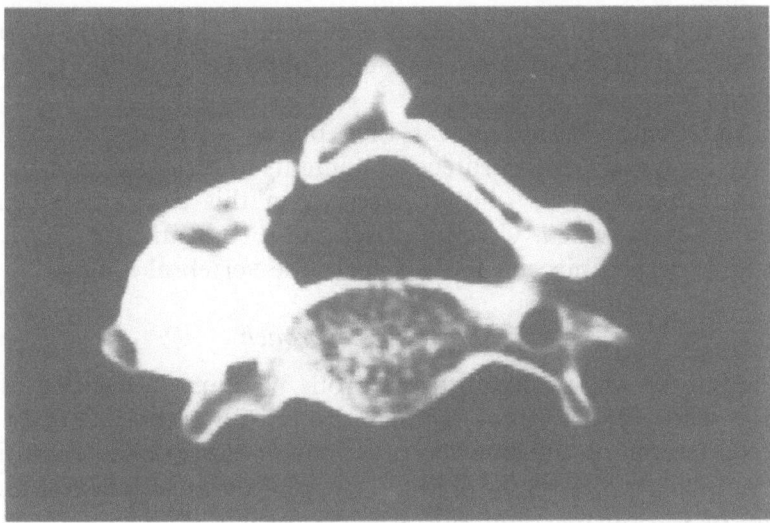

Fig. 2. CAT scan at C 6 level. The tumor involves the pedicle, lamina and transverse process. The defect in the right lamina is related to the previous surgery

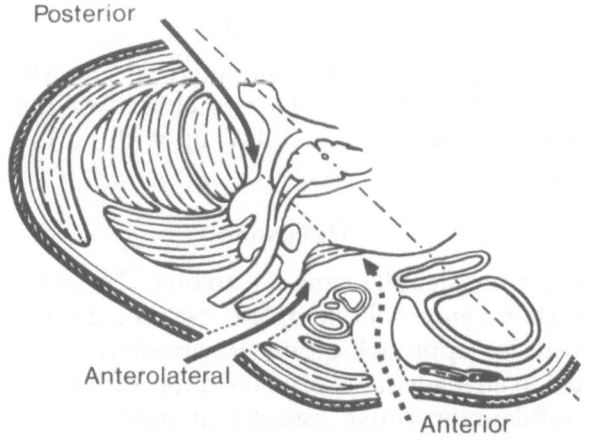

Fig. 3. Diagram of the combined approaches

confirmed radiographically. By subperiosteal dissection proceeding laterally, the longus colli muscle was detached from the anterior surface of the lateral mass.

Antero-lateral Approach

The posterior border of the sternomastoid was then released and the muscle and carotid sheath retracted medially to permit an antero-lateral approach to C 6 (Fig. 3). Beginning at the anterior tubercle of the transverse process and proceeding medially, the remaining muscle attachments to the anterior surface of the lateral mass were cleared. The C 6 and C 7 roots were identified and the upper root retracted gently to expose the lateral mass of C 6.

A McDonald's dissector was then placed anteriorly in the foramen transversarium of C 6 to protect its contents and the anterior lip of bone removed. The contents of the foramen, in this case small veins, were cauterized and divided. Using a chisel and a rongeur, the lateral mass of bone was resected piecemeal away from the vertebral body.

Posterior Approach

The patient was turned into the prone position and a vertical midline incision made to expose the laminae of C 5, C 6 and C 7 (Fig. 3). A solid posterior interlaminar fusion was present from the previous operation. This had not been obvious on the preoperative photographs. The resection of the lamina of C 6 on the right side was completed. The wound, which was continuous from front to back, was drained by a simple suction drain exiting posteriorly.

Follow-up

Radiography (Fig. 4 A) and computerized assisted tomography (Fig. 4 B) confirmed the extent and completeness of the resection. The patient remained asymptomatic at follow-up with no evidence of tumor recurrence.

Discussion

The tendency for osteoblastoma to involve the lateral and posterior elements of a vertebra may make complete resection difficult using either an anterior or posterior approach alone. Recurrence, in most instances, is probably related to an inadequate primary resection. If this problem is to be avoided, a careful preoperative assessment must be combined with an adequate exposure.

Bilateral vertebral angiography is essential in the preoperative assessment of these tumors. This investigation will demonstrate the course of the vessel and the level of entry into the foramen transversarium. Even if the vertebral artery, as in this case, enters the foramen transversarium at a level above the tumor, it is important to remember that the vertebral vein or accessory vertebral vein still needs to be considered. These may be ligatured without risk, but if not considered, may be a source of profuse hemorrhage. Evidence of a normal sized artery on the contralateral side provides some reassurance should intraoperative ligation of the ipsilateral artery be required.

Computerized axial tomography is a valuable adjunct in the pre-

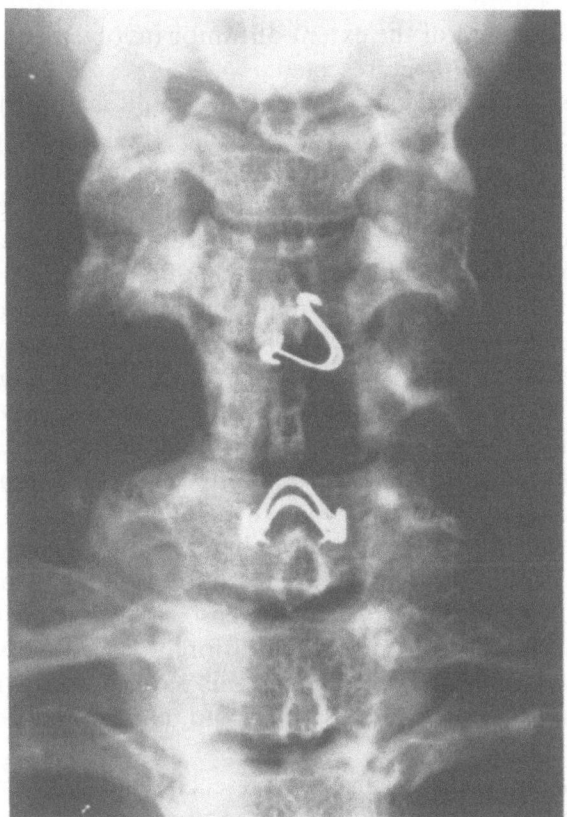

Fig. 4 A. Follow-up AP radiograph. There is a complete resection of the lateral mass of C 6

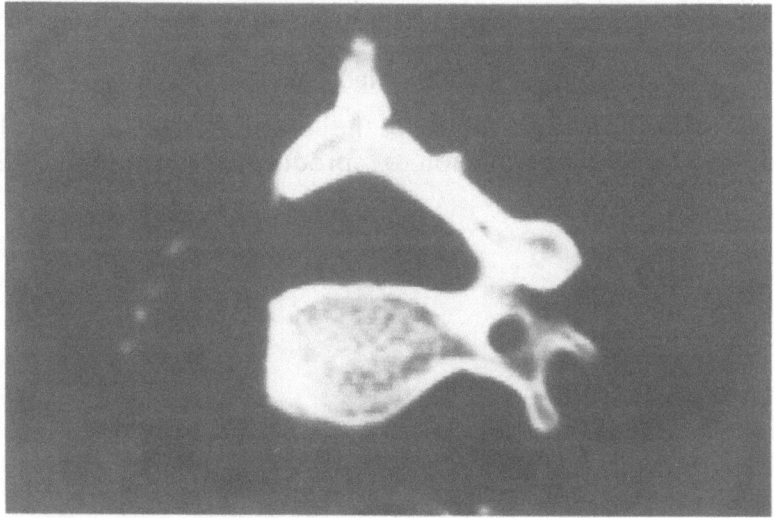

Fig. 4 B. Follow-up CAT scan at C 6 level

operative assessment of the extent of tumor involvement and, therefore, of the amount of bone to be resected.

Since these tumors occur in young people, it is important to avoid ugly scars. At the front of the neck, a transverse skin incision and a vertical split of the platysma provides adequate exposure and the best cosmetic result. Division of the sternomastoid is not required. Good access for the antero-lateral approach is easily obtained by liberating the posterior border of the sternomastoid and retracting the muscle anteriorly.

In the exposure of the lateral mass, prior to its resection, the nerve root above and below the involved vertebra should be clearly seen. The lower requires protection, but it is the upper root descending obliquely in the sulcus between the anterior and posterior tubercles of the transverse process that poses the greatest difficulty. This root has a very limited mobility at this juncture, and retraction should be limited in both extent and duration if permanent damage to the nerve is to be avoided.

Stabilization of the spine, by either an anterior or posterior fusion, should always be considered where resection is likely to give rise in the long run to secondary deformity. In this case, a sound posterior fusion was confirmed at operation and so an additional procedure was not necessary. The combined approach described in this paper affords the opportunity to fuse the spine anteriorly or posteriorly and to make this decision at the time of operation.

In conclusion, revision surgery to resect a recurrent osteoblastoma of the cervical spine might be avoided if a good initial preoperative assessment is combined with a flexible and adequate operative exposure. The approach described here provided the access for a radical, stable and safe procedure and might be used for other tumors in the same situation.

Acknowledgement

The authors wish to acknowledge the cooperation of the Journal of Bone and Joint Surgery for permission to reproduce the illustrations used in this text.

Cervical Spine I
© by Springer-Verlag 1987

4.3. Rheumatoid Spondylarthritis of the Cervical Spine
Prevalence and Surgical Treatment

R. Bauer, A. Giner, and F. Kerschbaumer, Innsbruck, Austria

Radiological changes in the cervical spine frequently occur in rheumatoid arthritis patients. Among others it was the aim of our inquiry to assess a relation between the radiological changes in the cervical spine in rheumatoid arthritis patients and the necessity of surgical treatment.

At the Department of Orthopaedic Surgery of Innsbruck University, standardized X-ray films of the cervical spine were made in 80 rheumatoid arthritis patients who were under stationary treatment between 1978 and 1983. The average age of these patients was 50 years (with a variation between 17 and 76 years). 67 patients were women (83.75%), 13 were men (16.25%). All patients listed in this study met the criteria of ARA. The following radiological changes in the cervical spine could be found:

1. Atlanto-axial subluxation (40%), 2. basilar impression (36.25%), 3. erosion of the dentoid process (51.25%), 4. subaxial subluxation (30%), 5. Demineralization (22.5%), 6. upper plate errosion (33.75%), 7. apophyseal erosion (18.75%), 8. apophyseal fusion (3.75%).

In 40% of the patients an atlanto-axial subluxation could be found radiologically. The distance between the anterior surface of the odontoid process and the posterior surface of the anterior arch of the atlas was taken as its measure. The pathological distance between the odontoid process and the arch of the atlas amounted—on an average—6 mm (4–12 mm, Fig. 1).

In 36.25% of the patients a basilar impression could be found. If the pallato occipital line = McGregor line was exceeded for more than 4.5 mm it was considered to be pathological. On an average, a pathological value of 8 mm (5–14) could be found (Fig. 2).

It appears from our investigations that the dislocations do not only occur in segment C 1/C 2 but also subaxially, with a maximum in the motion segment C 4/C 5 (Fig. 3). The curve diagram approximately corresponds to the diagram of summation of the range of motion in the cervical spine. It may therefore be assumed that the frequent occurrence of dislocating arthritis in certain levels—mainly C 1/C 2 but also C 4/C 5—is caused by an

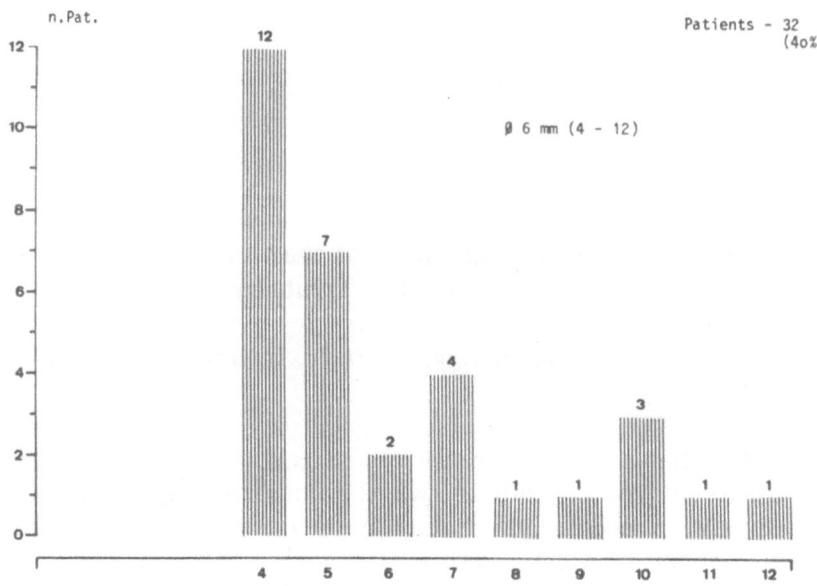

Fig. 1. Atlanto-axial subluxation, distance dens—atlas, mm

increased mechanical use of these segments. Altogether, surgical treatment was only required in 7.5% of the patients, but only with strict indication.

The patients involved were 4 women and 2 men, who were treated surgically. Postoperative follow-up comprised 3 to 8 years. Indication for surgical treatment was two-fold:

a) clinical: Nr.

Incomplete transverse syndrom   3
Radicular lesion   1
Pain   2

b) radiological: Nr.

Atlantoaxial subluxation   average 8 mm   4
Basilar impression   average 10 mm   4
Sublux C 3/C 4   4 mm   1
Sublux C 7/Th 1   5 mm   1

Operations:

4 Brattström   C 1/C 2 2 incomplete transverse syndrom
1 Dorsal decompression   C 3/C 4 1 incomplete transverse syndrom
  and anterior fusion
1 Anterior fusion   C 7/Th 1 1 radicular lesion

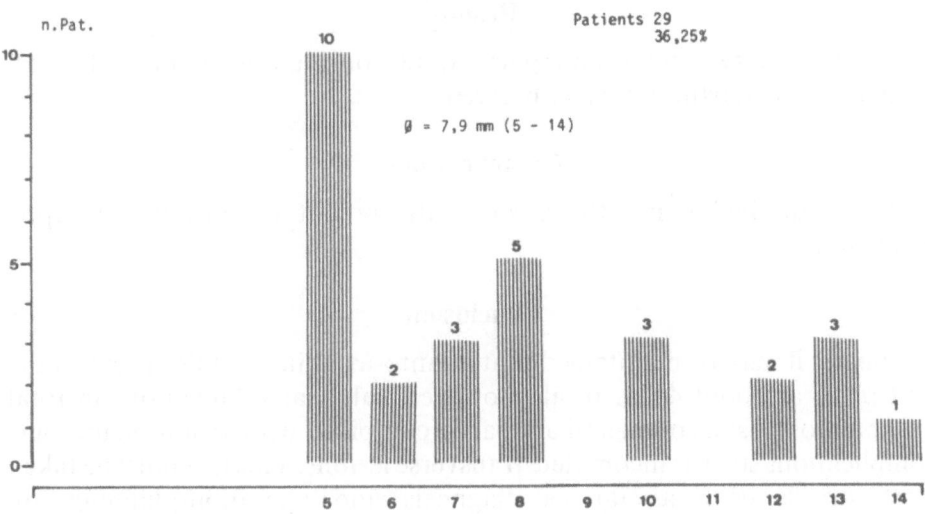

Fig. 2. Basilar impression. Number of patient, which exceeded McGregor line more than 4.5 mm

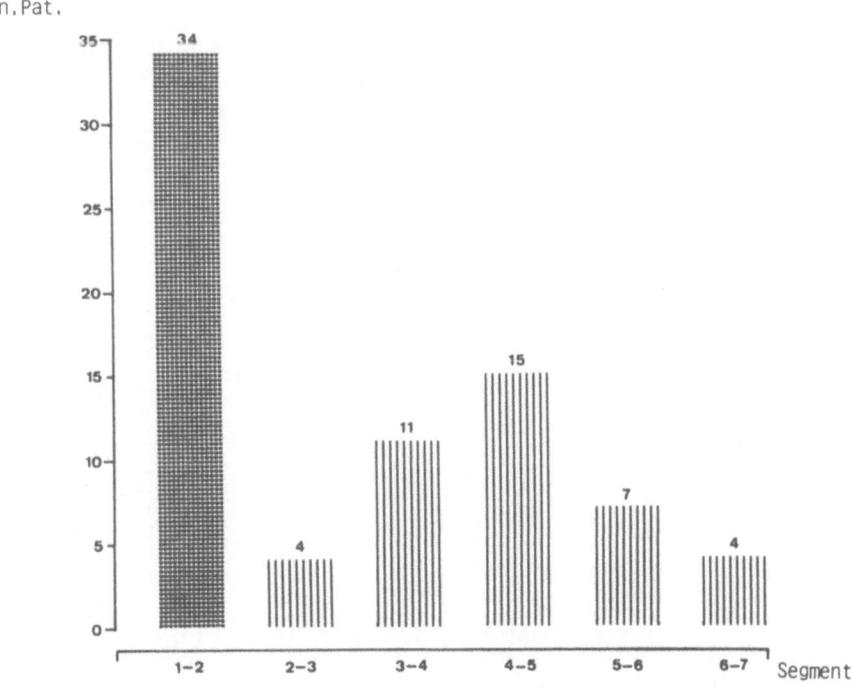

Fig. 3. Subluxation in rheumatoid arthritis at different levels of cervical spine

Results

Neurologic symptoms and pains were considerably improved in all cases. No pseudarthrosis was observed.

Complications

1 patient died 6 months postoperatively out of hospital of septic meningitis.

Conclusion

Finally it may be maintained that atlanto-axial instabilities occur in the first place at about 40%. In all, however, subaxial subluxations in total occur almost just as often and are partly combined with serious neurologic complications such as incomplete transverse lesions. This fact must be taken into consideration as far as diagnosis and operation-planning are concerned.

4.4. Anterior Interbody Fusion with Transdiscal Decompression in the Cervical Spine*

P.-S. Seemann, F. Magerl, and D. Grob, St. Gallen, Switzerland

Introduction

At the S.O.F.C.O.T. meeting in Paris in 1975, six types of cervical syndromes and their surgical treatment were discussed in a round table session. On this occasion Magerl presented two techniques for the treatment of cervical compression syndromes [1].

Technique 1 is a slight modification of the fusion described by Robinson and Smith [2]. The most important alteration concerning decompression is the widening of the intervertebral space prior to the insertion of the interbody bone graft using a bone spreader. Enlarging the vertical interbody distance tightens the protruding disc material and the ligaments and increases the space of the intervertebral foramen. Furthermore, if an anterolisthesis is present, this will be reduced simultaneously thus increasing the clearance of both the spinal canal and foramina. Experience has shown that this procedure is sufficient in the treatment of root irritation syndromes. The distraction fusion with simultaneous reduction is also adequate in cases in which cervical myelopathy is caused by either an anterolisthesis or kyphosis.

The second technique is indicated where nerve root compression (Fig. 1) or myelopathy are caused by either osteophytes at the uncovertebral joints or posterior spondylotic spurs. The purpose of this paper is to describe this technique and its results.

Surgical Technique

A standard anterior approach is used to expose the ventral aspect of the cervical spine. The musculature must be retracted further laterally than in the Robinson-Smith technique, in order to expose the anterior parts of the unco-vertebral joints. The disc is removed together with a thin layer of the corresponding end-plates (Fig. 2). Posterior spurs are now removed using fine chisels, curettes and ball-point air drills. When working with the chisel,

---

* This study was supported by research grants from the ASIF-foundation.

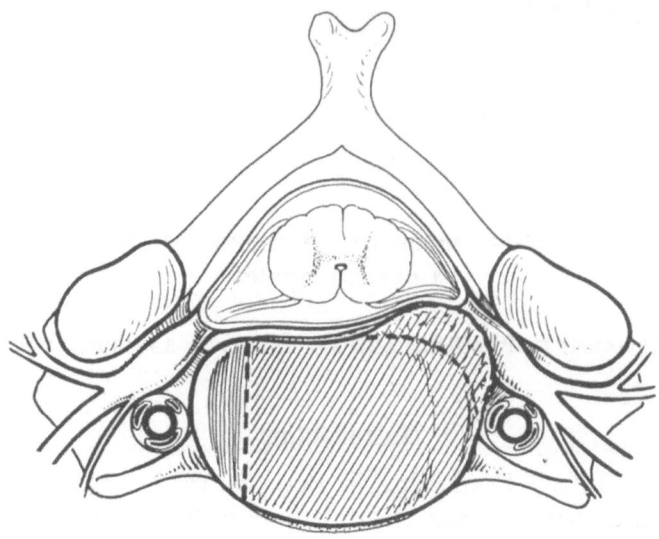

Fig. 1. Cervical nerve root compression by hypertrophied unco-vertebral joint. The dotted lines indicate the extent of the resection

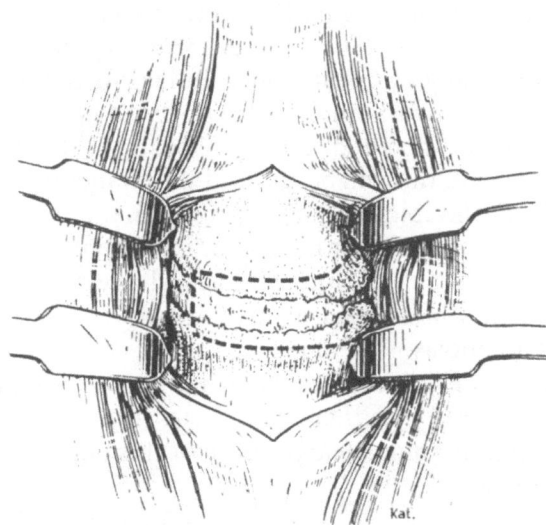

Fig. 2. Exposure of the intervertebral disc and the unco-vertebral joint. The dotted lines designate the extent of the excision

care is taken not to actually cut off the osteophyte but rather to fracture it off (Fig. 3). Using the same technique of removal the hypertrophied unco-vertebral joint is excised working from medial to lateral (Fig. 4). During the entire removal procedure a bone spreader is kept in place in order to facilitate the exposure and excision of the osteophytes.

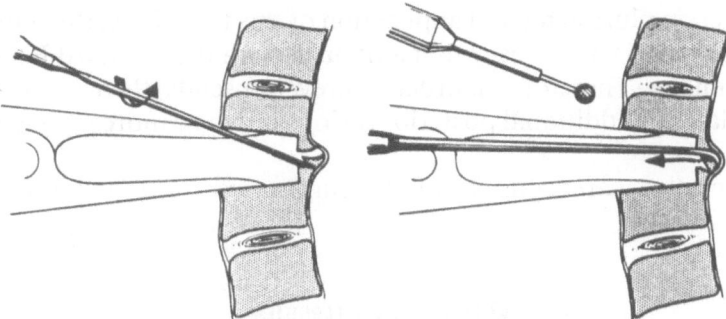

Fig. 3. The end-plates have been removed up to the posterior wall. With the bone spreader in place, the posterior spur is fractured off using a chisel and the fragments are removed with a curette. Instead of a chisel, a ball point air drill may be used

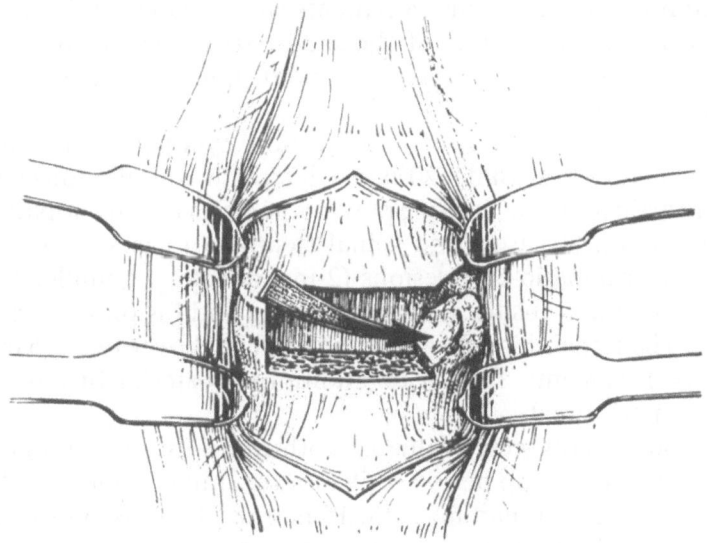

Fig. 4. After the removal of the disc, end plates, posterior spurs and upper portion of the unco-vertebral joint. The arrow shows the direction in which the unco-vertebral joint was excised. The bone spreader which would be in place at the contralateral side, is not shown

After decompression, fusion is carried out with two pressure resistant cortico-cancellous bone grafts from the iliac crest. When inserting the first graft, the bone spreader is kept in place in order to maintain the tightening of the soft tissues, which may then act as a tension band producing a compressive force at the level of the vertebral bodies, holding the grafts in place.

As a rule, anterior plates or additional posterior fusions were not thought to be necessary in monosegmental decompression fusions.

However, in plurisegmental application of this technique, the stability of the cervical spine is not as easy to maintain as with the standard Robinson-Smith technique. Therefore, in order to prevent pseudarthrosis, we applied anterior plates or additional posterior fusions if two or more segments were treated.

Postoperative care consists of wearing a semi-soft collar for three months.

Material and Results

From 1974 to 1984 a total of 107 anterior fusions of the cervical spine were performed. Of these, 34 cases were treated with transdiscal decompression and fusion. In 19 cases decompression was carried out by spondylectomy, the remaining 54 patients were treated by fusion alone.

We will discuss the results of those 34 patients (19 men, 15 women) treated with transdiscal decompression and fusion. The average age was 47 (range: 22–65 years).

Twenty-two cases had root compression syndromes due to hypertrophied unco-vertebral joints (20 cases), lateral disc herniation (1 case) and rheumatoid arthritis (1 case). Nine patients had cervical myelopathy caused by disc herniation (5 cases) and spinal stenosis (4 cases). Three patients suffered from traumatic cord lesions (2 incomplete, 1 complete).

Monosegmental transdiscal decompression and fusion were carried out in 16 cases. The remaining 18 patients were treated over two (15 cases) and three (3 cases) segments. In 8 cases, additional posterior fusion with plate fixation was performed.

In 1985, 30 patients were evaluated both clinically and radiographically after an average follow-up period of 59 months (range: 6 months–11 years). Of these 30 patients, 10 had no pain, 15 had residual discomfort but were very satisfied, while 5 experienced no improvement regarding pain.

Symptoms of root compression had been present in 22 cases (see above). In 18 patients the radicular signs have disappeared, in 3 patients they have improved and in one patient the signs remained unchanged.

Cervical myelopathy which had been present in 5 patients, improved in 4 cases and was unchanged in one.

In 2 cases of traumatic tetraparesis, neurologic signs regressed permitting working ability, while one case of complete tetraplegia persisted.

Complications

Two complications occurred in this series, both being pseudarthroses. Bony union was achieved by dorsal fusion in both cases.

Conclusions

In 1974 Magerl [1] presented a series of 37 cases treated with transdiscal decompression and fusion. This study already confirmed the efficiency of this technique in the treatment of root compression caused by hard hernias.

In the meantime however, an increasing number of plurisegmental decompressions were performed. Experience showed that in these cases decompression is more readily achieved by spondylectomy and that the stability of the fusion becomes increasingly important, as the number of segments to be decompressed grows. Anterior plating proved to be fairly unreliable in restoring stability. Therefore, in plurisegmental decompression we no longer use anterior plates, but rather perform an additional posterior fusion with plate fixation. The technique described above is presently used mainly for monosegmental decompression and fusion. Corresponding to the frequency of the initial symptoms, the main interest of the present study centered on the improvement of pain and root compression syndromes. Treatment was successful in reducing pain in all but five patients. Root compression syndromes were even more susceptible to improvement; only one case out of 22 remained unchanged.

References

1. Magerl F (1976) In: La chirurgie des syndromes cervicaux. Table ronde, Dir: A Jung. Rev Chir Orthop 62 [Suppl] II: 23
2. Robinson RA, Smith GW (1955) Anterolateral cervical disc removal and interbody fusion for cervical disc syndrome. Bull Johns Hopkins Hosp 96: 223

Cervical Spine I

4.5. Cervical Spondylotic Myelopathy:
The Results of Anterior Decompression and Stabilization

Th. S. Whitecloud, III, New Orleans, Louisiana, U.S.A.

Introduction

Cervical spondylotic myelopathy is the most common disease of the spinal cord developing during and after middle age.

There is no standardized surgical treatment for this condition. Numerous procedures are described in the literature which attempt to remove compressive forces, either anteriorly or posteriorly, or by stabilizing the involved segment. This report analyzes the results of the surgical management of a group of patients with cervical spondylotic myelopathy in which anterior spinal cord decompression has been carried out followed by stabilization.

Materials and Methods

Twenty-one patients with cervical spondylotic myelopathy were treated surgically by anterior decompression and fusion. There were thirteen men and eight women. Their ages ranged from 25 to 72, the average being 53 years. All patients in this series underwent vertebrectomy with removal of posterior and posterolateral osteophytes, followed by stabilization with cortical bone obtained from the fibula. The duration of symptoms prior to surgery ranged from four to 37 months, the mean being fifteen months. Follow-up averaged 32 months, the minimum being one year. No patient with acute disc herniation or major traumatic incident prior to the onset of symptoms is included. Grouped according to the functional classification of Nurick, seventeen had moderate to severe myelopathy, being in Grade III or above. Four patients were in Nurick Grade II classification.

Clinical Evaluation

All patients presented with a history of gait disturbance manifested as weakness or spasticity. All patients were spastic and hyperreflexic in the lower extremities. Twelve patients complained of upper extremity weakness. Eight patients had hyperactive reflexes in the upper extremities with positive pathological reflexes present; ten exhibited upper extremity radiculopathy. Nineteen had associated neck, intrascapular or shoulder pain. Three patients had bladder dysfunction.

All patients underwent myelopgraphy prior to surgery. Four demonstrated a narrowed spinal canal at two disc levels, thirteen at three disc levels, and four at four levels. The functional AP diameter of the spinal canal at the pathological levels was less than 12 mm in all patients.

Surgical Technique

All patients in this series underwent anterior decompression of the spinal cord with removal of posterior and posterolateral osteophytes followed by stabilization with cortical bone. Partial vertebrectomies were done between the disc spaces that were pathological. This allowed easier access to areas of osteophytic compression and allowed migration of the contents of the spinal canal anteriorly following decompression.

The surgical approach utilized was that of Robertson and associates. After exposure of the anterior portion of the vertebral column, discs overlying areas of spinal cord compression as shown by myelography were removed. Initially, removal is carried out only to the posterior aspect of the disc space, with no attempts being made to expose the posterior longitudinal ligament or remove osteophytes. A trough is then begun in the anterior aspect of the vertebral column with a rongeur and is deepened with a dental bur or air drill. With care the trough is deepened until the posterior aspect of the vertebral body is removed at its mid-portion. This exposes the posterior longitudinal ligament. To facilitate exposure of areas of osteophytic compression, more bone is removed from the posterior aspect of the vertebral bodies, utilizing angled curettes and punches. Thus rather than attempting to remove osteophytes throughout an area of limited exposure, adequate visualization is accomplished. At the time of surgery, the amount the contents of the spinal canal migrate anteriorly is determined by roentgenogram. After decompression, a radiopaque dye is layered into the area of removed bone and disc material and a lateral roentgenogram is obtained. The degree the dye is displaced anteriorly into the area of removed bone and disc represents the amount of anterior migration that has occurred. Following adequate decompression, a fibula strut graft is inserted to achieve stability and subsequent fusion.

Results

All patients underwent the operative procedure described. Thirteen patients had three levels decompressed and fused; four had four levels; and four had two levels. There was no progression of neurological symptoms in the immediate postsurgical period. All patients showed graft incorporation by one year. External immobilization was used approximately twelve weeks following surgery.

Sixteen of the twenty-one patients improved at least one functional grade following surgery. Of these sixteen, four had essentially complete resolution of their symptoms following surgery. These patients were all in Nurick Grade III categories, and had symptoms less than one year prior to undergoing operative intervention.

Three of the patients did not improve functionally following surgery. However, neurological symptoms seem to have stabilized following operation and the patients felt that surgery was beneficial. The remaining two patients showed functional improvement following surgery, only to slowly deteriorate within one year of operation.

Discussion

The exact pathophysiology of cervical spondylotic myelopathy is not yet defined. There are, however, several causative factors which have been delineated. Direct mechanical pressure on the spinal cord may result from disc degeneration with subsequent osteophyte formation or from congenital narrowing of the osseous canal. The functional diameter of the canal has been shown to be compromised when air-osseous canal width is less than 13 mm. Often a congenitally narrowed canal is associated with spondylotic changes and coexist in patients who develop this disease process.

Direct mechanical pressure can not only cause neural damage but also may induce ischemic changes secondary to vascular compromise. Experimental studies have shown that ischemia and compression can separately cause cord lesions that closely resemble those found in cases of human cervical myelopathy. It is known that the effects of compression and ischemia are additive, each separately having less profound effects on neurological function than when combined.

Additionally, motion of the cervical spine plays a role in the development of cervical myelopathy when associated with reduction in the sagittal diameter of the spinal canal. Flexion stretches the cord across the ventral spurs and extension may cause retrolisthesis of the vertebral body or in-buckling of ligamental flavum, further reducing the space around the cord. No standardized mode of treatment for cervical spondylotic myelopathy is available. Earlier reports in the literature indicating nonoperative modes of management produce results comparable to surgery. However, it should be noted that these reports were comparing nonoperative management to posterior decompressive procedures.

Numerous operative techniques have been described designed to either decompress the cord posteriorly thus allowing posterior migration of the dura and cord or to remove any areas of compression anteriorly. This may be done by direct surgical removal followed by fusion or by allowing remodeling to occur after segmental stabilization.

Generally the results of posterior decompression have not been gratifying. There is a real danger of further neural loss immediately following surgery. Improvement or at least stabilization of the patient's symptoms occurs only about 50% of the time.

Various reports in the literature indicate approximately 80% of patients undergoing anterior decompression and fusion are improved.

Because of the increased incidence of graft extrusion, collapse or nonunion when multiple level fusions are attempted, most anterior procedures for cervical spondylotic myelopathy are recommended for one or two level involvement.

In this series, however, seventeen of the twenty-one patients had three or more discs removed. The utilization of cortical bone for fusion helps eliminate the problems encountered with cortical cancellous graft material.

The results of the procedure described in this group of patients is similar to other series in which anterior surgery was performed. Sixteen patients were improved neurologically and functionally, and in three cases, the disease process appears to have been stabilized. Thus, in nineteen of twenty-one patients the course of the disease has been favorably altered by surgical intervention.

4.6. Extensive Posterior Fusion for Cervical Spondylotic Myelopathy *

J. F. Cusick, Milwaukee, Wisconsin, U.S.A.

The degenerative process of cervical spondylosis through acquired narrowing of the vertebral canal or segmental hypermobility of the vertebral column, either singularly or in combination, may increase to injurious levels the mechanical stresses acting upon the spinal cord or supportive vasculature. Determination of the most efficacious treatment for the individual case, therefore, requires evaluation of the relative importance of each possible causative mechanism. In the majority of cases, vertebral column narrowing acquired by laminal or ligamentous thickening or by osteophyte growth is usually predominant at lower cervical levels, whereas severe degrees of hypermobility or subluxation are more common at upper cervical levels, especially in patients with rheumatoid arthritis [4]. The long-term success of many routine surgical procedures with patients possessing this combination of mechanical abnormalities is frequently compromised by poor general health, advanced age, poor quality of bone and difficulty in maintaining immobilization. The failure to achieve fusion in the unstable cervical segments may result in a greater degree of spinal cord compromise through increased instability or accentuation of abnormal vertebral column curvature. A successful fusion may also be complicated by the additional strain upon adjoining vertebral column segments which have been previously compromised by degenerative changes or laminectomy and, therefore, accelerate instability at the adjoining unfused segments. Within this group of relatively high-risk surgical candidates who demonstrated subluxations of the upper cervical segments (C 1–C 3) associated with neighboring vertebral canal narrowing of the lower cervical segments (C 4–C 7), we have achieved significant resolution of myelopathy through a single-staged extensive stabilization of the entire cervical vertebral column.

* This research has been supported in part by Veterans Administration Merit Review no. 1655-03 P.

Clinical Material and Methods

During a recent 30-month period, a group of patients with severe and progressive cervical spondylotic myelopathy which had rendered them to an essentially bedridden status have had, as a single therapeutic procedure, posterior immobilization of all cervical segments. In two patients the fusion incorporated the occiput. The indications for this procedure include: 1. progressive cervical myelopathy associated with radiologic evidence of advanced spondylotic disease; 2. instability of one or more of the upper three cervical segments; and 3. radiologically significant narrowing of the neighboring cervical vertebral column. Although not a strict criterion, all patients were relatively high-risk subjects because of advanced age or poor general health.

The operative procedures were done with the patient in the prone position on a Stryker frame. The head was secured in skeletal traction to maintain the cervical segments in a neutral or slightly extended position. Operative technique consisted of exposure of the posterior elements of the vertebral column from C 1 through Th 1 as well as the occiput. Stabilization was initiated with posterior wiring of C 1 to C 2 with no. 18 wire. No. 20 stainless steel wires were passed through drill holes in the base of the spinous processes of C 3 through Th 1. When posterior occipitocervical stabilization was required (two cases), no. 20 wires were passed bilaterally in the squamous occipital bone through small trephines approximately 2 to 2.5 cm apart and secured to the C 1–C 2 wire fixation. In these cases, rib grafts were secured to the occiput and base of the spinous processes by the previously positioned wires. Prior to placement of the rib grafts the corresponding bony structures were decorticated. These patients with rib fusions were continued in skeletal traction and on a Stryker frame for the first seven days. In one case with acrylic fusion of C 1 through Th 1, the wires were woven about the spinous processes and methylmethacrylate was molded to include these wires and cover the lamina. During the molding process, copious saline irrigation was used to cool the exothermic reaction of the polymerizing acrylic. A rehabilitation program was initiated with external stabilization maintained with a removable Minerva cast when in the upright position. The criteria for patient selection and results of this treatment method are illustrated in the following selected case reports.

Illustrative Case Reports

Case 1: A 74-year-old female presented with a six-month history of progressive clinical deterioration exemplified by loss of unassisted ambulation. Neurologic examination revealed hyperactive deep tendon reflexes in the upper and lower limbs, bilateral extensor plantar reflexes, bilateral sustained clonus in the lower limbs, severe weakness in the upper limbs most marked in the intrinsic hand muscles, moderately decreased strength in hip flexors, mildly decreased position sense in the lower limbs and an absent vibration sense in both the upper and lower limbs. Plain cervical spine radiographs demonstrated severe degenerative changes resulting in narrowing of the sagittal diameter of the cervical canal most marked from C 2 through C 5, retrolisthesis of C 3–C 4 aggravated by cervical extension, mild anterolisthesis of C 2–C 3 and C 5–C 6 aggravated by cervical flexion. A gas myelogram showed obliteration of the subarachnoid space with associated spinal cord compromise from C 2 through C 4 and anterior osteophyte formation with spinal cord encroachment at C 5–C 6. Methylmethacrylate fusion reinforced with wire fixation was applied from C 2 through Th 1. After a five-month rehabilitation period, the patient achieved full self-care including independent ambulation. Subsequent examinations have revealed almost total recovery of motor strength and sensory functions with maintenance of clinical stability 26 months later.

Case 2: This 61-year-old female with a 20-year history of severe rheumatoid arthritis presented with inability to walk and progressive numbness of all extremities. Examination of the patient revealed severe quadriparesis with only minimal ability to lift the lower extremities against gravity and marked impairment of all sensory modalities up to the level of the clavicles. Cervical spine radiographs showed extreme disorganization of normal architecture including on flexion views, a 15 mm widening of the predental space with the resultant decrease to 8 mm diameter of the sagittal canal at C 1–C 2, as well as posterior dislocation of C 3 in relation to C 4 and anterolisthesis of C 5 on C 6. Gas myelography in the neutral position demonstrated obliteration of the subarachnoid space with associated spinal cord compromise at C 3 through C 4 and marked anterior osteophyte at C 5–C 6. An extensive posterior wiring and rib graft from occiput to Th 1 was performed. Nine months after surgery, the patient had significant resolution of her quadriparesis and was able to ambulate three blocks with intermittent assistance of a walker. All sensory modalities also demonstrated significant improvement with position and vibration sensation showing marked recovery at three months after surgery.

Discussion

Although the value of any specific surgical procedure for cervical spondylotic myelopathy remains a controversial issue, the markably debilitated condition of the patients in this series clearly demonstrates the failure of conservative therapy. These patients, who exemplify the predilection of cervical spondylosis to cause severe hypermobility or subluxation of the upper cervical levels (C 1–C 3) and vertebral column narrowing at the lower cervical segments (C 4–C 7), all have been reduced to essentially a bedridden status. The correction of these two different vertebral column abnormalities, however, presents a conflict between the usual methods of surgical resolution. Stabilization of the upper cervical segments will cause increased strain on adjoining vertebral joints with further vertebral column narrowing through acceleration of the degenerative process as well as increased risk of hypermobility or subluxation in the lower cervical levels. A laminectomy would offer an element of spinal cord decompression through a widening of the vertebral canal but also further weakens the integrity of the vertebral column making it more susceptible to local instability. The value of decompression and fusion by the anterior approach is a single procedure in this situation and is limited by the increased risk of spinal cord damage with a markably narrow vertebral canal and the difficulty of obtaining a solid fusion with a poor quality of vertebral bone, especially at the multiple levels required in these cases.

Total immobilization of all cervical segments, however, would reduce spinal cord exposure to the adverse forces induced by the excessive upper cervical motion and by the lower cervical canal arthrotic narrowing [1, 3, 5]. This complete restriction of cervical vertebral column motion as a consequence of total fusion does result in a compromise of functional characteristics of the vertebral column, but the clinical recovery through the marked resolution of the debilitating myclopathies in our patients indicates that this consequence of treatment is an acceptable occurrence. The adaptation to the loss of cervical motion has been enhanced by the limited social demands in these elderly patients. This consistent clinical improvement indicates that the stress as applied by motion of the cervical vertebral column upon a spinal cord compromised by narrowing of the vertebral canal is a major causative factor in the propagation of a myelopathy [2]. The rapid recovery of functional capacity over a four to five-month rehabilitation period also was an unpredictable event which lends additional credence to the marked sensitivity of a compromised spinal cord to motion. The use of multilevel fusions in the cervical region, including the total immobilization of the cervical spine, as a singular treatment of cervical spondylotic myelopathy has been shown to have special merit in our defined group of patients. The consistent beneficial results further emphasize the susceptibility of a compromised spinal cord to the stresses induced by excessive vertebral column motion originating at a site distant to the level of spinal cord compromise.

References

1. Breig A (1978) Adverse mechanical tension in the central nervous system. An analysis of cause and effect: relief by functional neurosurgery. Almqvist and Wiksell, Stockholm, pp 264

2. Cusick JF, Steiner RE, Berns T: Total stabilization of the cervical spine in cervical spondylotic myelopathy. Neurosurgery (in Press)
3. Ehni G (1984) Cervical arthrosis. Diseases of the cervical motion segments. Year Book Medical, Chicago, p 285
4. Menezes AH, VanGilder JC, Graf CJ, McDonnell DE (1980) Craniocervical abnormalities. A comprehensive surgical approach. J Neurosurg 53: 444–445
5. Reid JD (1960) Effects of flexion-extension movements of the head and spine upon the spinal cord and nerve roots. J Neurol Neurosurg Psychiatry 23: 214–221

4.7. Experiences With the Antero-medial Microsurgical Cervical Osteophyte Removal Without Interbody Fusion

L. Husag and Ch. Probst, Aarau, Switzerland

Introduction

The experiences of the last 25 years have shown that cervical disc disease may be adequately treated by anterior removal of disc or osteophyte without the need of formal interbody fusion. Omitting the bone graft which is not essential to the success of this operation, simplifies the procedure and eliminates graft related complications. This operation stresses a direct attack on the ventral osteophytes and provides the neural elements with immediate relief from pressure [1, 3, 7–9, 11]. On the other hand this method does not allow treatment of problems related to the size of the spinal canal and to the posterior elements. There is no ideal operation which can relieve the nerve roots and the spinal cord from pressure in all quadrants. The antero-medial microsurgery without interbody fusion is a surgical alternative for the treatment of spondylotic radiculomyelopathy. The lateral extent of the decompression is limited to 1–3 mm of nerve root in an anterior approach as compared to 3–5 mm exposure possible by facetectomy [10]. The operating microscope compensates for the restricted space in the surgical field and makes sufficient decompression possible [2, 4–6, 12]. The purpose of this paper is to present the method we use and our experiences with 102 operated cases.

Methods

The anterior cervical spine is approached in the standard fashion from the right side. Under the operating microscope the entire contents of disc space is removed leaving the cartilaginous plates intact. If the fragmented nucleus pulposus ruptures through the posterior longitudinal ligament to lie extradurally, this will be opened and partially removed on the side of the lesion. It is an essential part of the procedure to tilt the operating table 20° to the side of the lesion. In this way the lateral edge of the dural sac and 1–3 mm of nerve root can be seen free of encroachment (Fig. 1). The osteophytes on the posterior limits of the disc space are removed using angled high speed air

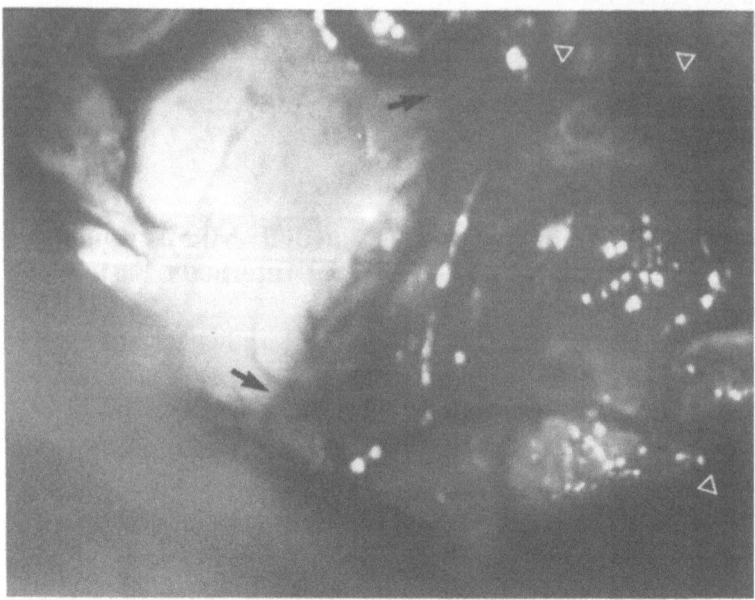

Fig. 1. Microscopic view of the lateral edge of the dural sac and the medial aspect of the nerve root after partial removal of the posterior longitudinal ligament

drill to gain adequate access to the soft tissue of the prolapsed disc which lies behind the vertebral body (Fig. 2). The spondylotically deformed neurocentral joint and the mutually adjacent dorsal edges of the vertebral bodies are drilled off in their posterior portion. Technically the removal of the osteophytes on the upper vertebra is as easy as the removal of the lower vertebral spurs.

Cases

Since January 1977 102 patients underwent antero-medial microsurgical disc or osteophyte removal without exogenous graft. The clinical, surgical and radiological results were analysed. The clinical appearance in all patients was that of a lateral or medial cervical disc compression syndrome refractory to appropriate conservative therapy. Neck pain alone was not considered as indication for surgery.

Results

The subjective estimate of the postoperative improvement and effect on working capacity was compared with the neurological findings and X-ray controls of the cervical spine. The overall results of surgery were categorized as *excellent* = 52% (complete subjective relief of symptoms, improved neurological signs and full activity), *good* = 26% (minimal

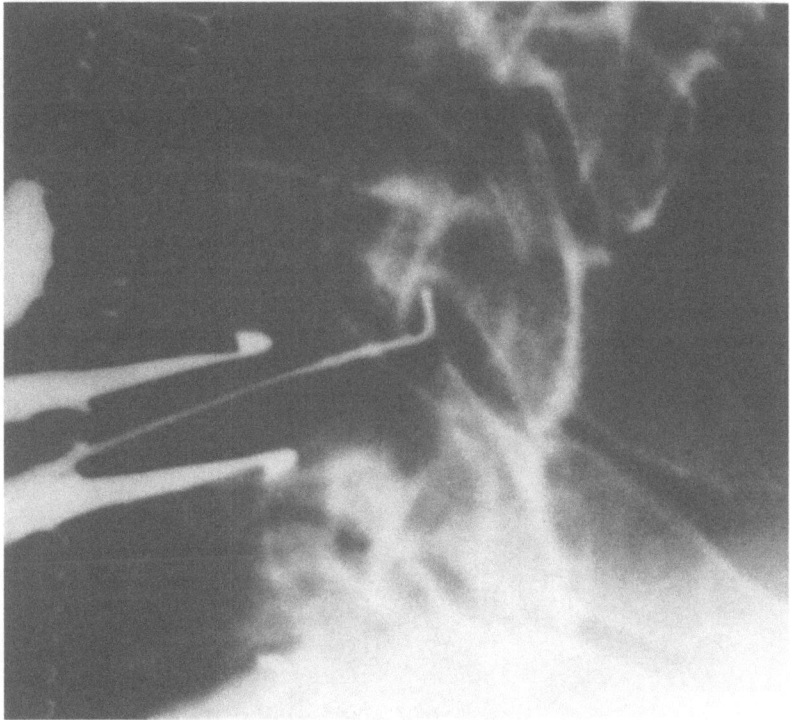

Fig. 2. Exploration of the epidural space after removal of the posterior osteophytes for free disc fragments lying behind the vertebral bodies

persistence of symptoms, unchanged neurological signs, full activity), *fair* = 17% (persistence of some symptoms, permanent limitation of activity) and *poor* = 5% (no improvement or deterioration after surgery). Adding up the positive results 95% of patients benefited from surgery. Comparing the long term results of soft discs to osteophytes, of one level to multilevel surgery and of radicular compression to spinal cord compression, no significant differences could be established. From the clinical point of view however the improvement of radiculopathies was constant and in myelopathies was less marked. The postoperative dynamic radiology indicates that in 77% of cases a normal cervical lordosis is present. An anterior angulation (5–15°) was without clinical significance. The movement of the operated level was abolished and good alignment was maintained with functional stability immediately after discectomy in 94% of cases. Bone fusion of the adjacent vertebral bodies followed in six months to one year in 70% of cases (Fig. 3). In all other patients there was a firm fibrous fusion present. It must be stressed however that there is no definite correlation between the radiological appearance and the clinical outcome. Plain X-ray films of the cervical spine reflect few if any of the anatomical

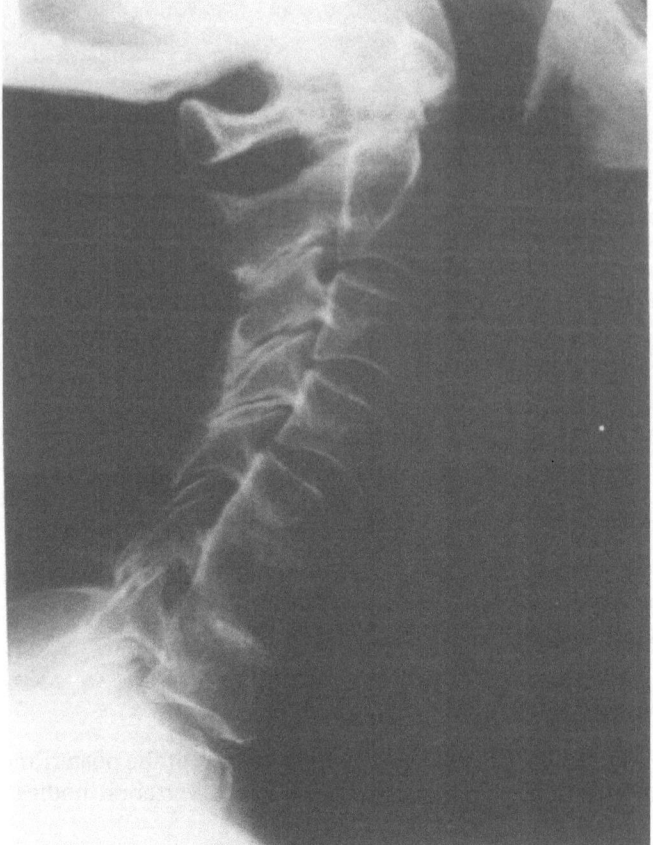

Fig. 3. Complete osseous fusion of the adjacent vertebral bodies 5/6/7 one year after anterior surgery without bone graft. The normal cervical lordosis is apparent

alterations accomplished by anterior decompression because the surgical foramen is inside the walls of the X-ray foramen. CT scan is valuable in confirming the diagnosis as well in the postoperative chek up. The extent of osteophytes removal is well demonstrated comparing the finding of axial CT before and after surgery (Fig. 4).

Complications and Recurrences

A few patients developed transient exacerbation of some neurological symptoms but no patient sustained nerve root, spinal cord or vertebral artery injury. No recurrence occurred on the operated site but three patients developed a new lesion on the adjacent level which required surgery several years after the initial procedure. One patient underwent an additional fusion procedure on three levels, because of persistent symptoms following insufficiently removed osteophytes.

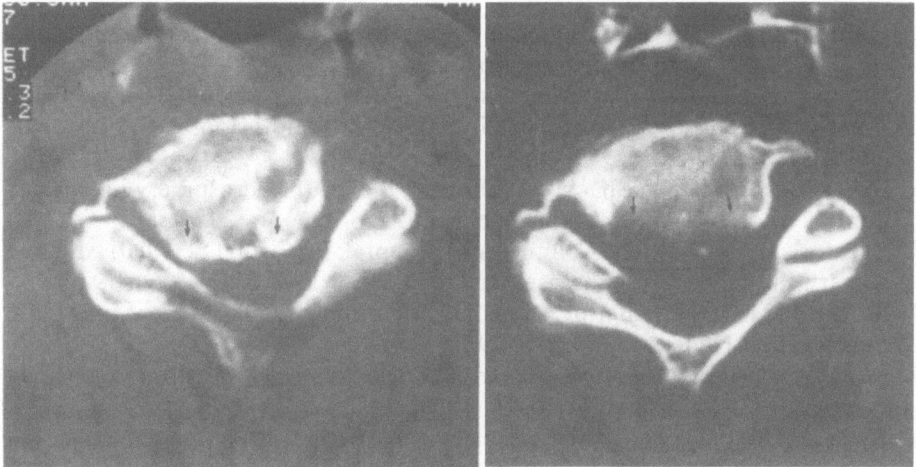

Fig. 4. Comparative axial CT before and after surgery demonstrates the extent of osteophyte removal

Conclusions

The presented method fulfills all the criteria of effective surgery—it provides ample exposure of neural elements through the disc space without great risk of damage to the underlying nervous structures or the vertebral artery,

— the visualisation is adequate through direct light and magnification of the operating microscope and through rotating the operating table to the side of the lesion,

— all types of cervical discs, medially or laterally placed, soft disc or osteophyte on one or multiple levels can be effectively treated to relieve radicular pain or spinal cord compression,

— the functional stability of the operated segment with collapse of the interspace is present immediately after discectomy, bony fusion follows gradually and is not prevented by retained cartilaginous plates,

— the method is simple and safe and as effective as the traditional procedures involving bone grafts, while carrying a lower morbidity, and can be recommended as the preferred treatment.

References

1. Dunkser SB (1977) Anterior cervical discectomy with and without fusion. Clin Neurosurg 24: 516–521
2. Hankinson HL, Wilson CB (1975) Use of the operating microscope in anterior cervical disectomy without fusion. J Neurosurg 43: 452–456
3. Hirsch C (1960) Cervical disc rupture. Acta Orthop Scand 30: 172–186

4. Husag L, Probst Ch (1981) Anterolaterale cervikale mikrochirurgische Discectomie. Schweiz Arch Neurol Neurochir Psychiatr 129: 47–59
5. Husag L, Probst Ch (1984) Microsurgical anterior approach to cervical discs. Review of 60 consecutive cases of discectomy without fusion. Acta Neurochir (Wien) 73: 229–242
6. Kosary IZ, Braham J, Shacked I, Shacked R (1976) Microsurgery in anterior approach to cervical discs. Surg Neurol 6: 275–277
7. Lunsford D, Bissonette DJ, Jannetta PJ, Sheptak P, Zorub DS (1980) Anterior surgery for cervical disc disease. Part I and II. J Neurosurg 53: 1–19
8. Martins AN (1976) Anterior cervical discectomy with and without interbody bone graft. J Neurosurg 44: 290–295
9. Murphy MD, Gado M (1972) Anterior cervical discectomy without interbody bone graft. J Neurosurg 37: 71–74
10. Raynor RB (1983) Anterior or posterior approach to the cervical spine: An anatomical and radiographic evaluation and comparison. Neurosurgery 12: 7–13
11. Robertson JT (1979) Anterior cervical discectomy without fusion: Long time results. Clin Neurosurg 27: 440–449
12. Spetzler RF (1982) The microscope in anterior cervical spine surgery. Clin Orthop 168: 17–23

4.8. Reoperative Cases After Anterior Spinal Decompressive Surgery for Cervical Spondylotic Myelopathy

Results and Adverse Effect

K. HIRABAYASHI, Tokyo, Japan

I. Material and Method

During 1963 to 1984, anterior decompressions followed by the intervertebral fusion were performed on 203 cases of cervical myelopathy due to the herniated soft disc and the cervical spondylosis involving less than three intervertebral levels, and of cervical myelo-radiculopathy (so-called Keegan type). Alternatively 56 cases had posterior decompression performed on cervical myelopathies due to spondylosis involving over four levels, and narrow spinal canal less than 12 mm of A–P diameter. Furthermore, combined posterior and anterior decompressions were performed on 11 cases having both anterior and posterior pathogenesis in the spinal canal.

The postoperative results were analysed using the score for the cervical spondylotic myelopathy by the Japanese Orthopaedic Association (JOA). The recovery rates of the JOA score after operation were calculated and were compared among each operative methods.

II. Results

The anterior decompression had the better recovery rate (71%) than the other two methods as showed in Table 1. This can be explained as follows.

Firstly, the anterior decompression group contained many cases of the soft disc herniation which afford good prognosis. *Secondarily,* in elderly patients, a less invasive posterior decompression tended to be preferred even if the lesion indicated anterior decompression.

Table 1. *Operative Results*

	Anterior decompression	Posterior	Reoperation	Stage ope.
No. of cases	101	24	7	4
Recovery rate	71.4%	52.2%	55.5%	61.6%

III. Adverse Effects of Anterior Spinal Fusion (ASF)

Of the adverse effects of the fusion of multiple disc spaces (Table 2), pseudoarthrosis was successfully resolved by use of an air drill and the subtotal excision of the vertebral body as reported by us in 1967. Actually, there has been no pseudoarthrosis in our cases since 1963.

Table 2. *Adverse Effect of Multi-level Fusion*

1. Rate of pseudoarthrosis ↑
2. Rate of sagittal malalignment ↑
3. Invasiveness ↑ (blood-loss, operation-time, bedrest period)
4. Effect on adjacent disc space

In face of malalignment, the author positions the neck in the neutral position during operation, then hollows a rectangular groove in the vertebral body and drives a matching iliac bone into the groove under light skull traction by hand, usually with good results.

An increase in invasiveness can be minimized by reducing blood loss and shortening the operation time through the use of an air drill and bone wax.

One of the unsolved problems is the adverse effect of fusion on the adjacent disc spaces.

IV. Reoperative Cases After Anterior Spinal Fusion

A. Soft Disc at Adjacent Space (Group 1)

The author had to perform a second anterior decompression on 3 cases due to the development of a hernia at the adjacent disc space (Group 1). In all the cases, the initial operation involved fusion of two levels, and the symptoms improved after the operation for a time, but aggravation set in at four to nine years after the operation, necessitating the second operation. Before the second operation, the hernia recurred at those disc spaces immediately above or below the fusion-level where the mobility was markedly high (Fig. 1).

A compensatory increase in range of motion (ROM) at the adjacent disc space prepared the grounds for recurrence of symptoms. Due to this, the author is forced to recognize the importance of long-term postoperative immobilization with a neck brace, and is inclined to think that fusion of two levels should be avoided, using fusion of one level or three levels instead.

B. Combined Spinal Canal Stenosis

Anterior decompression in 4 cases had been performed without regard to stenotic factors before the establishment of the concept of spinal canal stenosis (Group 2). In these cases, posterior decompression had to be done at one to four years after anterior spinal fusion but these results were unsatisfactory (Fig. 2).

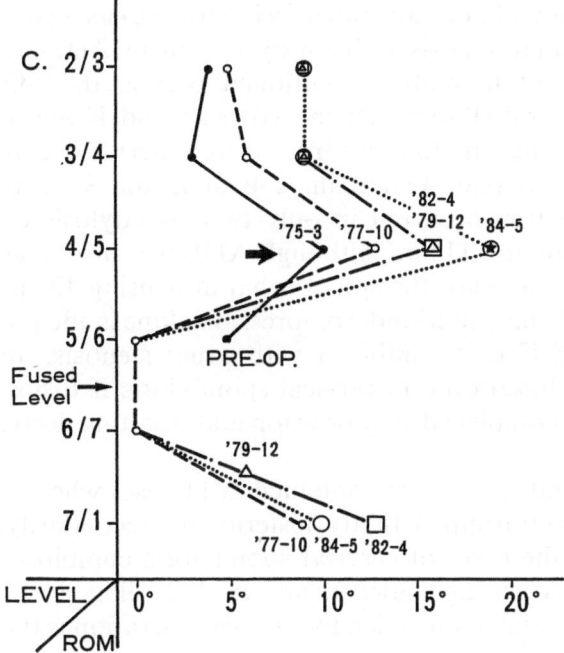

Fig. 1. Soft disc at adjacent space (case 2)

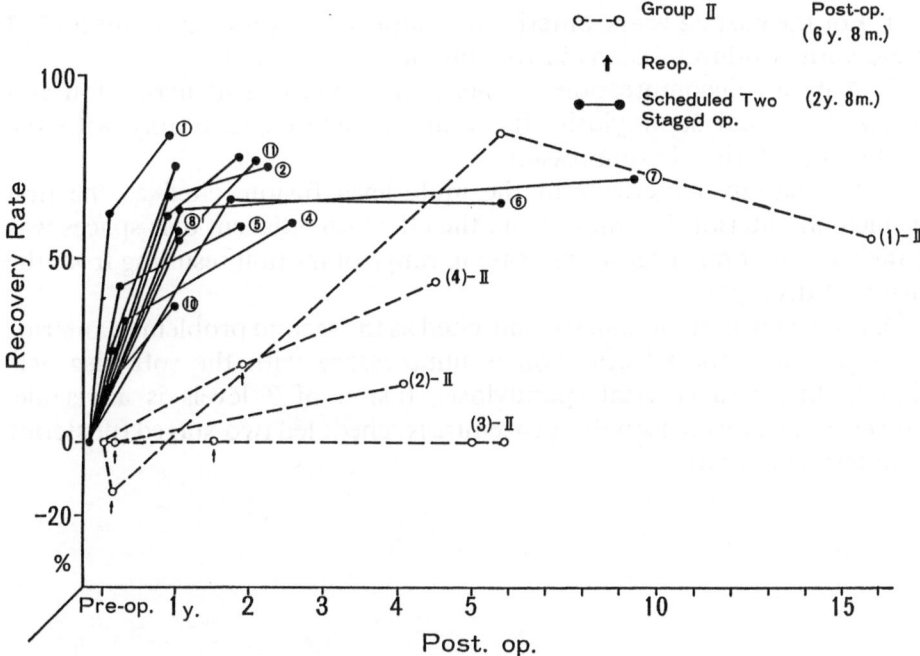

Fig. 2. Operative results of combined procedures

The application of anterior spinal fusion for the cases combined with the cervical spinal canal stenosis is obviously a problem. Actually, in three cases with recurrence of herniation mentioned before, the spinal canal was stenotic, 11 mm in A–P diameter in two cases and 12 mm in one case.

It was found that, in 35 cases treated by anterior decompression with spinal stenosis less than 13 mm in A–P diameter, 7 years later on, on average, aggravation occurred in only two spondylosis cases each with stenosis of 12 mm and 11 mm, although ADL was also aggravated due to old age in two cases with the spinal canal measuring 13 mm.

It may be said that anterior decompression alone is adequate for soft disc herniation, even if it is combined with canal stenosis, and the risk of recurrence is reduced even in cervical spondylosis if fusion of 3 levels is carried out with complete decompression and resulting decrease in range of motion.

However, good results were obtained in 11 cases where scheduled two-staged operations (Group 3), firstly posterior and secondarily anterior, were carried out for the cases of cervical spondylosis combined with a spinal canal stenosis measuring under 12 mm in A–P diameter. Therefore, the author considers that a scheduled two-staged operation is the best choice in such conditions.

V. Conclusion

1. For the past 22 years, anterior decompression was carried out on 203 cases, with two-level fusions in roughly half of the cases.

2. Anterior decompression is chiefly indicated in soft herniation and localized cervical spondylosis. Its results compared favorably with the results of posterior decompression.

3. Of the adverse effects of the multi-level fusion, cited as the first problem in anterior decompression, the effect on adjacent disc spaces was manifested as compensatory increase in range of motion resulting from the fusion of disc space.

4. For stenosis of the spinal canal, cited as the second problem in anterior decompression, special attention is unnecessary with the soft disc herniation, but with cervical spondylosis, fusion of 3 levels is advisable. However, the most reasonable procedure is scheduled two-staged (posterior → anterior) operations.

Cervical Spine I
© by Springer-Verlag 1987

4.9. Combined Anterolateral and Anteromedial Approaches of the Lower Cervical Spine

Method, Indications, Results in 55 Cases

P. KEHR, Strasbourg, France

Progresses are often the outcome of ideas opposed at the beginning. We have thus for a long time advocated anteromedial approaches exclusively and thought that arthrodèsis was to be an exceptional solution. Our reasoning was based on the fact that the arthodesis adds a new pathological state to the preexisting arthrosic pathology.

On the contrary, other authors were of the opinion that the arthrodesis was the ideal solution and that it was unnecessary to free the vertebral artery or the nerve roots; the simple immobilization appearing to them as being sufficient.

Later on, the works of Verbiest, Robinson, Cloward, Dereymaker, Magerl [1, 3], were to show that the freeing of the anterior part of the dura mater and/or the nerve root by transdiscal approach was possible, realizing an osteophytectomy and even a posterior uncusectomy by transdiscal approach, obligatorily followed then by a fusion.

After the Congress of the Orthopaedic Swiss Society held in 1972 at Chur where we had organized a Symposium on the cervical syndromes with Friederich Magerl, we were to perfect step by step the combined technique of the anteromedial and anterolateral approach.

The approach allows to perform at the same time: the discal curetting, the freeing of the anterior part of the dura mater and the spinal cord by removal of the osteophytes, be they discogenic or corporeal on the one hand, and the freeing of the vertebral artery either by transversectomy and uncusectomy, or the frontal opening of the intervertebral foramen by uncal foraminectomy on the other hand (Fig. 1).

This combination presents only advantages:

— double opening of the intervertebral foramen, the transdiscal medial approach coming close to the anterolateral one;

— permanent control of the vertebral artery, avoiding it to be injured, its compression or straining during the intervertebral spacing.

If one places himself on the standpoint of one carrying out only anteromedial approaches, the additional freeing of the vertebral artery and the opening of the intervertebral foramen by uncal foraminectomy may appear as being a difficult technique.

Nevertheless this is the only way a total freeing and a complete fusion can be carried out without any risk for the vertebral artery when on the contrary the lateral scooping-out of the uncarthrosis by the only transdical medial approach implies that the surgeon comes very dangerously close to the vessel without knowing it. More over, the vertical gap secondary to the technique of fusion increases the uncarthrosic compression of the artery if this last one has not been freed previously. If, at last, one used to carry out only anterolateral approaches, and who, as we did, condemned arthodesis, the realization of a combined operation appears to be a betrayal or a challenge. It is in fact a compromise justified by two arguments:

— the anatomic necessity to sacrifice the disc if one wants to free efficiently the anterior side of the dura mater;

— the advantage brought by the double access to the intervertebral foramen.

In fact, two types of combinations are possible:

— the combination of transdiscal osteophytectomy with fusion according to Robinson and simple freeing of the vertebral artery by transversectomy or by uncusectomy. This technique has been used in 25 cases from 1967 to October 1983 (Figs. 2 and 3);

— the combination of transdiscal osteophytectomy and arthrodesis of Robinson on the one hand, and uncal foraminectomy of Jung on the other hand, or operation of Kehr [2], which allows in only one surgery the treatment of the complex cases existing simultaneously: an uncarthrosis with compression of the vertebral artery and narrowing with compression of the vertebral artery and narrowing of the intervertebral foramen. We used it in 43 cases, since 1973 until September 1984 (Fig. 4).

On a technical point of view, the combination is the simultaneous addition of both approaches which are each described in separate chapters. We shall only insist on both following points:

— the necessity to cut down very gently a first fragment of the posterior osteophyte with the use of a chisel which will attack the osteophyte staring from the vertebral plate, the instrument being directed from front to back and obliquely either upwards (for the osteophyte of the above lying vertebral body) or downwards (for the osteophyte of the vertebral body underneath). The chisel will be inclined at an angle of about 30°. This position, perpendicular to the spinal cord, may seem dangerous but in fact it is not, as we shall hit only very slightly the chisel with the mallet and after two or three hammerings, we shall use a movement of lever in order to weaken and, after several attempts, to break the posterior rim. This will take

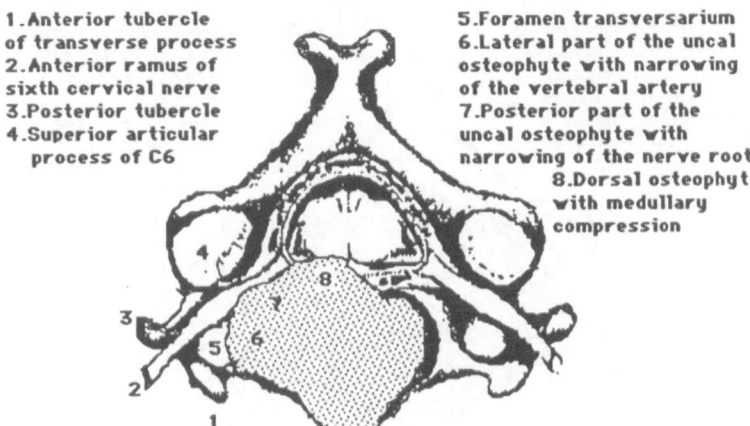

1.Anterior tubercle
of transverse process
2.Anterior ramus of
sixth cervical nerve
3.Posterior tubercle
4.Superior articular
    process of C6

5.Foramen transversarium
6.Lateral part of the uncal
osteophyte with narrowing
of the vertebral artery
7.Posterior part of the
uncal osteophyte with
narrowing of the nerve root
8.Dorsal osteophyte
with medullary
compression

Fig. 1. Drawing of a C 6 cervical vertebra osteoarthritis of the right uncovertebral
joint (uncarthrosis) and posterior osteophyte

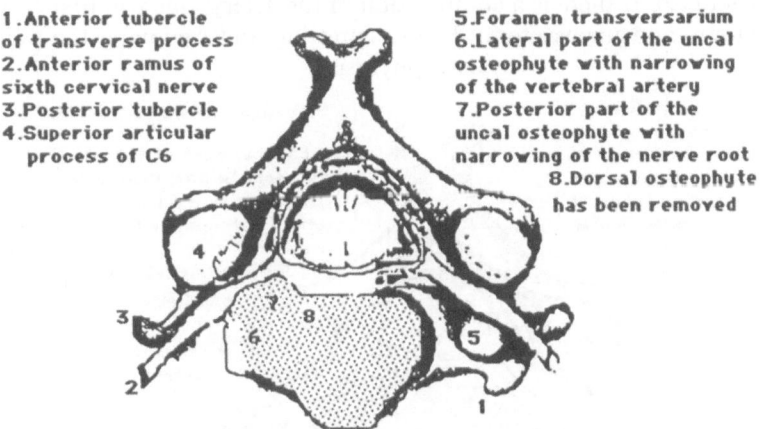

1.Anterior tubercle
of transverse process
2.Anterior ramus of
sixth cervical nerve
3.Posterior tubercle
4.Superior articular
    process of C6

5.Foramen transversarium
6.Lateral part of the uncal
osteophyte with narrowing
of the vertebral artery
7.Posterior part of the
uncal osteophyte with
narrowing of the nerve root
8.Dorsal osteophyte
has been removed

Fig. 2. Drawing of the transversectomy associated with transdiscal osteophytectomy. These has been a resection of the anterior bridge of the right transverse
process of C 6 on the one hand, and the removal of the posterior osteophyte which
was compressing dura mater and medulla on the other hand. These still remain,
nervertheless, the lateral and posterior part of the uncarthrosis and, therefore,
neither the vertebral artery, nor the nerve root are totally freed yet

off a small piece of osteophyte which will be extracted. Through the hole
thus created, a bent probe and a punch gouge will be successively
introduced; the use of this latter one allows to wear away progressively the
osteophyte (Fig. 5). It is possible to go from here laterally in the
intervertebral foramen and to remove the posterior part of the uncarthrosis.
Depending on the origin (corporeal or discogenic), of the osteophytosis, the
common posterior vertebral ligament, situated behind the osteophyte, will
be intact or on the contrary in holes when the osteophyte is the consequence

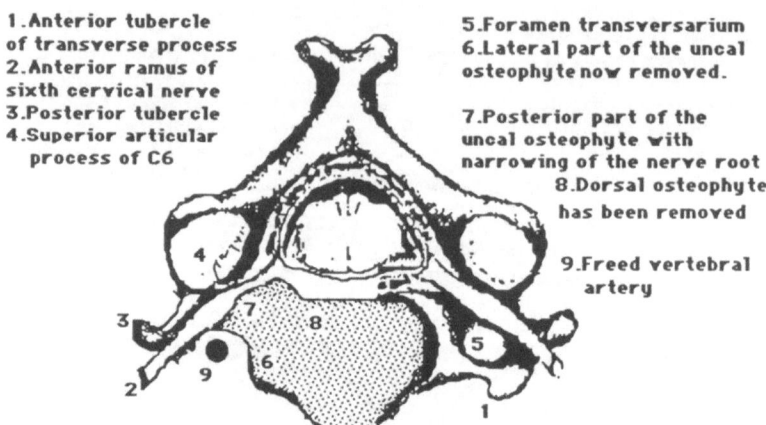

1.Anterior tubercle
of transverse process
2.Anterior ramus of
sixth cervical nerve
3.Posterior tubercle
4.Superior articular
process of C6

5.Foramen transversarium
6.Lateral part of the uncal
osteophyte now removed.

7.Posterior part of the
uncal osteophyte with
narrowing of the nerve root
8.Dorsal osteophyte
has been removed

9.Freed vertebral
artery

Fig. 3. Drawing of the uncusectomy. It has been performed after the transversectomy. Transdiscal osteophytectomy is usually realized after having freed the
vertebral artery (9). If there is a compression of the artery, one will first carry out
transversectomy and uncusectomy before curetting and removing the posterior
osteophytosis

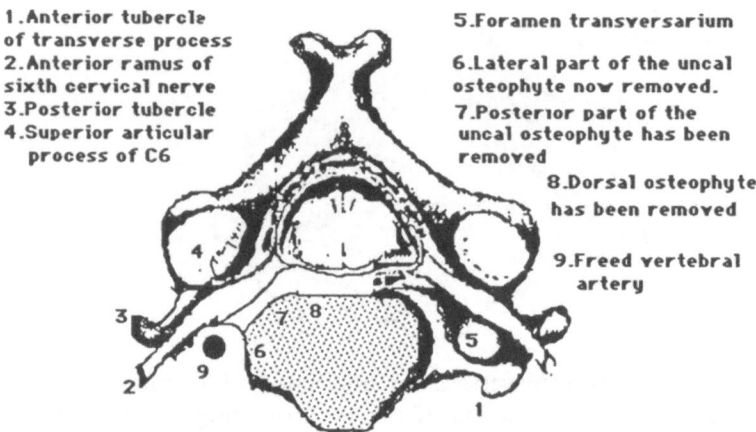

1.Anterior tubercle
of transverse process
2.Anterior ramus of
sixth cervical nerve
3.Posterior tubercle
4.Superior articular
process of C6

5.Foramen transversarium

6.Lateral part of the uncal
osteophyte now removed.
7.Posterior part of the
uncal osteophyte has been
removed

8.Dorsal osteophyte
has been removed

9.Freed vertebral
artery

Fig. 4. Drawing of Kehr operation (combination of Jung uncoforaminectomy with
transdiscal osteophytectomy). Vertebral artery, nerve root and spinal cord are
totally decompressed

of a former discal hernia. In this second case, one will have to be extremely
careful with the gouge because one will come in close contact with the
epidural veins.

The ideal operative sequence is, for us: 1 freeing of the vertebral artery by
transversectomy and uncusectomy; 2 discectomy; 3 transdiscal osteophytectomy; 4 posterior uncusectomy through a transdiscal approach; 5
perfection of the foraminectomy by a final anterolateral uncal foraminectomy (Fig. 6).

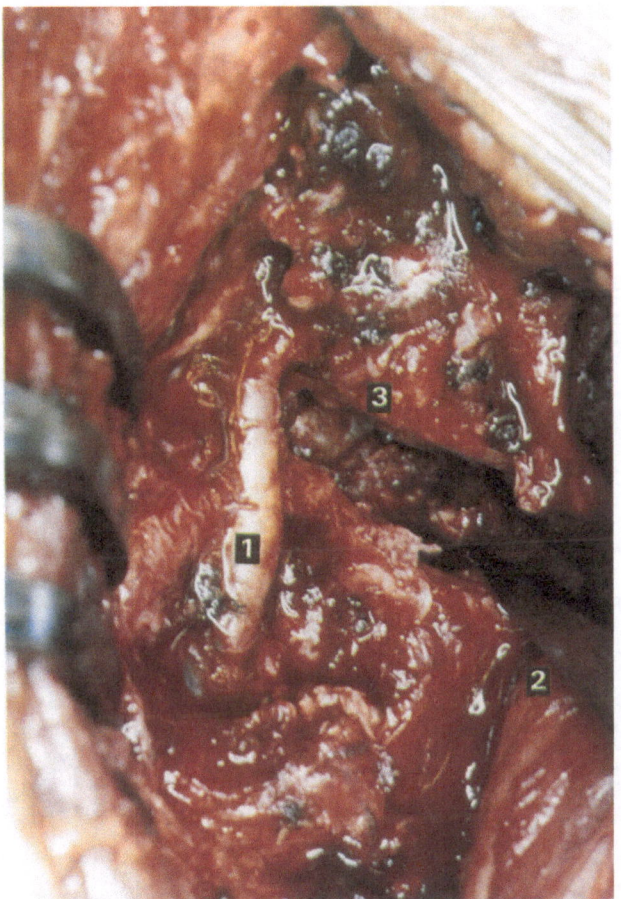

Fig. 5. Intraoperative photography of a combined operation of uncusectomy and transdiscal osteophytectomy. The vertebral artery is completely freed (*1*); the C 5/C 6 disc has been excised and removed and the intervertebral space is kept aside by an autostatic retractor (*2*). The posterior osteophytosis has been extirpated bit after bit with a punch gouge and in the background the dura-mater can be seen, recognizable to its bluish colour (*3*)

Out of the 68 operations carried out, the follow-up is 1 to 14 years in 55 cases. Overall results are excellent and good in 28 cases, fair in 15 cases, that is to say 78% of successes on the 55 cases. The success rate is of 83% for the operations of Kehr and only 68% for the combination fusion with freeing of the vertebral artery alone.

The indication of the combined operation is the simultaneous presence of an acquired spinal stenosis and an uncarthrosis, both being pathogenic. The pathogenicity of these lesions requires the showing-up of such structures as spinal cord, nerve roots and arteries through CT, myelography

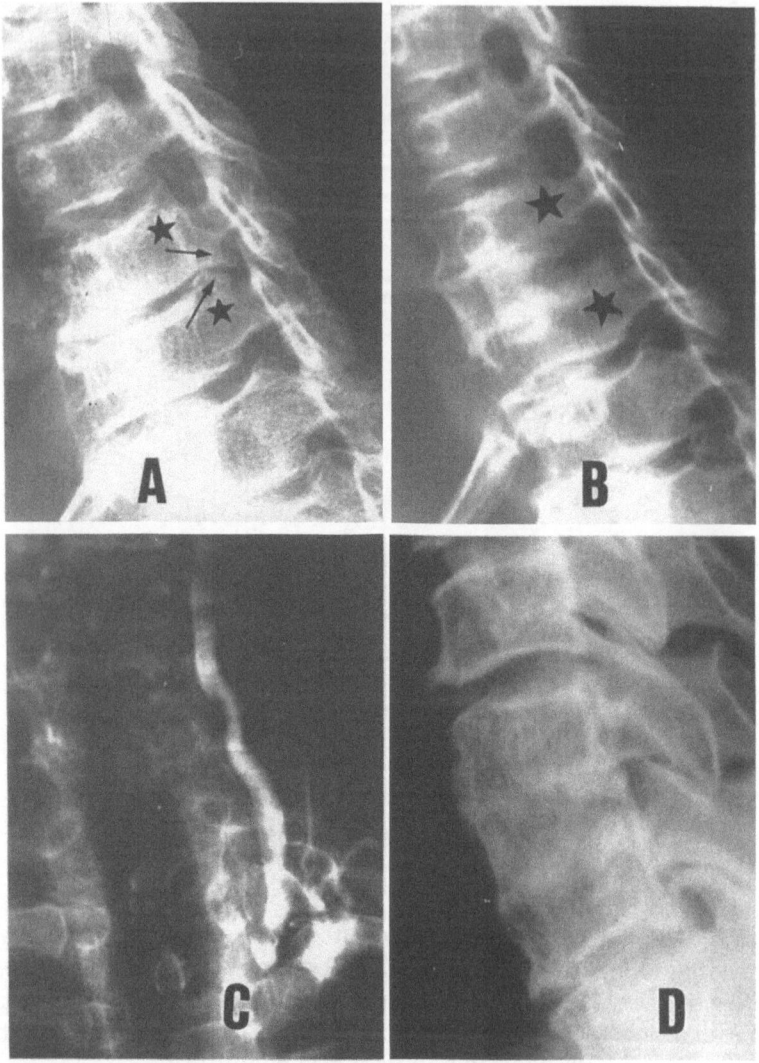

Fig. 6. Example of a combined operation. Mr. E., aged 56. Has been suffering for many years from left C 7 cervicobrachialgia with aggravation since a few months and appearance of vertigos induced by the head rotation to the right together with lower limbs parestheses brought about by flexion of the head (Lhermitte). The various examinations show: a narrowing of the C 6/C 7 left intervertebral foramen, visible on "A"; a pronounced narrowing of the left vertebral artery due to C 6/C 7 uncarthrosis; this uncarthosis is so invading that it compresses the artery when this one enters quite naturally the foramen transversarium of C 6 (operative observation) and should therefore be still away from the spine; this is seen on "C"; a stenosis of the rachidian canal at C 6/C 7 on a myelography, not shown here because of the low contrast of the X-rays due to the shoulders' forward position.

The patient is operated on in June 1979 by triple freeing, of the vertebral artery, and angiography. The clinical starting point lies in the coexistence of a cervicobrachialgic syndrome possibly a cervico-medullary syndrome, and a syndrome of vertebrobasilar insufficiency. As all these syndromes have an important subjective expression on the one hand, and as they have numerous differential diagnoses on the other hand, the putting forward of indisputable objective signs is a major necessity. Spinal cord and/or roots have to be impaired and compressed by the osteophytosis or uncarthrosis; the vertebral artery has to be narrowed by the uncarthrosic compression.

When comparing the results shown above, we come to the conclusion that it is nevertheless preferable to avoid the arthrodesis when the freeing alone of the vertebral artery is concerned and neglect then possibly a posterior osteophyte even if there are objective neuroradiological signs but no clinical symptoms. On the contrary, we are of the opinion that one has to add systematically a discectomy and a transdiscal uncusectomy to each uncal foraminectomy when vertebral artery and root are to be freed and even if there is no posterior discal osteophyte.

What to do when facing a cervicobrachialgia due to an uncarthrosis and to a posterior discal osteophytosis when the angiography shows a normal vertebral artery? Has it to be freed nevertheless? We are of the opinion that it has not, as in this case there is no risk of any iatrogenic suffering and one may be contented with a transdiscal medial uncal foraminectomy.

References

1. Jung A, Kehr P, Magerl F, Weber BG (1974) The cervical spine—primary and posttraumatic disorders. Advances in surgical management. Huber, Bern Stuttgart Vienna
2. Kehr P (1984) Anterolateral approaches to the cervical spine for management of cervical vascular and radicular syndromes. Contemporary Neurosurgery 6: 24, 1–6
3. Kehr P, Jung A (1985) Chirurgie der Arteria vertebralis an den Bewegungssegmenten der Halswirbelsäule. Funktionelle Pathologie und Klinik der Wirbelsäule. Die Halswirbelsäule. Fischer, Stuttgart New York

---

of C 7 left root and of the medulla. The opening of C 6/C 7 intervertebral foramen on the left side is visible on "B". Fusion according to Robinson is visible on "D".

Patient seen again for a check-up in 1985: very good result concerning cervicobrachialgia, vertigos and medullary signs; all signs having disappeared with the operation; reappearance of some neckpains due C 5/C 6 discarthrosis; Follow-up: 6 years.

4.10. Transdiscal Osteophytectomy and Fusion According to Robinson's Method

P. Kehr and G. Lang, Strasbourg, France

Spinal stenosis acquired by medial and/or lateral osteophytosis provokes a cervicobrachialgia or symptoms of spinal cord compression. The neckpain is generally localized in the lower part of the neck, on the medial or paramedial line. A thoracic or interscapulary irradiation is frequent. During exacerbations, there exists a limited mobility and palpation encouters acute painful points on the transverse processes, in particular on those of C 6. The origin of this cervicalgia can be discal, uncovertebral or on articular processes. The uncarthrosic origin is certainly the most frequent. The radiculalgia spreads itself in the whole metameric territory.

The medial osteophytosis can also provoke spinal cord compression and the clinical expression can go from increasingly from the simple Lhermitte syndrome to the genuine spastic paraplegia. But one should know that the clinical expression of such a medial osteophytosis can also take a radicular aspect. The characteristic feature of such a cervicobrachialgia lies in frequency of motor deficits, particularly the abolition of reflexes, but also of sensitive deficits. In a pathogenetic point of view, the osteophytosis itself takes place as much as the possible congenital narrowness of the vertebral canal, as the ischemia of a territory of the anterior spinal artery and of its branches during cervical movements. One has to add veinous troubles, the pathogenetic role of which is not to be underestimated either.

Facing ourselves the pathology of the vertebral artery and of the roots in the intervertebral foramen, it rapidly appeared to us that uncarthrosis, in spite of its determining role in the "uncoarterioradicular crossroads", did not play an exclusive role in the etiology of cervicobrachialgia. The systematic use of cervical amipaque myelography, then of CT, led us to distinguish two types of cervicobrachialgia:

1. those where the vertebral artery is not involved and where a median discal osteophytosis exists or an uncarthrosis with a development posterolateral only;

2. cervicobrachialgia by uncarthrosis, postero-lateral osteophytosis or median osteophytosis, but where there is, in addition, a lateral development of the uncarthrosis leading to a discomfort of the vertebral artery.

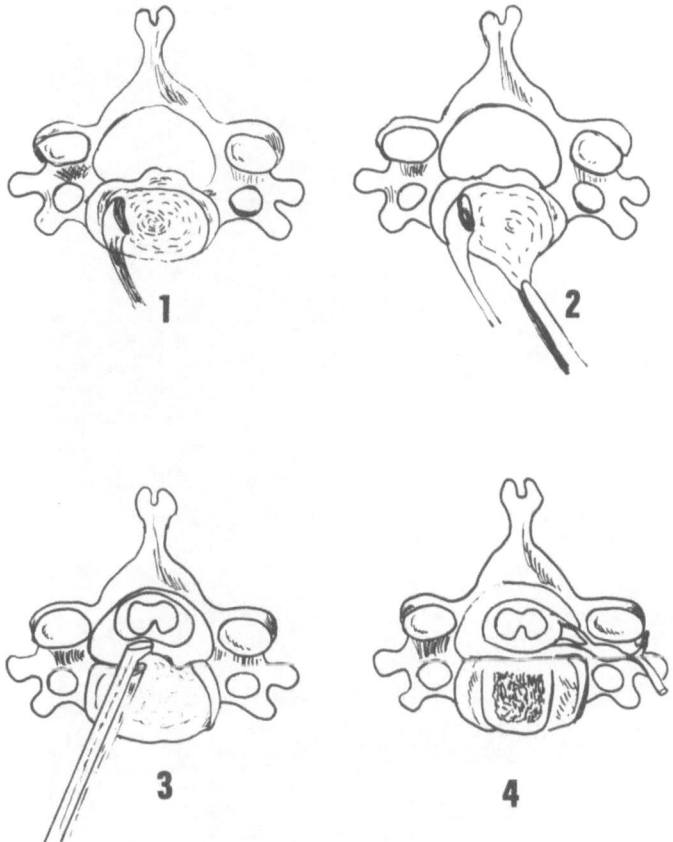

Fig. 1. Drawing of the operation: discal curreting on *1* and *2*; transdiscal osteophytectomy on *3*; tricortical iliacal bone graft fitted in on *4*

In the first type it is not necessary to free the vertebral artery and therefore needless to approach the intervertebral foramen antero-laterally; we think that the transdiscal approach with transdiscal osteophytectomy followed by fusion is the good technique.

The surgical technique we use is consequently as follows: freeing of the prevertebral level through a presternocleidomastoidal approach. Personally we prefer the oblique incision rather than the transverse incision, as this allows to extend eventually the approach upwards and downwards easily and not to be limited to an only level. We then locate the pathological disc with an intra-operative X-ray control. The disc is than totally excised (Fig. 1, *1–2*). An intervertebral retractor is set in. Then a progressive transdiscal osteophytectomy is performed by cutting down the vertebral

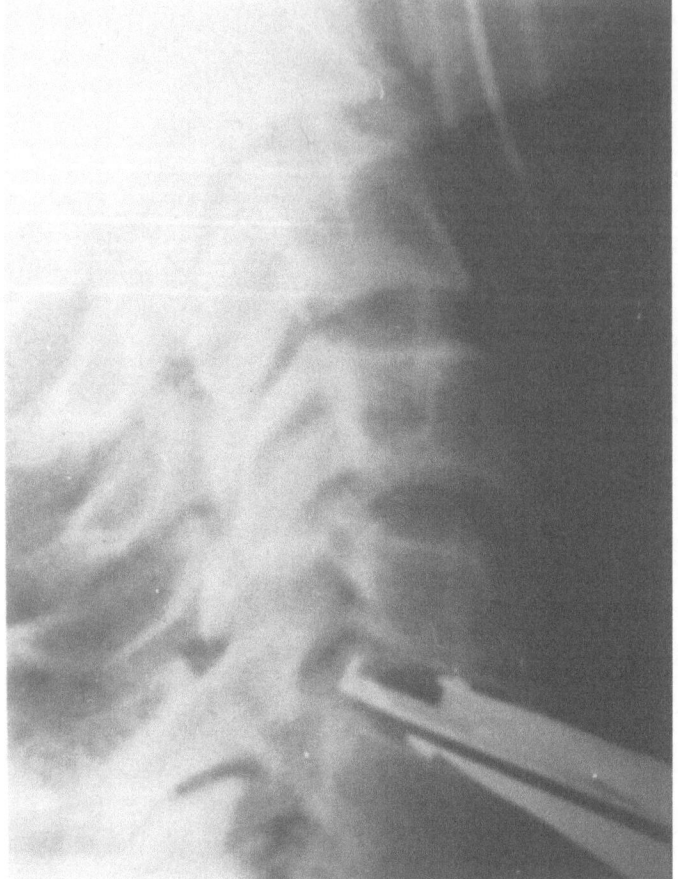

Fig. 2. Intraoperative lateral roentgenogram showing the punch gouge in place (see
3 on Fig. 1)

plate with a chisel and by cutting into the posterior rim and the posterior
osteophytosis with little knocks of chisel, then by breaking the posterior rim
with little lever movements.

As soon as a breach is made, a punch gouge is inserted, which allows then
to widen that breach and to carry out an osteophytectomy (Fig. 1, *1–3* and
Fig. 2). Depending on the cases, this osteophytectomy leaves at the same
place the posterior common vertebral ligament or, if is already torn, frees
the anterior side of the dura-mater. A tricortical iliacal bone graft is then
inserted and fitted (Fig. 1, *4* and Fig. 3).

We are of the opinion that an osteosynthesis of the AO plate type has to
be added under three conditions:

— impairment on two levels;

— traumatic instability;

— postoperative instability after a first surgery.

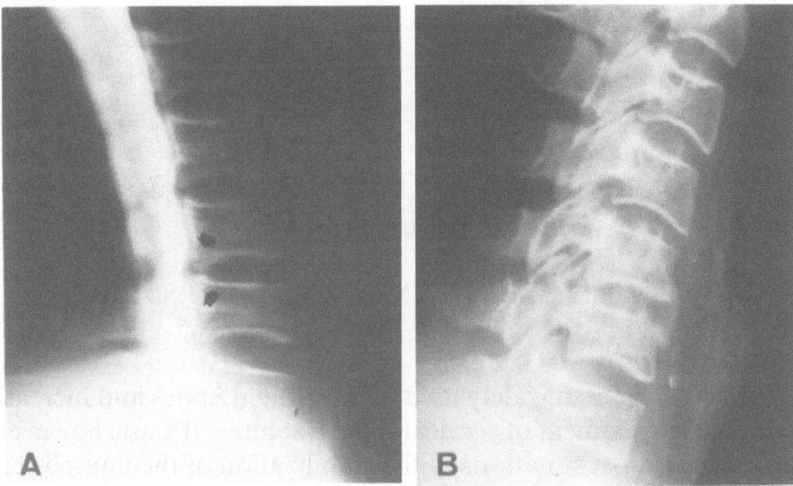

Fig. 3. Example of a transdiscal osteophytectomy because of a posttraumatic discogenic osteophytosis easily noticeable on the myelogram (A). Postoperative state on (B). Complete recovery; follow-up: 6 years

38 operations of this type have been carried out between April 1974 and January 1985, out of which 28 since January 1983. The overall results are 32 successes and 6 failures. The 32 successes are divided up in 29 excellent and good results and 3 fair results.

The 6 failures include an early postoperative complication, tetraplegia in a case of myelopathy and 3 cases of posttraumatic pension-neurosis.

The best indication is a syndrome being cervicobrachialgic or cervicomedullar through a acquired stenosis with a monometameric osteoarthritis occurring to a patient aged between 40 and 50 years. The indication is based on clinical examination data as well as electromyography, cervical amipaque myelography and above CT-scanning or myelo-CT, which show at best the pathogenetic role of the stenosis.

Cervical Spine I
© by Springer-Verlag 1987

4.11. Halo Vest Indications

D. S. Pierce, Boston, Massachusetts, U.S.A.

The halo vest has been widely used in the United States and increasingly in Europe for the treatment of cervical spine fractures. It's use, however, has been restricted in most situations to the stabilization of the injured cervical spine during a healing period without surgical intervention or during and after surgical intervention. The alignment of the fracture having been achieved at the time of application of the halo vest or halo cast. Our experiences at the Massachusetts General Hospital between 1969 and 1985 where there were three hundred applications of the halo vest has shown that it is possible to manipulate the fracture or dislocation of the cervical spine intraoperatively either with the patient intubated awake, manipulation of the fracture being carried out while the patient is conscious and able to respond to tell the surgeon whether or not there is any neurological changes as a result of fracture manipulation or with the patient asleep under general anesthesia manipulation of the fracture would have been too painful otherwise. The ability to carry out such manipulation greatly expands the value and use of the halo vest in the surgical treatment of cervical spine injury.

The type of vest used is that manufactured by the Ace Company, Los Angelos, California. The reason for its selection is that the device which is mounted on the plastic jacket consists of four upright bars with two horizontal bars which are mounted by vertical traction screws which are coupled to the halo allowing the device to be moved in flexion extension, traction applied to it, and to move and translate the head and neck in anterior or posterior direction. The versatility of this device makes possible the manipulation for the proper positioning of the fracture prior to surgery from either an anterior or posterior position.

Case 1. An eighty year old white female fell down stairs suffering a Type II odontoid fracture which was initially treated in a collar because of the patient's age and adversion to the use of the skeletal fixation. The odontoid fragment slipped into an anterior position with compression of the spinal cord. The patient was placed in a halo vest, intubated awake, placed face down on the operating table and the posterior half of the halo vest removed.

Surgical exposure of the C 1–C 2 was carried out and the arch of C 1 grasped with a Coker Clamp. Traction was then applied by an associate from underneath the operative drapes and at the direction of the operating surgeon holding C 1 the head was gently extended and the halo device moved back on the horizontal bars of the halo vest until excellent reduction had been obtained. A Galley-Fusion was then carried out with iliac crest graft. Patient was held in the halo for a period of three months until excellent healing of the fusion had been obtained.

Case 2. A twenty-two year old white female was thrown against the roof of an automobile in which she was riding striking her head over the left eye causing her, thereafter, to hold her head in a position deviated, angulating severely to the right and severe pain on any attempted motion initially. Decreasing pain after the first week postinjury brought a fixed position of the head with severe angulation to the right and rotation of the chin downward. When she was seen six weeks after her injury and X-ray was taken for the first time at that time. X-rays with tomography revealed a dislocation of the skull on C 1 and the dislocation of C 2 on C 3. In other words C 2 was rotated out from under the skull in a clockwise manner and rigidly fixed in this position.

Because of the extreme danger of manipulation of such a dislocation and the possibility of lethal cord damage, she was placed in a halo vest in the position which her head was normally held. She was taken to the operating room, intubated awake, turned into the prone position with the posterior half of the halo removed. With suitable prepping of the skin the surgical intervention was undertaken with exposure of the arch of C 1 at the base of the skull and C 2 and C 3. The arch of C 1 was securely grasped with a Coker clamp. Traction was applied by an associate from underneath the drapes and the arch of C 1 was manipulated into position. Initially it tended to move back while the Coker clamp was still held and with further traction applied it was rotated in a counter clockwise position until it snapped into place and was clearly stable and obviously aligned properly. X-rays confirmed the proper position. A fusion from the occiput to C 2 was then carried out. The patient was held in the halo device for three months until union occurred.

Case 3. A thirty-five year old male which suffered an injury to the cervical spine falling from a roof ten years before. He had undergone the rare condition of disappearing bone disease following his cervical spine injury with complete lysis of C 4 and C 5. Severe subluxation of the cervical spine with quadriplegia had ensued prior to his being seen by the author. He has been in a halo cast for approximately seven years prior to his having come under the author's care.

The halo device was continued and an attempt at massive tibial crest graft, although away from the spine itself, with manipulation of the cervical spine into satisfactory position intraoperatively with the halo device was carried out. Despite the fact that the graft was not directly lying on the spine itself, it had some soft tissue interposed and was wired at both ends, lysis of the graft occurred after two months opposite the area of the disappearing bone disease. The tibial graft remained intact. Measurements were taken and a device was manufactured which appropriated a plate for the back of the skull, a special plate for the spine sockets on them into which could be placed a rod. Opposed to this anteriorly were two rods inserted with specially made plates and cemented to the mastoid processes with rods running through the mastoid muscle and inserting onto socketed plates which fitted over the sternum. Manipulation of the cervical spine intra-operatively with the halo vest was carried out with insertion of all three rods and the plates which where cemented in place with fixation by bone screws as well.

Significant realignment of the spine was obtained at the time of the operative manipulation with the halo device, good stability was obtained by the internal fixation device making it possible for the patient to live for the first without a halo.

Conclusions

The intraoperative manipulation of cervical spine fractures, were appropriate with the halo device and clearly an advanced treatment of cervical spine fractures as this manipulation can be very carefully carried out without the danger of going too far and the fracture can be stabilized during a surgical procedure or appropriately stabilized during a healing process where surgery is not indicated.

Cervical Spine I
© by Springer-Verlag 1987

4.12. Freeing of the Vertebral Artery by Uncusectomy of Jung
Method, Indications, Results in 114 Cases

P. Kehr and T. Trensz, Strasbourg, France

It was in 1962, in Strasbourg (France), that the first uncusectomy, or more precisely, uncal foraminectomy of Jung was performed [1, 3].

Uncusectomy constitutes one of the three anterolateral approaches of Jung which are, respectively, transversectomy, uncusectomy and uncal foraminectomy. Transversectomy frees the vertebral artery by opening one or several foramina transversaria, but does not have any action at all on the uncus. The uncusectomy can be performed by us only after having first opened the foramina transversaria and after having performed a transversectomy. The uncal foraminectomy, at last, in the first description by Jung, is strictly achieved by an antero-lateral approach and necessitates therefore first a transversectomy and an uncusectomy. These three operations can be performed as such or each of them can be possibly combined with a medial approach of discectomy, of transdiscal posterior osteophytectomy and finally of arthrodesis in which case we prefer Robinson's technique [2].

With A. Jung we advocated for the 12 first years the only anterolateral approaches, performing only exceptionally an arthrodesis. Our conceiving changed since 1974 and we now think that the antero-lateral approach keeps an important and irreplaceable position. When the aim is freeing the vertebral artery by transversectomy or uncusectomy, the quality of the disc and of the mobile segment should always be carefully examined. One should not leave behind an instability, source of recurring and residual neck pains. In the case of an uncal foraminectomy, the antero-lateral approach of the foramen intervertebrale after an uncusectomy, does not appear to us to be sufficient any more and we do not use it in a pure and isolated way since April 1978. We think that if there is any indication for the intervertebral foramen to be opened, in all cases one has to combine the antero-lateral approach with the antero-medial approach as this combination is the only way to see and open perfectly the intervertebral foramen and to free the nerve root.

Surgical Technique

The incision is made on the anterior side of the sternocleiodomastoideus muscle which allows the easy approach from C 3 to C 7. The approach of the prevertebral level is realized between the visceral sheath and the vascular sheath (carotid common artery and jugular vein trunk). Incision of the middle cervical fascia and cutting of the omohyoideus muscle. Cutting of the inferior thyroid artery, if it is visible, in order to avoid an elongation of the recurrent nerve. Incision of the deep cervical fascia, retracting cautiously the sympathetic trunk outwards. Recognition of the carotid tubercle (C 6) and isolation of this tubercle by cutting all the muscular insertion, fibers by fibers. Tracing of the vertebral artery which usually enters the sixth transverse foramen, covered by its vertebral vein which is generally located in front of the artery. This stage is very delicate and can be greatly facilitated under magnification. It should be noted that this entrance of the vertebral artery to the C 6 transverse foramen happened in 218 times out of 234 operations (93%) but it entered C 5 *11* times (4.7%), C 7 *4* times (1.7%) and C 4 once. The entrance of the artery at C 5 or C 4 is to be feared, as in this case the artery comes in front of the transverse foramen, thus in front of the transverse process.

Once the entrance of the artery is carefully checked at C 6, the transverse process is completely freed from C 6 in its anterior part until the junction with the vertebral body. The same maneuver is then repeated at C 5 level and if necessary at C 4 level. We always start at C 6 in order to follow the artery anatomically, upwards. Once the transverse foramina are opened, the uncarthrosis and the compression of the vertebral artery became clearly visible. This uncarthrosis is most often located at C 5/C 6 level, then, following an order of decreasing frequency, at C 6/C 7 and C 4/C 5. The vertebral artery is now carefully freed from the adhesions which connect it to the uncarthrosis, using the subperiosteal separation technique. Once the artery is freed from the bony adhesions, it can be protected and moved aside with a blunt dissector and the uncusectomy can be carried out, either with the chisel or with the rongeur (Fig. 1). At this stage, the uncusectomy will also benefit from the possible use of magnifying glasses.

Venous bleeding is the major intraoperative problem. Indeed, the antero-external vertebral vein is the visible part of a real peri-arterial network of thin ramifications communicating with veins of the intervertebral foramen and veins coming from the vertebral body. All these veins adhere to the periosteum of the transverse foramen and the uncus and it is easy to have an hemorrhage during this stages of bony freeing. In order to prevent them, one always has first to free the adhesions with a blunt instrument "dissecteur" type, and then remove bony fragments only if the forceps chisel cuts sharply; otherwise the fragment will have to be seized

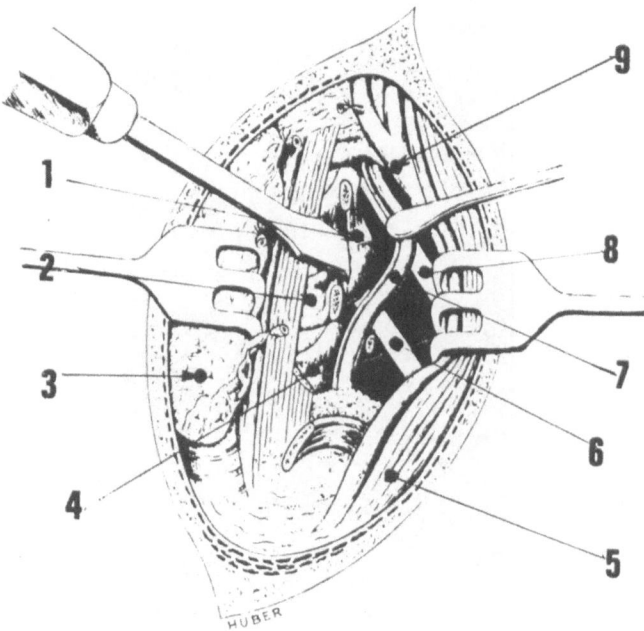

Fig. 1. Drawing of the uncusectomy: A chisel digs out a trench facing the uncarthrosis (*1*) and the vertebral artery is protected meanwhile (*7*) with a blunt instrument. This is made possible by opening of the foramina transversaria C 6 and C 5 which allows the mobilization of the vertebral artery (*7*). One recognizes the roots C 5 (*8*) and C 6 (*6*), the vertebral bodies C 6 (*2*) and C 7 (*4*), the thyroid gland (*3*), the sternocleidomastoidal muscle (*5*) and the carotid common artery (*9*) with its parting

with a pair of tweezers and cut closed to the bone. If despite these precautions, a venous hemorrhage occurs, it is often impressive. Several measures have then to be taken: raising of the patient's head to facilitate the venous draining off, avoid venous stasis, bipolar coagulation, application of hemostatic agents and compression for a few minutes. We use suction only when the hemorrhage impaires the course of the operation and when the bony fragments are still compressing the veins.

A second extremely rare problem (3 cases of 266 operations) is caused by the injury of the vertebral artery itself. In this case of course the intensity of the bleeding is very important and the aspirator must be then used and should always be close at hand. A fine suture can be attempted, or a parietal coagulation with the bipolar coagulation. One may also use silver clips that pinch laterally the vessel.

The indications of this uncusectomy are the uncarthosic cervico-cephalic syndrome (also called syndrome of the vertebral artery) due to a spontaneous osteo-arthritis (unco-disc-arthrosis) or a posttraumatic unco-disc-arthrosis.

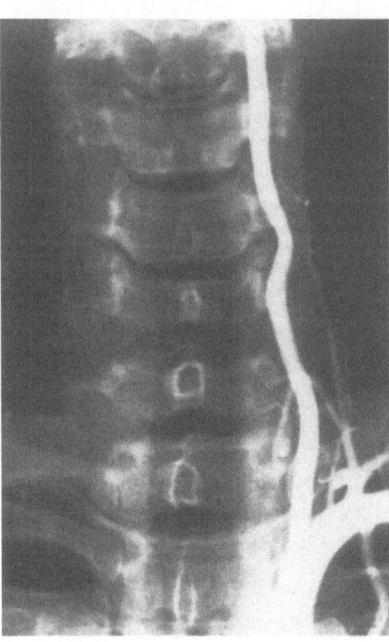

Fig. 2. Example of vertebral artery lesion. The artery is forced back and narrowed by the C 5/C 6 uncarthrosis, its diameter is reduced almost at its half where the narrowing is at its most. It is easily conceived that such a lesion impairs the sliding of the vessel during cervical spine movements

One has nevertheless to insist on the importance of the conservative treatment in cervico-cephalic syndromes and only resistant cases are surgically treated on active people.

The indication is based on a cervico-cephalic syndrome consisting of neckpain, headaches generally occipito-parietal, vestibular troubles of the rotatory vertigo type, cochlear troubles (hypacousia-like and tinnitus), visual troubles (scotoma-like or eye watering-like), drop-attacks and psychic troubles of the psychasthenia type. All these troubles may exist at the same time or just partially. The most frequently encountered grouping is: neckpain, headaches and vertigo. Important is to determine if these troubles are related to head or neck movements and in this last case, extension and contralateral rotation provoke the symptomatology or at least aggravate it.

The diagnosis relies on suspicion examinations such as Doppler ultrasonography of the vertebral arteries and cochleo-vestibular examinations, in particular the electro-nystagmography and of course the cervical X-rays when they show an unco-disc-arthrosis especially when this unco-disc-arthrosis is monometameric. The confirmation of the diagnosis is the vertebral arteriography only (Fig. 2). The pathognomonic signs of the

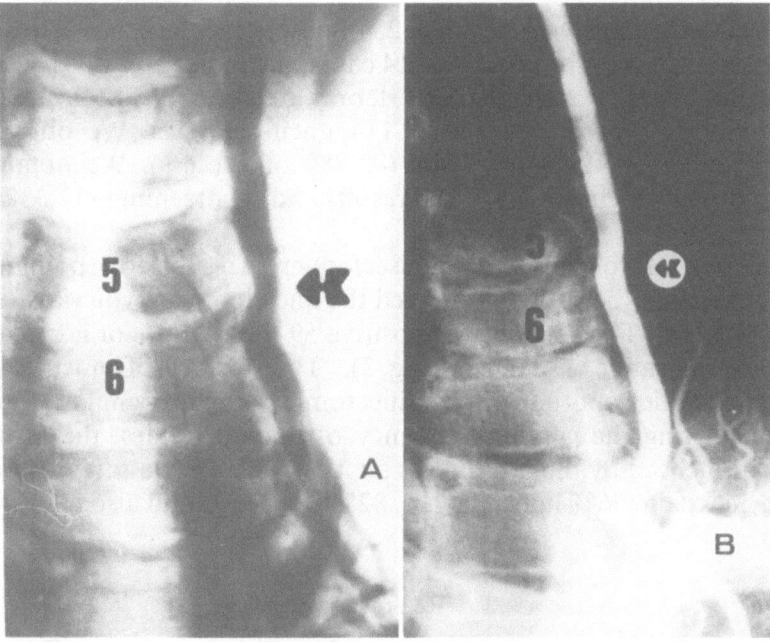

Fig. 3. Pre- and postoperative arteriograms of a patient aged 50 years presenting a complete cervico-cephalic syndrome after a road accident. (A) Note the left artery narrowing facing the C 6 uncus, (B) postoperative arteriogram taken two years after the uncusectomy and witnessing the vascular decompression effect of the operation. Good result; follow-up: 9 years

vertebral arteriography are the narrowing, associated or not with a deviation, whereas the deviation achieved by alone does not appear to us as being a sufficient reason to explain the symptomatology.

Results

Since 1962 we have carried out 117 uncusectomies and 41 transvers-ectomies (we will not talk about here but we mention them as they possibly constitute a stage in the uncusectomy).

It has been possible to analyze 114 uncusectomies. These operations took place between June 1963 and May 1983 and correspond to 103 patients (11 were operated on both sides). The operations have been carried out 66 times on male patients and 48 times on female patients. 11 patients (12 operations) died not related to surgery. 80% of the operations were carried out on patients aged between 40 and 59 years. The approach was in 56 cases on the left side and in 58 cases on the right side. The preponderance of the left vertebral artery is thus not encountered. For these 114 uncusectomies, 273 foramina transversaria have been opened, out of which 112 times C 6 and 109 times C 5.

The uncusectomy was decided 23 times because of a posttraumatic cervico-cephalic syndrome. In the 114 cases, the indication was based in all cases on an arteriography of the vertebral artery. It has been possible to analyze the results of 98 of these 114 uncusectomies. We obtained 28 excellent, 32 good, 21 fair results (82.7% of success). We obtained 17 failures, out of which 12 unchanged results and 5 worsenings (17.3% failure rate).

It was possible to analyze 76 uncusectomies on a subjective point of view, that is to say that the patient answered the question: "are you satisfied with the operation?". This answer was positive 59 times, more or less positive 4 times and negative 13 times (Fig. 3). The results of uncusectomies, transversectomies and uncal foraminectomies only are similar. Nevertheless, considering the greater frequency of uncusectomies, the results are mainly influenced by them. We thus see that we obtain a rate of success of 74% in neckpain, 76% in headaches, 82% in vertigo and also 82% in drop-attacks.

References

1. Jung A, Kehr P, Magerl F, Weber GG (1974) The cervical spine. Primary and posttraumatic disorders. Advances in surgical management. Huber, Bern Stuttgart Vienna
2. Kehr P (1984) Anterolateral approaches to the cervical spine for management of cervical vascular and cervical radicular syndromes. Contemporary Neurosurgery 6: 24, 1–6
3. Kehr P, Jung A (1985) Chirurgie der Arteria vertebralis an den Bewegungssegmenten der Halswirbelsäule. Funktionelle Pathologie und Klinik der Wirbelsäule. Die Halswirbelsäule. Fischer, Stuttgart New York

4.13. An Isolated Congenital Narrow Canal of the Atlas

T. Itoh, Toyama, Japan

We experienced a case of cervical myelopathy due to an isolated narrow spinal canal of the atlas whose myelopathy recovered after C 1 laminectomy. The condition of congenital cervical canal stenosis is well known and reported in the literature, but only few of these papers describe a narrow spinal canal including the level of C 1.

I. Case Presentation

A 69-year-old male had sensory and motor disturbances of right upper and lower extremities. His past history and family history were not particular. Six months prior to the hospitalization, he felt a paraesthesia in his right trunk and became clumsy with concomitant muscle wasting of the right arm and leg. He had some difficulty in feeding himself and putting on clothes, and also complained of a gait disturbance. His neurological summary at the time of hospitalization was a Brown-Séquard syndrome below C 2 level with no symptoms referable to the medulla oblongata.

The most remarkable finding in the radiographs was the isolated spinal canal narrowing of the atlas. The A–P diameter of the spinal canal at C 1 was extremely narrow, only 12 mm, while those from C 2 to C 7 were around 18 mm (Fig. 1). Furthermore, the atlas-dens interval was 4 mm resulting from osteo-arthritic changes of C 1/C 2 joints. An ossiculum terminale persistence was found at the top of the odontoid process in the frontal tomogram. Degenerative changes in atlanto-axial joints were also noted. Computed tomogram at the level of C 1 showed a narrow spinal canal with a rather hypertrophic condition of the atlas ring (Fig. 2). No congenital abnormality was found radiographically in the thoracic and lumbar spine other than hyperostotic condition.

Metrizamide barely passed through C 1 level in a flexion position and the A–P diameter of subarachnoid space measured only 8 mm in the myelogram. A normal subarachnoid space was observed below C 2. In extension, a complete block was noted (Fig. 3).

Resection of the posterior arch of the atlas was carried out. During the

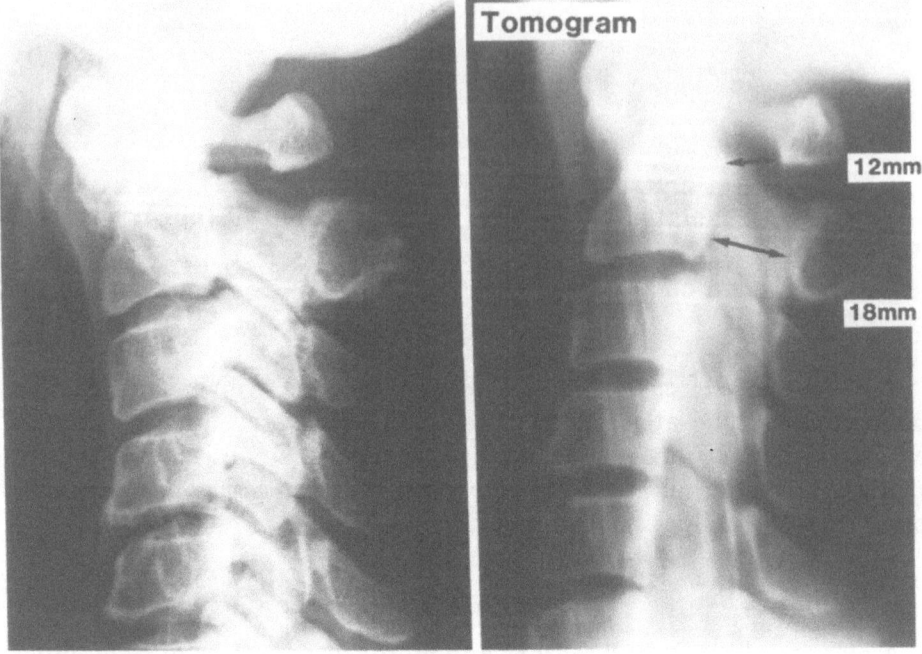

Fig. 1. Plain X-ray view and tomogram of an isolated congenital narrow canal of the atlas

surgery, the C 1 neural arch which was thick and hard was situated extremely anteriorly compared to the C 2 lamina and the foramen magnum, and compressed the dural tube.

Three years after C 1 laminectomy, the clumsiness and dysesthesia of his right upper extremity and gait disturbance were improved, but paresthesia of the left leg still remains at present. At this point in time he can use chopsticks and walks smoothly.

II. Discussion

The morphological anomalies of the atlas have been classified into 2 categories, namely, 1. a segmentation anomaly comprising fusion with the occiput or the axis, and 2. aplasia, hypoplasia or dysplasia. These anomalies are often associated with structural lesions such as basilar impression, C 1/C 2 instability and Klippel-Feil syndrome, and/or neural lesions such as Arnold-Chiari malformation. However, in the text books the concept of an isolated narrow canal of the atlas is not found in the classification of congenital malformations and deformities of the upper cervical spine.

Radiological study of the upper cervical spine was carried out to get the normal values of the sagittal diameter of the atlas ring and the spinal canal at both C 1 and C 2 levels. The subjects were 105 Japanese adult males who

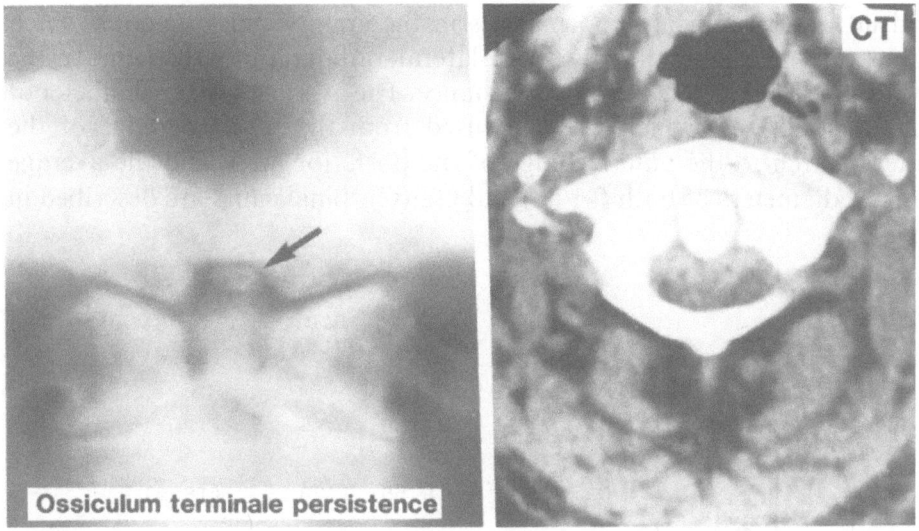

Fig. 2. A–P tomogram showing an ossiculum terminale and CAT scan demonstrating hypertrophic condition of the atlas ring in case of a narrow canal of the atlas

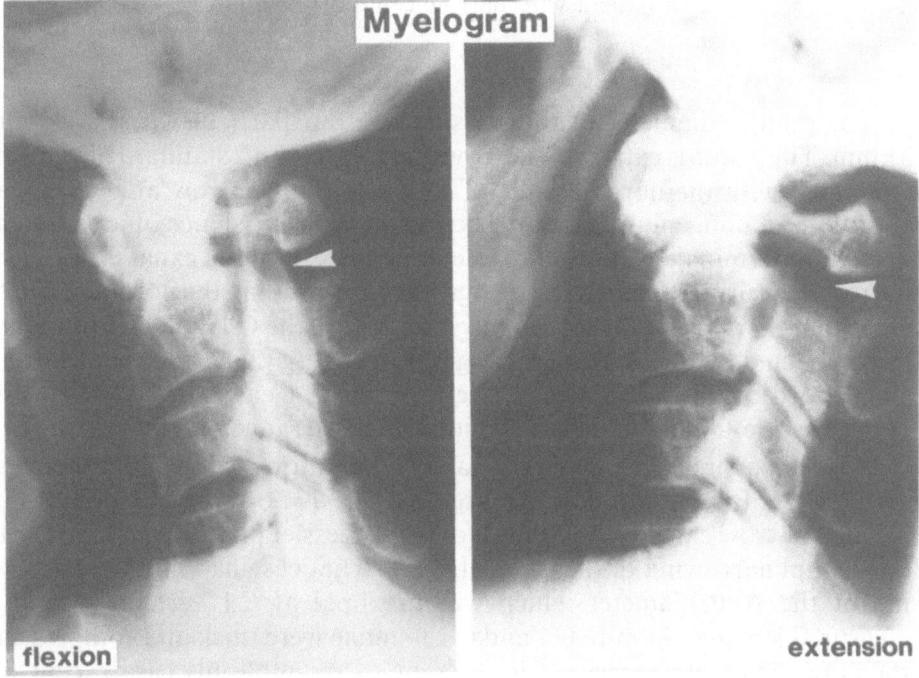

Fig. 3. Myelogram in flexion/extension of the patient with a narrow canal of the atlas. In extension complete block at C 1 level

had no radiographical abnormalities in the cranio-spinal junction. Each value was measured directly from lateral radiographs taken under the condition of 1.5 meters film-focus distance. The average sagittal diameter of the atlas ring (A) which was measured from the posterior edge of the anterior arch to the anterior edge of the posterior arch, and the average sagittal diameters of both C 1 (B) and C 2 (C) spinal canal are described in Fig. 4.

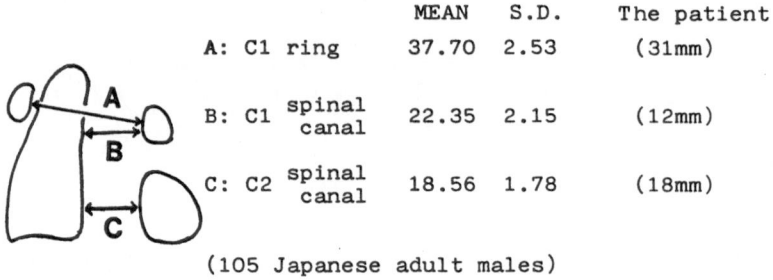

	MEAN	S.D.	The patient
A: C1 ring	37.70	2.53	(31mm)
B: C1 spinal canal	22.35	2.15	(12mm)
C: C2 spinal canal	18.56	1.78	(18mm)

(105 Japanese adult males)

Fig. 4. Values of the sagittal diameter at different levels in normal individuals and in a patient with narrow canal of the atlas

The sagittal diameter of the atlas ring in this particular case was only 31 mm. This value is extremely narrow and is less than 2 standard deviations compared with the normal value of 37.7 mm. This narrow atlas ring was considered a congenital anomaly because of the coexistence of a persistent ossiculum terminale. The A–P diameter of the C 1 spinal canal is also very narrow measuring 12 mm which is significantly less than the normal value of 22.35 mm. In addition to the narrow ring of C 1, the C 1 canal was thought to be affected by degenerative changes. Greenberg [2] has determined that spinal cord compression always occurs if the C 1 canal is 14 mm or less. However, the C 2 spinal canal is within normal range of 18 mm.

Several papers have reported a narrow condition of the cervical spine as a whole. As far as we could investigate, there is no report describing the isolated narrow canal of the atlas. However, Kessler [4] reported a case with congenital narrowing of the cervical canal. That case had marked narrowing of the A–P diameter which was maximal at C 1 vertebra where it measured less than 11 mm. C 1 and C 2 laminae were thick and compressing the cord. The case presented is thought to resemble his case except for having a normal canal below C 2. The concept of the isolated congenital narrow canal of the atlas is not included in the classification of upper cervical anomalies. However, this condition should be noted as one of the anomalies of the atlas which has a potential risk of causing myelopathy.

References

1. Fuller DJ (1970) Surgical relief for spastic tetraplegia due to cervical cord compression. J Bone Joint Surg 52-B: 465–467
2. Greenberg AD (1968) Atlanto-axial dislocations. Brain 91: 655–684
3. Hashimoto I, Tak Y (1977) The true sagittal diameter of the cervical canal and its diagnostic significance in cervical myelopathy. J Neurosurg 47: 912–916
4. Kessler JT (1975) Congenital narrowing of the cervical canal. J Neurol Neurosurg Psychiatry 38: 1218–1224

Cervical Spine I
© by Springer-Verlag 1987

4.14. Stable Posterior Fusion of the Atlas and Axis by Transarticular Screw Fixation*

F. Magerl and P.-S. Seemann, St. Gallen, Switzerland

Introduction

Various methods have been described for the surgical treatment of acute or chronic atlanto-axial instability. Anterior techniques (Cloward [4], Fang and Ong [7], Estridge [6]) have well known disadvantages connected with the approach. Both the lateral (Barbour [1], du Toit [5], Simmons [11] and the combined techniques Boehler [2]) require two approaches. Posterior techniques (Gallie [9], Brooks [3]), while having the easier approach rely on the integrity of the posterior atlas arch and their stability is not at the best in treatment of dens pseudarthrosis (Boehler [2]).

In 1979 a new method of atlanto-axial fusion was developed by Magerl [10] in which the C 1–C 2 facet joints are blocked by transarticular screws and posterior fusion.

Surgical Technique

A midline approach is used and the neural arches are exposed from the occiput to C 7. By careful subperiostal dissection, the cranial surface of the isthmus of C 2 is exposed bilaterally to the facet joints. The facet joints of C 1–C 2 are opened and the posterior surfaces of the inferior articular processes C 1 are exposed by approximately five millimeters. K-wires are inserted into these processes and used to retract the soft tissues containing the greater occipital nerve and its accompanying venous plexus (Figs. 1 and 2). The C 1–C 2 joints are visible. Reduction may be visually verified and the direction of the screws determined. The screws are inserted in a sagittal direction entering C 2 close to the lower edge of the caudal articular process of C 2 (Figs. 2 and 3) crossing the isthmus close to its posterior surface and exiting C 2 at the posterior rim of the upper articular surface. The screws are placed through the facet joints into the massae laterales. The length of the screws may be checked using an image intensifier. Following screw fixation, a Gallie type posterior fusion is added (Fig. 3).

---

* This study was supported by research grants from the ASIF-foundation.

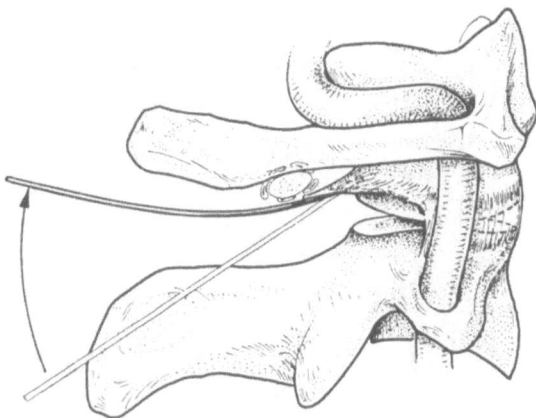

Fig. 1. Lateral view of C 1 and C 2 with the vertebral artery. The K-wire reflects the soft tissue containing the occipital nerve and its accompanying venous plexus

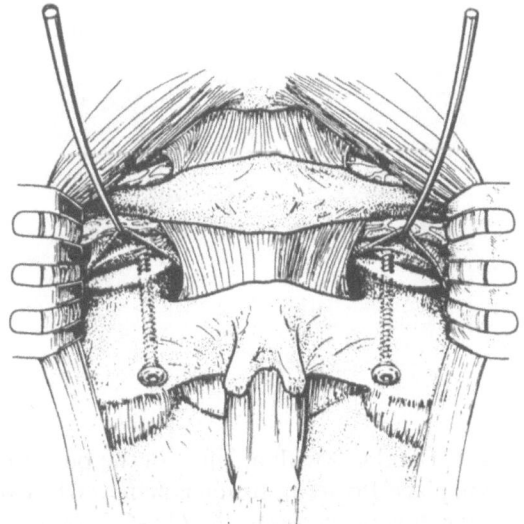

Fig. 2. Dorsal view of C 1 and C 2. The K-wires hold back the soft tissue permitting visualization of the C 1–C 2 joint. The screws are inserted sagitally and may be observed as they go through the joint

Complete reduction of an anterior displacement of C 1 on C 2 may prove difficult since no fulcrum is available. Using the transarticular screws as lag screws, C 1 may be pulled dorsally over C 2, thus facilitating and completing reduction. Initial reduction is performed by pulling the wire which is placed around the atlas arch.

Unlike other techniques, if there is a defect in the posterior ring of C 1, this technique can still be used. In these cases the subchondral bone of the

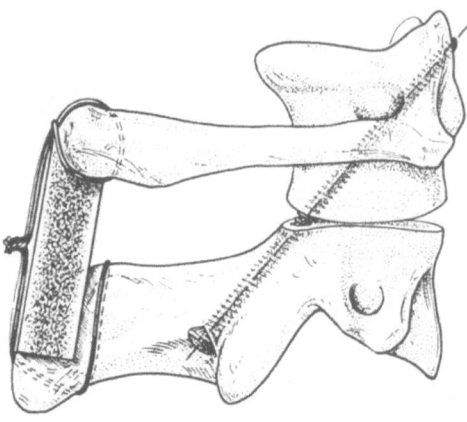

Fig. 3. Lateral view of C 1 and C 2 with the transarticular screw in place and the standard posterior fusion using cortico-cancellous bone graft and wire loop

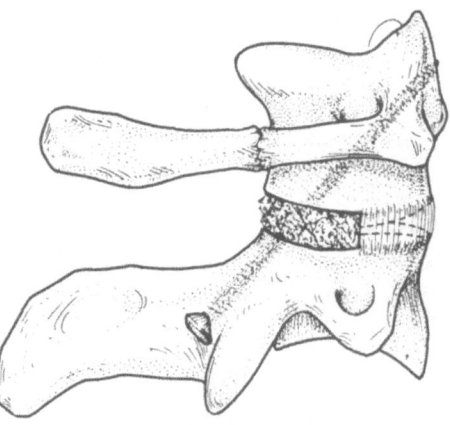

Fig. 4. Lateral view of C 1 and C 2 with a defect in the posterior arch of C 1. The transarticular screw is in place. Posterior fusion is achieved by cancellous bone graft which is packed into the C 1–C 2 joint

posterior half of the facet joints is exposed using a fine chisel before screw fixation. The resulting gap is packed with a cancellous bone graft (Fig. 4).

The oblique caudal-cranial direction of the screws may cause problems, because the soft tissue of the base of the neck may obstruct the positioning of the drill and screw driver. The following three measures will be of help: 1. head and neck should be in slight flexion, 2. the incision should reach down to C 7, 3. as a last resort the spinous process of C 2 may be lifted cranially using a towel clamp.

In cases of atlas assimilation compensatory hypermobility and instability may occur at the C 1–C 2 joints. In these cases the C 1–C 2 facet joints are stabilized in the way described above. However, the posterior graft is placed between the occiput and the spinous process of C 2. The broad cortico-cancellous bone graft is shaped like a clothes-peg which rides on the spinous process of C 2 and is inserted into a nut at the occiput. A tension-band wire loop is additionally attached to the occiput and around the spinous process of C 2.

Postoperatively the patients wear a semi-soft collar for 10–12 weeks.

Results

Since 1980 a total of 23 patients have undergone transarticular stabilization and posterior fusion. The average age was 43. Approximately a third of the patients had injuries, while the remainder had chronic instabilities (Table 1). 5 patients had neurologic deficits Grade D (Frankel *et al.* [8]).

Table 1. *Indications for Transarticular Screw Fixation C 1–C 2* (n = 23)

Acute Injuries

Odontoid fractures	3
Jefferson fracture	2
Combined odontoid and Jefferson fracture	1
Hangman's fracture	1
Rotatory subluxation	1
Neurologic symptoms	2 patients

Chronic Problems

Odontoid pseudarthrosis	5
Rheumatoid arthritis	4
Os odontoideum	3
Occ.-cervical abnormalities	2
Post traumatic incongruency C 1–C 2	1
Neurologic symptoms	3 patients

All of the 23 patients were followed until consolidation of the fusion. Of the original 23 patients 3 died after fracture healing from unrelated causes. 4 have returned to their respective native countries. The remaining 16 patients were evaluated in 1985. The average period of follow-up was 17.2 months (range: 8 months to 5 years).

12 patients were free of symptoms. The remaining patients had slight discomfort. Of those 5 patients who had presented with neurologic signs, each experienced complete recovery. All fusions healed without secondary displacement.

Complications

Two complications developed: One low-grade infection healed after debridement and removal of the screws. In another case the screws had been placed incorrectly into the massae laterales. These screws were removed and replaced correctly. Fusion and healing followed. There were no neurologic or vascular complications.

Discussion

Gallie [9] advocated surgical treatment in atlanto-axial instability because "although no neurological signs may be present, they are altogether likely to develop later". Various methods for the stabilization of this segment have been described.

Transarticular screw fixation and fusion of the C 1–C 2 joint offers secure stabilization requiring a single, namely the easier posterior approach.

Since the screws are anchored in the massae laterales the fixation as a whole does not rely on the integrity of the posterior arch of the atlas.

The anchorage of the screws also allows fixation of the massae laterales of the atlas to the axis in unstable Jefferson's fracture while sparing the atlanto-occipital joint. Reduction of this fracture is achieved by skull traction and may be supported by manipulating the K-wires inserted in the massae laterales.

Transarticular screw fixation C 1–C 2 and posterior fusion from the occiput to C 2 is a dependable method in the treatment of instabilities between the atlas and axis in atlas assimilation.

References

1. Barbour JR (1971) Screw fixation and fractures of the odontoid process. S Australian Clin 5: 20
2. Boehler J (1979) Nonunion of the Dens axis. In: Chapchal G (ed) Pseudarthroses and their treatment. Thieme, Stuttgart, p 196
3. Brooks AL, Jenkins EW (1978) Atlanto-axial arthrodesis by the wedge compression method. J Bone Joint Surg 60-A: 279
4. Cloward RB (1970) Air instrument surgery. Hall Publishing, Inc. Springer, Heidelberg Berlin New York
5. Du Toit G (1976) Lateral atlanto-axial arthrodesis, a screw fixation technique. S Afric J Surg 14: 9
6. Estridge MN, Smith RA (1967) Transoral fusion of odontoid fracture: case report. J Neurosurg 27: 462
7. Fang HSY, Ong GB (1962) Direct anterior approach to the upper cervial spine. J Bone Joint Surg 44-A: 1588

8. Frankel HL, Hancock DO, Hyslop G, Melzack J, Michaelis LS, Ungar GH, Vernon JDS, Walsh JJ (1969) The value of postural reduction in the initial management of closed injuries of the spine with paraplegia and tetraplegia, part I. Paraplegia 7: 179

9. Gallie WE (1939) Fractures and dislocations of the cervical spine. Am J Surg 46: 495

10. Magerl F (1982) Spondylodesen an der oberen Halswirbelsäule. Acta Chir Austriaca [Suppl] 43: 69

11. Simmons EH, du Toit G (1978) Lateral atlanto-axial arthrodesis. Orthop Clin North Am 9: 1101

4.15. Mandibular Splitting Approach to the Upper Anterior Vertebral Canal

E. S. STAUFFER, Springfield, Illinois, U.S.A.

Adequate exposure of mass lesions behind the vertebral bodies of the second and third cervical vertebrae may be difficult to achieve through the standard anterolateral approach, due to limitations at the superior margins of the exposure. Adequate exposure at the superior end of the anterolateral approach requires division of the superior thyroid and lingual and facial branches of the external carotid artery and places the superior laryngeal nerve in jeopardy. This nerve innervates the vocal cords and is responsible for shouting and singing high notes. The standard exposure through the open mouth transpharyngeal approach is frequently hampered due to the limited range of motion of the temporal mandibular joint and the depth of the wound as one approaches the posterior aspects of the vertebral bodies. It is also difficult to get caudad to the C 2–C 3 intervertebral disc. On occasion, particularly with patients who have been operated on previously, wider exposure is necessary to adequately remove mass lesions from the anterior vertebral canal which are producing progressive myelopathy.

The mandibular tongue pharyngeal splitting approach to the upper cervical vertebrae affords wide exposure of the cervical bodies from the clivus to C 6. This is indicated for exposure of the anterior vertebral canal behind the upper cervical vertebrae from the clivus to C 6, and adequate excision of vertebral body, disc, tumor, or other pathologic tissue can be performed without special instrumentation or tension on tissue.

Case Report: E. H., a 65-year-old white female, developed an upper cervical myelopathy consisting of burning pain and weakness in her right hand and clumsiness of her legs in 1979. An X-ray revealed an osteoblastic lesion of C 3 vertebral body. This was biopsied through a right side anterolateral extrapharyngeal approach with removal of the dense sclerotic bone and replacement by a tibial graft. The biopsy revealed no tumor, only dense sclerotic bone. Her myelopathy increased, and six months later she underwent a posterior decompressive laminectomy, which relieved her symptoms. Four years following decompressive laminectomy in June 1984, her symptoms returned. She could not knit or sew or walk over 50 meters.

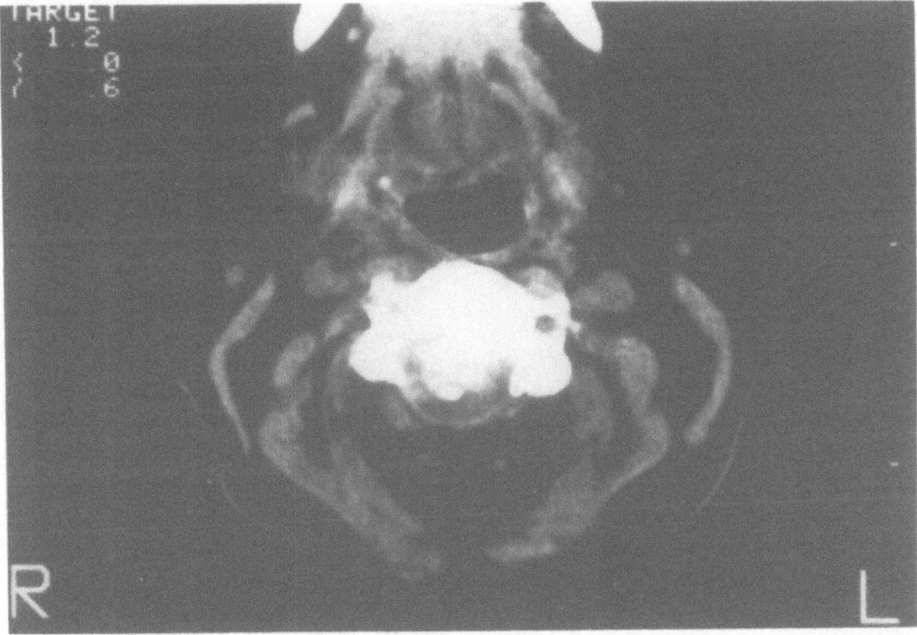

Fig. 1 A. Computerized axial tomogram of bony lesion in spinal canal behind cervical 2

Physical examination revealed bilateral ankle clonus, bilateral positive Babinski signs, and weakness of both hands. X-rays revealed a solid fusion of the previous tibial graft from C2 through C3 to C4. Myelogram and computerized tomography revealed a large bony lesion posterior to the body of C2 and C3 (Figs. 1 A–C). Excision of the central portions of the vertebral bodies of C2, C3, and C4 and the previous bone graft was accomplished by the mandibular tongue splitting direct anterior approach (Fig. 2). Exposure was accomplished from the clivus to C6 (Fig. 3). The previous fusion mass, remaining sclerotic bone, and large osteochondroma was removed from the posterior aspect of the bodies of C2 and C3. This was replaced by a fibular strut graft from the odontoid to C5. Postoperatively, the patient's neck was immobilized in a halo for six weeks and a cervical orthosis for six weeks. At follow-up one year postsurgery, all symptoms were relieved, clonus and Babinski were absent, and there was mild residual atrophy of the right hand; the bone graft appeared consolidated on X-ray (Fig. 4) and there were no alterations of the function of the tongue or taste and no malocclusion of the teeth.

This approach has been carried out on two other occasions by the otolaryngology service for resection of extensive pharyngeal tumors with similar results and no infection or other complications. One patient had a

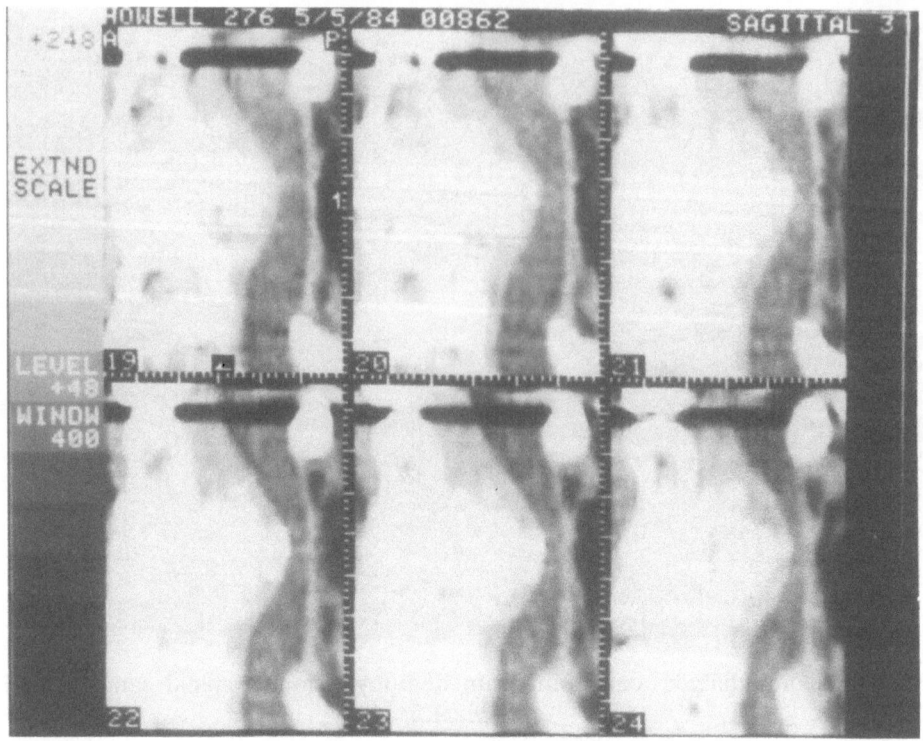

Fig. 1 B. Sagittal reconstruction demonstrating impingement on spinal cord

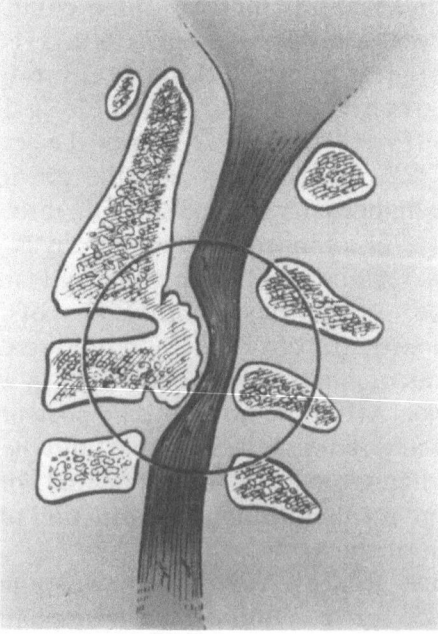

Fig. 1 C. Drawing of bone lesion in spinal canal

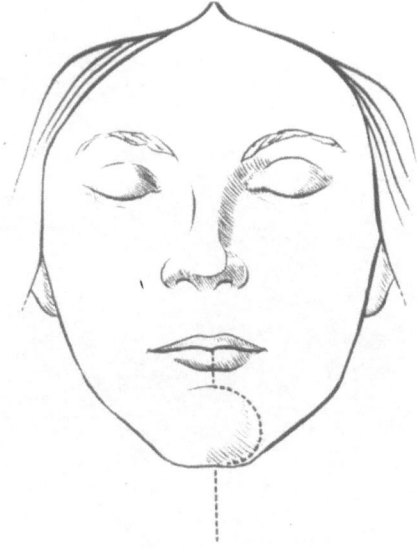

Fig. 2. Chin incision for mandible splitting approach

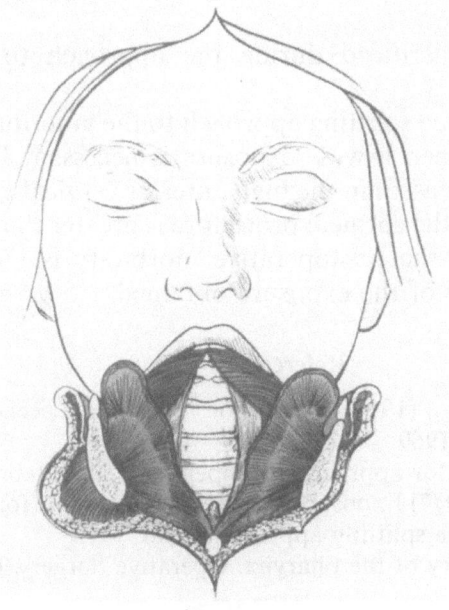

Fig. 3. Exposure of vertebrae from clivus to cervical 6

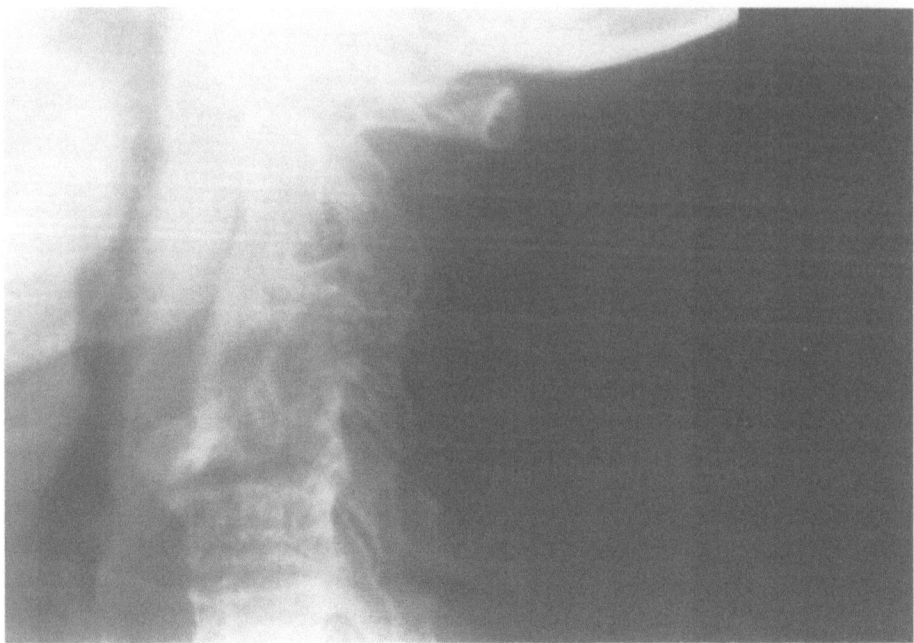

Fig. 4. Lateral X-ray one year following interbody fusion from cervical 2 to cervical 5

single central incisor sacrificed during the approach to facilitate the mandibular repair.

The mandibular tongue splitting approach to the anterior cervical spine should be considered when a wide exposure is necessary for removal of myelopathy producing masses in the high anterior cervical vertebral canal. While the magnitude of the surgical procedure is greater than the standard anterolateral approach, the postoperative morbidity is minimal for the improvement and safety of the exposure obtained.

References

1. DeAndrade, McNab (1969) Anterior occipital cervical fusion—extrapharyngeal. JBJS 1969
2. Fang Ong (1962) Anterior approach to upper cervical vertebrae. JBJS
3. Hall, Denis, Murray (1977) Exposure of upper cervical spine for decompression by mandible and tongue splitting approach. JBJS
4. Kocher T (1911) Surgery of the pharynx. Operative Surgery/Black

Thoracic and Lumbar Spine and Spinal Cord Injuries

Managing Editor: **Ph. Harris**

Editorial Board: J. C. Christensen, G. J. Dohrmann, S. El-Gindi, J. W. Glowacki, B. Ramamurthi

1986. 64 figures. Approx. 230 pages.
Cloth DM 110,-, öS 770,-
ISBN 3-211-81928-2

(Advances in Neurotraumatology, Volume 2)

Owing to their frequency and possible consequences, traumatic lesions of the thoraco-lumbar spine represent a special point of interest within the field of neurotraumatology. Traffic accidents are the commonest cause, which accounts for the high peak between 15 and 24 years of age. According to previously published statistics nearly 50% of the cases affect the thoraco-lumbar junction.

After an introduction on epidemiology and the biomechanical properties, the clinical aspects of these injuries are discussed in detail. The radiological chapter stresses the generally available techniques as X-ray and CT scan and points out the future possibilities of MRI. The intraoperative use of ultrasound and medullary evoked potentials allows a more precise localisation and appreciation of the extent of the lesion as well as a better evaluation of the prognosis and the choice of treatment in the acute phase.

As regards treatment, there is still conflict between those in favor of conservative treatment, the indications of which are well known, and those advocating surgery at a fairly early stage. In all cases, the aim is to reduce and stabilize osseous lesions, lessen the risk of complications and facilitate rehabilitation. Chapters on revascularisation of the spinal cord and an appendix on head injuries complete the volume.

Prices are subject to change without notice

Springer-Verlag Wien New York

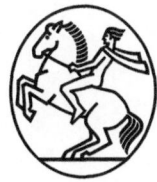

Moelkerbastei 5, P.O. Box 367, A-1011 Wien
175 Fifth Avenue, New York, NY 10010, USA
Heidelberger Platz 3, D-1000 Berlin 33
37-3, Hongo 3-chome, Bunkyo-ku, Tokyo 113, Japan